FURTHER STUDIES ON FAMILY FORMATION PATTERNS AND HEALTH

The World Health Organization is a specialized agency of the United Nations with primary responsibility for international health matters and public health. Through this organization, which was created in 1948, the health professions of more than 150 countries exchange their knowledge and experience with the aim of making possible the attainment by all citizens of the world by the year 2000 of a level of health that will permit them to lead a socially and economically productive life.

By means of direct technical cooperation with its Member States, and by stimulating such cooperation among them, WHO promotes the development of comprehensive health services, the prevention and control of diseases, the improvement of environmental conditions, the development of health manpower, the coordination and development of biomedical and health services research, and the planning and implementation of health programmes.

These broad fields of endeavour encompass a wide variety of activities, such as developing systems of primary health care that reach the whole population of Member countries; promoting the health of mothers and children; combating malnutrition; controlling malaria and other communicable diseases, including tuberculosis and leprosy; having achieved the eradication of smallpox, promoting mass immunization campaigns against a number of other preventable diseases; improving mental health; providing safe water supplies; and training health personnel of all categories.

Progress towards better health throughout the world also demands international cooperation in such matters as establishing international standards for biological substances, pesticides and phamaceuticals; formulating environmental health criteria; recommending international nonproprietary names for drugs; administering the International Health Regulations; revising the International Classification of Diseases, Injuries, and Causes of Death; and collecting and disseminating health statistical information.

Further information on many aspects of WHO's work is presented in the Organization's publications.

FAMILY FORMATION
PATTERNS AND HEALTH
Further Studies

An international collaborative study
in
Colombia, Egypt, Pakistan, and the Syrian Arab Republic

STUDY COORDINATORS AND EDITORS

A. R. OMRAN
Chapel Hill
USA

C. C. STANDLEY
WHO
Geneva

PRINCIPAL INVESTIGATORS

Colombia
G. Ochoa
A. Gil

Egypt
H. Hammam
F. El-Sherbini

Pakistan
Batul Raza
Talat Khan

Syrian Arab Republic
F. El-Boustani

WORLD HEALTH ORGANIZATION
GENEVA

1981

ISBN 92 4 156070 3

PRINTED IN ENGLAND

79/4619—Spottiswoode Ballantyne Ltd.—5000

CONTENTS

PART III: AN OVERVIEW OF THE STUDY

INTRODUCTION

A. R. Omran & C. C. Standley

In 1976 the World Health Organization published *Family formation patterns and health,* reporting the results from 5 of the 10 centres that collaborated in these epidemiological studies. Their purpose was to determine the extent to which certain components of family formation, particularly the age of the mother at pregnancy, pregnancy intervals, parity and family size, affected the health of the mothers, their reproductive performance, and the health and development of their children.

The 1976 volume presented the findings from the centres in India, Iran, Lebanon, Philippines, and Turkey. This volume contains the results from centres that joined the study later, and were located in Colombia, Egypt, Pakistan and the Syrian Arab Republic. The findings from the centre in China (Province of Taiwan), that withdrew from the study in 1972, are being published separately by the centre.

For ease of reading, we have sought to make this volume independent of the preceding one, although following the same format. We have therefore repeated, with the required modifications, the methodological sections, i.e., the chapter on the design of the collaborative studies and the introductions to the substantive chapters. The review of the literature, with which the first volume opened, has not, however, been reproduced. It has been replaced by an update of the review, focusing mainly on publications that have appeared since 1976, but nevertheless giving a general indication of earlier findings.

COLLABORATING CENTRES

NATIONAL SCHOOL OF PUBLIC HEALTH, THE UNIVERSITY OF ANTIOQUIA, MEDELLÍN, COLOMBIA

PRINCIPAL INVESTIGATORS

Angelina Gil, Statistician, Assistant Professor of Statistics and Demography, Department of Basic Sciences

Esneda Gil, Nurse, Assistant Professor, Department of Medical Care and Hospital Administration

Augusto Hernández, Paediatrician, Professor, Department of Medical Care and Hospital Administration

German Ochoa, Emeritus Professor, Chairman, Medical Care and Hospital Administration Section

Luz E. Vásquez, Sociologist and Social Worker, Assistant Professor, Department of Basic Sciences

OTHER STAFF INVOLVED IN THE STUDY

Jairo Algate, MD
Miriam Arias, Interviewer
Elvia Bedoja, Auxiliary Nurse
Marta C. Betancourt, MD
Gustavo Castrillon, Data Processing
Cristina Echeverri, MD
Francisco Echeverri, MD
Hernando Escobar, Mapping, Listing dwelling units
Aracelly García, Interviewer/Supervisor
Cecilia Gaviria, Interviewer/Supervisor
Mindy Goldweit, Translator
Gaston Gómez, ICD Coder
Romelia Guisado, Outreach Worker
Lillian Henao, Interviewer
Consuelo Isaza, Laboratory Technician
Ariel Marina, MD
Gloria Murillo, Interviewer
Rolando Ortíz, MD
Marta L. Ospina, Interviewer
M. Victoria Ospina, Bilingual Secretary
Carmen Pavon, Interviewer/Supervisor
Soledad Posada, Interviewer

9

Cecilia Puerta, Interviewer
Celime Puerta, Interviewer
Teresita Restrepo, Bilingual Secretary
Esmeda Robledo, Outreach Worker
Antonio Rodriguez, MD
Mercedes Saldarriaga, Interviewer
Juan F. Sierra, MD
Miguel A. Suarez, Accountant
Julia Uribe, Nurse L.C., Field Supervisor
Neyda Vargas, Interviewer

ACKNOWLEDGEMENTS

The investigators wish to express their gratitude for the leadership and guidance given by Dr Luis F. Duque, who was the coordinator for the study at the initial stages of design and planning

**FACULTY OF MEDICINE, ASSIUT UNIVERSITY, EGYPT
HIGH INSTITUTE OF PUBLIC HEALTH, ALEXANDRIA
UNIVERSITY, EGYPT
POPULATION AND FAMILY PLANNING BOARD, EGYPT**

PRINCIPAL INVESTIGATORS

Dr A. Bindary, Chairman, Executive Board, Population and Family Planning Board

Dr M. H. El Sammaa, Coordinator and Central Supervisor, Deputy Director, Population and Family Planning Board

Dr A. F. El-Sherbini, Director of Alexandria Study, Department of Family Health, Alexandria High Institute of Public Health

Dr H. M. Hammam, Director of Assiut Study, Chairman, Department of Preventive Medicine, Assiut Faculty of Medicine

Dr A. F. Moustafa, Head of the Computer and Statistical Analysis Team, Assistant Professor of Statistics, Zagazig University

OTHER STAFF INVOLVED IN THE STUDY

From Assiut:

Fathy Abdel Hamid Dardeir, Field Supervisor, Department of Epidemiology and Public Health

Mohsen El Arkaan, Lecturer, National Institute of Social and Criminological Research

Mohammed Ali El Torky, Lecturer, Department of Epidemiology and Public Health

10

Dr Mahmoud Fathalla, Department of Obstetrics and Gynaecology

Abdel Hamid Ibrahim Guinena, Associate Professor, Department of Epidemiology and Public Health

Abdel Hamid, Gussein Gad, Technologist

Dr Farouk S. Hassanein, Chairman, Department of Paediatrics

Laila Mohammed Hassanein, Lecturer, Department of Epidemiology and Public Health

Ramzy Ibrahim M. Ismail, Lecturer, Department of Epidemiology and Public Health

Hosam Sabet Salem, Assistant Professor, Department of Obstetrics and Gynaecology

Ali Hussein Ali Zaraour, Lecturer, Department of Epidemiology and Public Health

From Alexandria:

Dr Mohammed El Amine

Dr Emad El Din Eid, Associate Professor, Department of Family Health, High Institute of Public Health

Dr Sawsan I. Fahmy, Department of Family Health, High Institute of Public Health

Dr M. E. Abdel Fattah

Dr Enayat Abdel Kader

Dr Amal Khairy

Dr Ahmed Wasfi

Dr Mohammed Yassin

Dr Ahmed Zaher Zaghloul, Department of Public Health Administration, High Institute of Public Health

From the Computer Centre:

E. S. Khashaba

Mr S. M. Abdel Maksoud

NATIONAL RESEARCH INSTITUTE OF FERTILITY CONTROL, KARACHI, PAKISTAN

PRINCIPAL INVESTIGATORS

Dr Talat Khan

Mohammad Saeed Qureshi

Dr Batul Raza

OTHER STAFF INVOLVED IN THE STUDY

Miss Taskeen Abidi

Dr Farhat Ajmal

Syeda Farooqi

Kaniz Fatima

S. H. Fatima
Nighat Haqui
Mr Feroz Y. Hayat
Irshad Hussain
Sohail Imam
Miss Farhana Irum
Shamim Izhar
Mr Abidi Jaffar
Mussarat Jehan
Sami Ahmad Khan
Zar Khan
Aquila Khatoon
Tahira Najma
Shahnaz Niazi
Dr Afroze Qazi
Mrs Rafiq
Sahnaz Safder
Mumtaz Sajjad
Dr Shaheen
Malahat Shaheen
Dr Azra Shaikh
Mrs M. Siraj
Mehboob Sultana
Mr Ehsan M. Syed
Miss Razia Wahid
Dr Hafez Zaidi

CENTRAL BUREAU OF STATISTICS, DAMASCUS, SYRIAN ARAB REPUBLIC

PRINCIPAL INVESTIGATORS

Aref Alyafi, Ministry of Health
Farid El-Boustani
Ahmed Radjai, Former Director

OTHER STAFF INVOLVED IN THE STUDY

Ahmed Dahman
Ahmed Dashash
Muti El Din Mamish
M. El Jabi
Sadek Feroun
Nabih Ghabra
M. Gharib
G. Ghebe

Adnan Habbat
Nader Hallak
N. Hanbali
Anton Houmsi
Lyla Shark

WHO COLLABORATING CENTRE FOR EPIDEMIOLOGICAL STUDIES OF HUMAN REPRODUCTION

Alan Johnston, Research Associate
A. R. Omran, Professor of Epidemiology, School of Public Health and Director of the Collaborating Centre, University of North Carolina, Chapel Hill, USA

OTHER STAFF INVOLVED IN THE STUDY

Mary Kay Falconer, Research Assistant
Victoria Fontenot, Research Assistant
Mahmoud Riad, Statistical Consultant
Ibrahim Salama, Statistical Consultant
Jennifer Terrenoire, Research Assistant
Madeline Walker, Secretary

WORLD HEALTH ORGANIZATION

P.-C. Kaufmann, Statistician, Health Statistical Methodology
C. C. Standley, Scientist, Special Programme of Research, Development and Research Training in Human Reproduction
H. Woodward, Secretary, Special Programme of Research, Development and Research Training in Human Reproduction

CONSULTANT

A. M. Woolman, Consultant Editor, Eastbourne, East Sussex, England

These studies were in part supported by the United Nations Fund for Population Activities

13

PART I: BACKGROUND TO THE STUDY

Chapter One

REVIEW OF THE EVIDENCE—AN UPDATE

A. R. Omran

INTRODUCTION

In the first volume of this series reporting studies in India, Iran, Lebanon, the Philippines, and Turkey (Omran & Standley, 1976), a chapter was devoted to a review of the evidence in the world literature relating family formation patterns and health. The purpose of the review was to assess the findings of other studies and to supplement our own findings with those obtained in different settings.

The present chapter is an update of the previous review and includes primarily studies published since the preparation of the preceding volume or not included in it for other reasons. Attention is drawn to studies considered milestones in this field of inquiry. Important findings mentioned in the first volume of the WHO Family Formation Study are also included. The chapter is divided into several sections corresponding to the principal family formation variables. Each section opens with a summary statement of the cumulative evidence from the literature, followed by a review of selected studies. Previously, the evidence was drawn largely from studies in the more developed countries. Fortunately, an increasing number of reports from developing countries are now becoming available, and these are given priority in this update. Special attention is also given to national surveys, surveys of large communities, and longitudinal studies with repeat surveys providing comparative data from the same area.

Here it should be noted, that family health is usually taken to be synonymous with the health of the mother and younger child. Only a few studies have addressed themselves to the health of the family as a whole. A number of recent reports have tended to contest the accepted relationships of family health with parity, maternal age, and birth interval. While this review does not include a comprehensive analysis of the different methodological issues, a note at the end outlines some of these issues.

Finally, it must be noted that the literature on family formation has grown rapidly and this review can only include a selection of published reports. For further information, the reader is referred to a number of reviews on these topics that have been published elsewhere (Omran, 1971; Wray; 1971; Omran, 1975; Lesinski, 1976; Watson et al., 1979).

I. IMPACT OF FAMILY SIZE AND BIRTH ORDER

Fetal and Child Mortality

Summary The general pattern that emerges from studies in both industrialized and developing countries indicates that the risk of late fetal death (stillbirths) is relatively high for first births, decreases for second and third births, rises slightly for fourth and fifth births, and increases much more sharply for later order births. Such a pattern is frequently described as a J-shaped or parabolic curve. When the risk of late fetal death for first births is very high, the curve becomes U-shaped.

The relationship between neonatal mortality rates and birth order shows a similar U-shaped or J-shaped pattern. Post-neonatal and total infant mortality rates either follow the same pattern or increase steadily with increasing birth order, as do the mortality rates for early childhood (1–4 years). If maternal age is considered simultaneously, infant mortality rates continue to show a steady increase with parity, or they may take the form of a U-shaped curve, especially for older mothers.

Some of the more detailed studies indicate that, although a strong inverse relationship exists between mortality and social class, the variations in mortality with birth order are maintained within each social class. These patterns also occur among all cultures and racial groups and persist over long periods, despite a considerable decline in mortality levels.

Finally, the effects of birth rank on health may be mediated through the size of the family or the total number of pregnancies (gravidity) in the biological family.

In repeated national studies, several British researchers have utilized the linkage of birth and death records (thus constituting reconstructed cohort or prospective studies) to investigate the effect on infant and childhood mortality of birth order, maternal age, and social class. This approach was carried out in England and Wales first for the years 1949 and 1950 (Heady & Morris, 1955), then for 1963 and 1964 (Spicer & Lipworth, 1966), and most recently for the years 1975–1977 (Davies, 1980). Each of these studies confirmed the well-known patterns described above, despite the dramatic declines in mortality risks between 1949 and 1977. (Infant mortality per 1000 live births in England and Wales declined from 327 in 1949 to 19.9 in 1964 and down to 14.0 for 1976.) For example, the lastest report (Davies, 1980) included records of more than 98% of the 25 639 infant deaths occurring in England and Wales during 1975–1977 linked to their corresponding birth records. As in the two earlier reports, the lowest stillbirth, perinatal, and neonatal mortality rates were found for second-order children of mothers in their 20s and early 30s (particularly late 20s) and the highest rates for first-born or births of higher orders (3+) to mothers aged 35 and over. The study also showed an inverse association between mortality and social class (i.e., the higher the social class the lower the mortality). Although detailed cross-classification by social class and family formation is not yet available for the latest study, the earlier reports demonstrated consistently that the relationships of mortality risks with maternal age and parity were independent of social class effects.

18

Another national study on perinatal mortality in the United Kingdom not belonging to the above series was reported by Chamberlain et al. (1975) and depicted the same patterns. A subnational British study is also worthy of special mention. The British Perinatal Mortality Survey used a carefully designed longitudinal approach and included 7117 deaths among single, legitimate births in Great Britain in the three months from March through May 1958 (Butler and Bonham, 1963; Butler & Alberman, 1969). The findings again revealed that the lowest perinatal mortality rates were associated with second-order births and the highest rates with higher-order births.

A series of national studies in the USA since 1937 has likewise demonstrated the typical relationships described above. These studies include, for example, (a) analysis of records of all births and stillbirths in the USA during the period 1937–41 by Yerushalmy (1945), (b) studies of all births and child deaths during the first three months of 1950 by Loeb (1965) and Shapiro (1954), (c) a study of infant, perinatal, maternal, and child mortality during 1960–61 by Shapiro et al. (1968), (d) a study of the 1960 live birth cohort by Armstrong (1972), and (e) a comparative study of linked records from the first quarters of 1950 and 1960 by Chase (1972).

Another series of subnational studies, particularly of large cities in the USA, also provides evidence for these relationships. Such studies were carried out, for example, in New York State and/or New York City by Yerushalmy (1938), Chase (1961, 1962, 1973) and Kessner et al. (1973), and in Baltimore by Shah & Abbey (1971) and Gendell & Hellegers (1973). These studies not only confirmed the general patterns of relationships of mortality with birth order, maternal age, and birth interval but also demonstrated that these patterns occur among all racial groups and social classes.

An indication that similar patterns may exist even for women under relatively good medical care comes from a study by Shapiro et al. (1970) of approximately 12 000 women belonging to the Health Insurance Plan (HIP) of Greater New York. These women were under medical care throughout their pregnancies. Fetal death within the first 20 weeks of gestation occurring among births to that cohort of women increased progressively with pregnancy order, while the rates for late fetal loss (20 weeks or more of gestation) followed the typical J-shaped curve with pregnancy order.

Supporting evidence is continuing to accumulate from industrialized countries. To mention a recent example, a national study in Norway by Bakketeig et al. (1978) covered 464 067 births registered during the period 1967–1973. Perinatal mortality rates during the seven-year period were lowest for mothers aged 20–29, were somewhat higher for mothers aged less than 20 and 30–40, and were highest for mothers aged 35 or over. In regard to parity, the lowest perinatal mortality occurred for second-order births. Mortality was higher for first- and third-order births, and was highest for birth orders four and over.

Finally, an international collaborative study in eight countries initiated by the World Health Organization examined the effect of social and biological factors on perinatal mortality. Data collected in 1973 in Austria, Cuba, England and Wales, Hungary, Japan, New Zealand, Sweden, and the USA consistently showed a lower risk of perinatal death for second-born than for first-born infants, with the risk progressively increasing for third, fourth, and subsequent births (World Health Organization 1976, 1978).

It is indeed encouraging to witness the increasing interest and flow of documentation from the developing countries. Unfortunately, community-based studies are relatively few and far between, while hospital-based studies are relatively more abundant. It should be emphasized, moreover, that some of these studies, especially those based on hospital deliveries, should be examined with considerable caution. Because in many developing countries only a small fraction of deliveries occur in hospitals, such samples are highly selective and include mainly emergency or complicated deliveries from undefined catchment areas. Differences in admission policies between areas often make comparisons difficult.

A large body of evidence on the determinants of infant mortality has been collected by the Inter-American Investigation of Mortality in Childhood organized by the Pan American Health Organization. Data for various periods between 1968 and 1971 are available from surveys in five countries: Chile, El Salvador, Mexico, and, for Pan-American comparisons, Canada and the USA (Puffer & Serrano, 1975). Although neonatal and infant mortality levels in the USA and Canada were much lower than those in the Latin American countries (infant mortality rates ranged from 21.2 per 1000 in one Canadian project to 133.5 in one Latin American project), in each case a rising trend with ascending birth order was evident. In all centres, both neonatal and total infant mortality rates were more than twice as high for birth orders of five or more as for first- or second-order births. Analysis by maternal age and birth order for Chile and El Salvador showed infant mortality rates increasing with ascending birth order in each maternal age group.

A more recent report from Chile (Cabrera, 1980) corroborates the above evidence in a national study of all births and infant deaths in Chile during a five-year period (1969–1974) as taken from the Civil Registry records. During the study period, the infant mortality rate declined from 85.3 per 1000 live births in 1969 to 69.4 in 1974. Neonatal, post-neonatal, and total infant mortality rates were lowest for maternal ages 20–34 and highest for ages under 20 years and 35 and over. In addition, a steady rise in mortality was observed with increased birth order for each of the three mortality categories. The observed patterns of variation in infant mortality by maternal age and birth order persisted over the five-year period. A tabulation of the patterns in urban areas by social class demonstrated an increase in infant mortality with birth order in the low social status neighbourhood, while a J-shaped relationship was apparent in the high social status neighbourhoods.

In the WHO Family Formation Study in India, Iran, Lebanon, the Philippines, and Turkey (Omran & Standley, 1976) evidence was examined on the relationship between pregnancy order and pregnancy outcome. For most cultural and residential groups pregnancy wastage rates (stillbirths and abortions) described a U-shaped or J-shaped pattern when related to pregnancy order. This pattern was quite consistent for stillbirths, whereas abortion rates tended to increase steadily with pregnancy order in Iran and Turkey. In

Lebanon, the Philippines and India a relatively high risk of losing the first pregnancy was found; this may have been, in part, a reflection of the fact that many such pregnancies occurred several years before the study when health risks were much higher.

One of the earlier studies in Asia was the Khana Longitudinal Study conducted in 11 Punjab villages in India and reported by Wyon & Gordon (1962). Pathak (1978) re-analysed data from the Khana study for evidence of the relationship between infant mortality and birth order. Pathak's study covered 1479 births during 1955–1958 and reported that infant mortality was high for first-order births (153 per 1000), reached a minimum for second- and third-order births (93 and 97 per 1000, respectively), increased slightly for fourth-order births (113 per 1000), and increased sharply for fifth- (153 per 1000), sixth- (161 per 1000), and seventh- and higher-order births (170 per 1000).

In Bangladesh, birth and death reports were collected in 132 villages (total population 117 000) of Matlab Thana between May 1967 and April 1969 through repeated household visits by local female residents (Stoeckel & Chowdhury, 1972). Neonatal mortality rates described a clear reversed J-shaped relationship, both with maternal age and with birth order. The post-neonatal mortality rate was high for young mothers (under 20 years of age) and highest for mothers aged 35–39 years, with fluctuations for other maternal age groups. In relation to birth order, post-neonatal mortality rates generally followed a J-shaped curve, the highest risks being observed for birth orders of 8 and above. A striking finding was the comparatively low infant mortality rates among children born to mothers who had large families and who either had no previous child losses or had lost only one child.

A more recent analysis of the data from the Matlab area for the period 1966–69 (Swenson & Harper, 1979) found that early fetal wastage and stillbirths rates were lowest for second and third pregnancy orders and high for first order and for fourth and higher orders. An increased risk was also particularly apparent among pregnancies following two or more fetal deaths.

In China (Province of Taiwan), the Vital Demographic and Registration Survey collected data on births and infant deaths from a stratified sample of 57 townships out of 361 administrative districts from the period May 1966 to February 1969 through household visits (with 5-month intervals) Sullivan, 1972). Over 200 000 persons were surveyed. Neonatal mortality rates followed a U-shape in relation to birth order and post-neonatal mortality rates bore a linear relationship to maternal age, but a steady rise in both neonatal and post-neonatal mortality was observed as birth order increased. Higher rates were found in rural areas than in urban areas, although under-reporting—especially of neonatal deaths—may have affected the results in rural areas. Higher mortality rates were also associated with lower education and were attributed partly to less adequate medical care.

Adlakha & Suchindran (1980) are currently analysing 1975 World Fertility Survey Data from Sri Lanka. Initial results show a minimum infant mortality rate for second-order births, a fluctuating pattern between birth orders 3 and 6, and a greatly increased rate for birth order 7 and over. When both birth order and maternal age are considered, a pattern of steadily increasing risk with birth order is shown for mothers aged less than 20, while older mothers have a J-shaped pattern of risk with the minimum risk for second-order births.

Blacker (1979) has reported on data obtained from the birth histories compiled in the Kenya Fertility Survey of 1977–78 which showed that first-order births were associated with an infant mortality rate 35% higher than second-, third-, and fourth-order births. Additional study of higher-order births from this and similar surveys is needed.

Additional evidence is available from several African sample registration areas. Cantrelle & Leridon (1971) reported on 8456 births in the Sine-Saloum region of Senegal from 1962 to 1968. Infant mortality was at a minimum at intermediate parities and formed a U-shaped curve with excess risk for first births and seventh- and higher-order births. Grouping of parities 4–6 prevented a more detailed description of the pattern. Ayeni & Oduntan (1978) analysed corrected registration returns from a rural area in Nigeria for the period 1971–75. Infant mortality rates increased consistently from 72.4 per 1000 for birth order one to 126.5 per 1000 for birth orders seven and over. The authors also reported a J-shaped pattern of risk with maternal age and noted that these two factors are closely interrelated. In a survey of 3700 households in a rural area of Kenya, Voorhoeve et al. (1979) found that, while maternal age was an important factor, parity was not associated with differences in the outcome of pregnancy.

Many hospital-based studies have also been reviewed and several will be reported here. Reference was made in the previous review to certain earlier hospital studies in developing countries. Bajpai et al. (1966) examined 1000 consecutive births in a hospital in Lucknow, India and found that the risk of death per 1000 live births before or immediately after birth was 130 for first-born babies, 50 for second-born, 110 for third-, fourth- and fifth-born, 160 for sixth- to ninth-born, and 250 for tenth- or later-born. Similar studies by Mehdi et al. (1961) for 13 634 consecutive deliveries in Hyderabad hospitals, India; by Radovič (1966) of 569 patients at Tema General Hospital, Ghana over a ten-month period; and by Roberts & Tanner (1963) of records of 1624 births over the period 1952–57 for the Hangaza, a Bantu-speaking people in Tanzania, all found similar patterns of risks with parity and maternal age. The number of hospital-based studies has been increasing in recent years. The following are only a few examples.

A prospective study of 1595 live births at Kenyatta National Hospital during 1975 was reported by Meme (1978). Neonatal mortality depicted the typical J-shaped relationship, both with age and with parity.

Gebre-Medhin et al. (1976) examined the records of 9070 deliveries in a hospital in Addis Ababa, Ethiopia during the five-year period 1964–68. While there was a steady increase in the stillbirth rate with maternal age, no significant change with parity was revealed. Reinhardt et al. (1978) likewise examined 7433 delivery records at Adjamé Maternity Hospital in Abidjan (Ivory Coast) and found a distinct U-shaped relationship of spontaneous abortion and stillbirth with parity. In particular, parities 1, 2 and 8 or over had the highest risks.

22

In a recent study of 12 262 deliveries in Zaria, Nigeria, during 1976–77, Harrison (1979) found that perinatal mortality was related to both age and parity. Higher rates were found for both younger women (under 20) and older women (over 30). For parity, the lowest risk was found for third-order births with higher risks for earlier births, especially the first, and for fifth and later births. Omran (1978) analysed data collected from 14 maternity centres and covering 45 957 deliveries in the 1970s (Bangladesh 2017; Egypt 6459; Indonesia 6936; Iran 19931; Nigeria 2849; Sri Lanka 2903; and Sudan 4862). Centres in two developed countries (Italy and Sweden) were included for comparison. Uniform procedures and a standard maternity record were used by all centres. Analysis revealed that perinatal mortality[1] (except in Ibadan) described the typical J-shaped relationship with both maternal age and parity. In Ibadan, the rate was higher for teenage women than for older women, while no change with parity was observed. It should be emphasized that although uniform methods were used, the data were based on selected samples and, further, the degree of representativeness differed greatly from one centre to another.

Child Health and Development

Summary Several studies describe a detrimental effect of large family (or sibship) size and high birth order on physical and intellectual development. However, in view of the many competing variables (genetic and environmental) and the difficulties of assessing intellectual attainment in developing societies, these data must be interpreted cautiously.

Birth weight and prematurity provide measures of infant physical development. Controversy exists about the relationship of birth weight and prematurity to birth order. Mean birth weight seems to increase with birth order (although not consistently), while the rates for prematurity (defined as birth weights of 2500 g or less) have either a linear increase with both orders or a J-shaped relationship to birth order.

As measured by weight, height, and sexual maturity, the physical growth of children from large families compares unfavourably with that of children from small families. The difference, however, is small and is evident mainly in large studies.

In regard to intellectual development, increasing evidence shows that children from large families obtain relatively lower intelligence scores than those from small families. Mental retardation also is positively associated with family size. This area, however, will require further research, especially in the developing world.

A number of child health conditions have also been linked to family size and birth order (as well as to maternal age). Included are congenital malformation, physical handicaps, malnutrition, dental problems, infectious diseases, emotional problems, and mental illness. Some conditions—like malnutrition—are probably directly related to increased strain on family and maternal resources with each additional child; in the case of common infections, larger family size may simply lead to more frequent exposure to infectious agents through other family members.

---

[1] This should actually be called "paranatal mortality" since it related to stillbirths and deaths of infants within the first 48 hours before the mother was discharged from the centre.

Birth weight

While some studies show no clear-cut relationship between birth weight (or prematurity) and parity, the pattern emerging from several other investigations indicates that mean birth weight and prematurity rates (which are crucial in relation to child survival) differ in their relationship to birth order. These patterns were established, for example, in a national study of all births in the USA in the first quarter of 1950 (Loeb, 1965) covering 837 786 births. Among children included in the study, births of premature infants occurred most frequently among first births and births of fifth and higher orders (7.7%). The lowest incidence of prematurity was found among second births (6.9%) and each subsequent birth order brought a slightly increased proportion of premature infants. The changes in median birth weights with birth order did not accord completely with differences in the incidence of premature birth, however. Despite the rise in the proportion of small babies (2500 g or less) at birth orders above the second, the median birth weight increased at each successive birth order.

These patterns were later demonstrated in a study of all births in the USA in 1976 (Taffel, 1980), despite considerable demographic changes since 1950. For example, the proportion of children born to teenagers increased from 12 to 18% of all births in the period 1950–1976, whereas, at the same time, the proportion of infants born to mothers aged 35 years and over fell from 11 to 4% of all births. There was also an increase in the proportion of first-order births from 32 to 42% of all births, while fourth- and higher-order births declined from 21 to 11% of all births. The study noted that 18% of the overall decline in prematurity rates among whites in the USA was due to changes in the age–birth-order distribution of births. Among the non-white population, other causes of the decline played a more important role. While the incidence of low birth weight described the familiar J-shaped curve when age and parity were considered independently, the study noted that the lowest incidence of low birth weight for any age-parity group was recorded for women aged 25–29 years bearing their second child (5.1%). The highest rates were for teenagers under 15 years of age having a second child (30.5%) and for those aged 15–19 years having a fourth- or higher-order birth (20.3%).

Similar patterns were also found in a study by Selvin & Garfinkel (1972) of over 1.5 million birth certificates in New York City, which showed both an increase in median birth weight with parity (and maternal age) and a J-shaped relationship between premature birth rates and birth order.

An increase in mean birth weight by parity was also found in Great Britain by Karn & Penrose (1951) and in Italy by Fraccaro (1956). Other studies of sibships did not agree completely with these findings, however. James (1969) in England found birth weights increasing only up to the fifth birth order, and Bonarini (1979), using regression analysis of birth history data from Verona, Italy, found that birth weight "probably does not increase with birth order".

The pattern of an increase in mean birth weight with parity has also been found in a large number of studies in developing countries. These include, for example, studies by Gebre-Mehdin et al. (1976) in Ethiopia, Mbise & Boersma

(1979) and Roberts & Tanner (1963) in the United Republic of Tanzania, Reinhardt et al. (1978) in the Ivory Coast, Simpkiss (1968) in Uganda, Lewis (1974) in the United Republic of Cameroon, Rehan & Tafida (1979) in Nigeria, Millis & Seng (1954) in Singapore, and Namboodiri & Balakrishnan (1959) in India.

In regard to prematurity, two studies in Africa provide some evidence. In a study of 7433 deliveries in Abidjan, Ivory Coast, Reinhardt et al. (1978) found a reversed J-shaped relationship between prematurity and birth order. There was an extremely high incidence for first births, a lower incidence for intermediate births, and a subsequent rise for higher birth orders. Re-analysis of data from a study in Dar-es-Salaam, United Republic of Tanzania (Mbise & Boersma, 1979, Table III) revealed a U-shaped relationship.

Finally, the analysis by Omran (1978) of data from several centres in developing countries and two centres in developed countries likewise showed a U-shaped relationship between prematurity and parity in Bangladesh, Indonesia, Italy, and Sweden; a steady increase in prematurity with parity in one maternity centre (Egypt); and a small decline in prematurity with parity in Nigeria and Sudan.

Physical growth and development beyond infancy

In almost all of the studies reviewed, it was found that both family size and birth order influenced the physical growth of children, as measured by height, weight, and sexual maturity. The most detailed studies include those of Scott (1962), Grant (1964), and Douglas & Simpson (1964) in England, as reviewed in the previous volume.

In the WHO Family Formation Study (Omran & Standley, 1976) data for four centres, India, Iran, Lebanon, and the Philippines, were tabulated classifying children as of low or high pregnancy order in relation to maternal age. In almost all the age groups and in most of the cultural and residential groups examined, children of mothers who had a large number of pregnancies for their age had lower mean heights, weights, and haemoglobin levels than those of mothers with fewer pregnancies for the same age.

Several of these studies indicate that in addition to having an influence on the weight and height of children, family size and birth order may also influence sexual maturation of boys and girls, particularly the age at menarche. Stukovsky et al. (1977), for example, examined this issue in a large study in Romania and found that age at menarche was delayed by an average of 2.1 months for every additional sibling. Tanner (1968) and Douglas & Simpson (1964) found similar relationships in the United Kingdom.

Intelligence

The relationship between intelligence and family size or birth order continues to be an area of considerable debate. The debate centres on the relative influence of biological, social, and genetic factors on intellectual development.

In the earlier review, reference was made to eight major studies that indicate collectively that the intelligence quotient (IQ) tends to decline for later born children and for large family size. Prominent examples include the study of 386 114 nineteen-year-old military recruits in the Netherlands (Belmont & Marolla, 1973) and the study in England by Record et al. (1969) among 50 172 Birmingham children. Both of these studies indicated that the decline in IQ with birth order persists within each social class.

Additional evidence on the relationship between intelligence and family size or birth order is becoming available from both developed and developing countries. For example, in examining the average scores of nearly 800 000 candidates on the National Merit Scholarship Qualification Test in the USA, Breland (1974) found that the scores generally declined with increasing family size. Within each family size, the scores declined with birth order, the rate of decline decreasing with successive birth orders.

Three examples can be given from the developing countries. In a large study in Colombia, Velandea et al. (1978) examined test scores, family information, and socioeconomic variables from over 36 000 college applicants. They found almost no family size effects for the lower socioeconomic group, and inconsistent birth order effects across family sizes, and concluded that socioeconomic status was the more important variable affecting mental ability. A recent study was conducted by Fan & Omran (1981) among 20 000 school-age children in China (Province of Taiwan). This study showed a decline in IQ for birth order four and over, a decline that occurred among both sexes in both urban and rural areas, and among all social classes.

In the WHO Family Formation Study (Omran & Standley, 1976) the Cattell & Cattell Culture–Fair Test was used by all centres to measure the IQ of children age 8–14 years. No clear pattern by birth order could be found in the Iranian study of 696 children, while the Indian study, including 2310 children, indicated some decline in the mean IQ for children of sixth or higher birth order, or for children of family size 6 or over. In both the Philippines and Turkey, however, including 2199 and 2293 children, respectively, a tendency for IQ scores to decrease with increasing birth order and family size was evident. In all areas, the mean IQ of children from low social status families was relatively lower than that of their counterparts from high social status families, but controlling for social status did not change the negative association between IQ scores and family size.

Recently, there has been a growing debate over whether the interval between siblings is a more important factor than birth order or family size. Zajonc & Markus (1975), Zajonc (1976), and Zajonc et al. (1979) introduced and developed the "confluence model" for studing the importance of birth intervals. This model predicts that the effects of birth order are mediated entirely by the age spacing between siblings, and that with large enough gaps between siblings to allow sufficient time for the earlier born to mature the negative effects of birth order can be nullified and even reversed. This concept has been contested by Velandea et al. (1978) and Bahr & Leigh (1978).

Readers particularly interested in this field may consult an extensive review of the subject by Wagner & Schubert (1979).

Congenital malformations and handicapping conditions

Study of the effect of birth order on congenital malformation and other handicaps is fraught with methodological problems and hampered by lack of sufficient data. Not only are we dealing with very rare conditions requiring very large samples, but most studies depend on birth records that are available, with few exceptions, only for the developed countries. The problem is compounded by the fact that not all congenital malformations are recognizable at birth.

Evidence for the effect of birth order on the incidence of congenital conditions has been equivocal. A major infant mortality study referred to earlier (Heady & Morris, 1955) found no discernible relationship between congenital anomalies and birth order. Other studies have found an increasing incidence with higher birth order.

Extensive studies by Newcombe (1964) and Newcombe & Travendale (1964) demonstrated a high risk of handicapping conditions for infants of "young" mothers (under 20 years) and "old" mothers (over 35 years) and for those of first-order or high-order births. The risks were accentuated by "unusual" combinations, such as high-order births to young mothers and first-order births to older mothers. The authors suggested that the association, especially of mental and related disorders, including Down syndrome, with older maternal age may result from a high rate of degenerative change in the ova of older mothers. It was also suggested that the risks associated primarily with high birth order, particularly handicaps of infective origin, might be environmental rather than congenital.

Hay & Barbano (1972) calculated incidence rates for selected categories of congenital malformation reported on birth certificates from a population of more than eight million registered white, single, live births in 29 states and two large cities in the USA from 1961 to 1966. While most of these categories of malformation exhibited increasing incidence as maternal age increased, none of the conditions showed a consistent increase with increasing birth order once maternal age was held constant.

More recently, a major study on congenital anomalies was based on data from 46 states and the District of Colombia in the USA for 1973–1974 (Taffel, 1978). For all anomalies combined, the incidence of congenital defects was highest for fourth and higher order births. Most of the increase, however, was related to the relatively greater number of older women having high-parity births. The relationship with age was J-shaped, with a relatively lower incidence at ages 20–24 (804.1 per 100 000 live births) and ages 25–29 (780 per 100 000). The highest incidence was for mothers aged 35 years and older (1175 per 100 000). Taffel emphasized that "due to the high degree of association between age of mother and birth order of child, it was not possible to determine which of these variables had a greater effect on the overall congenital anomalies rates".

Malnutrition

Among families with comparable income, family size becomes one of the important determinants of the nutrition of family members. Both the mother's nutritional status and that of the children themselves have important effects on children's growth and development, and on their resistance to infection. Two studies that illustrate this point are those of Wray & Aguirre (1969) among preschool children of Candelaria, Colombia, and of Gopalan (1968) in India. Wray & Aguirre found a steady increase in the incidence of protein-energy malnutrition, from 32.0% of only children to 46.2% of children from families of 8 or more children. Gopalan studied preschool children in India and found a higher prevalence of malnutrition (32%) among children of birth orders four or higher compared with 17% for lower birth orders. The differences between these two groups were highly significant for both protein-energy malnutrition and vitamin-A deficiency.

Similar results have been found in a number of studies in Africa. Morley et al. (1968) in Nigeria, El-Behairy et al. (1976) in Egypt, and Khan & Gupta (1979) in Zambia found relationships between large family size and the incidence of malnourished children.

The relationship between child health, maternal nutritional status, and parity was investigated also by Hefnawi et al. (1972). They studied milk yields in 238 lactating Egyptian women (1–12 months postpartum) randomly selected from lower socioeconomic classes and aged 18–36 years. It was found that milk yields were better for women aged 21–30 with parity of 2–4 than for either younger or older women who were primiparous or of parity greater than 4.

Infection

In a longitudinal study of Cleveland (Ohio) families, Dingle et al. (1964) found an increasing incidence per person-year of common respiratory diseases and infectious gastroenteritis with increasing family size. This increase seemed to be attributable to the greater likelihood of direct exposure of family members to infections. Similar findings were reported earlier in two extensive British studies, one by Spence et al. (1954) and one by Douglas & Blomfield (1958).

The WHO Family Formation Study (Omran & Standley, 1976) included a medical examination of children under five which showed that, while parasitic infection, as revealed by stool examination, was severe regardless of family size, the prevalence of infection in children increased with family size in most areas.

Maternal Mortality

Summary   Several studies, both early and recent, have found that multiparity, especially grand multiparity, carries increased risks of maternal mortality and morbidity. The classical triad of maternal mortality in industrialized countries used to be toxaemia, haemorrhage, and sepsis. These conditions have been on the decline in recent years and are being displaced by complications of anaesthesia and amniotic fluid embolism, with toxaemia continuing to be a problem.

Maternal mortality and parity

Increased risks of maternal mortality with high parity, especially grand multiparity—defined in older studies variously as parities of 6 or over and in others as those of 8 and over—were recognized by early gynaecologists. During these early years, the classical triad—toxaemia, haemorrhage, and sepsis—led the causes of maternal mortality. Within the last 50 years, maternal mortality has declined dramatically. During the same period, the prevalence of high parity also declined to the extent that grand multiparity is now defined in the West as parities of 4 or 5 and over. Despite the apparent decline in the absolute risk of mortality among multiparas, it is still possible to demonstrate the relatively high risk of grand multiparity, though only in large samples.

Community-based or national studies confirm the increase of mortality with parity. For example, Jaffe & Polgar (1964) showed that for 348 393 live births in the USA between 1951 and 1961 maternal mortality generally increased with parity and age. When age was controlled, mortality for women with high parity was still more than twice as high as mortality at lower parity.

Reports on sizable series of the grand multipara exist in the literature and interest in those series has not disappeared. One example of long-term studies is a 26-year series at a hospital centre in Pittsburgh, PA, USA, for the period 1937 to 1973, published in two reports, Phillips et al. (1965) and Guha-Ray (1976). The 1965 report revealed that the leading causes of maternal deaths from 1937 through 1945 were haemorrhage and toxaemia; the latter continued to be a leading cause through 1962, but anaesthesia complications displaced haemorrhage during that time. In more recent years (the 1976 report), the single most common cause of maternal mortality was amniotic fluid embolism during labour or the puerperium. In both reports, maternal mortality was known to increase with parity.

In the developing countries, maternal mortality is still very high and is related to the high prevalence of grand multiparity. Grand multiparity carries the greatest risk of mortality, not only from the three classical causes, but also from obstructed labour leading to uterine rupture, a condition that has become extremely rare in Western hospitals. One important report by Rao (1975) gives an account of a 13-year experience in a teaching hospital in South India where 1245 maternal deaths occurred among 74 384 deliveries for a maternal mortality rate of 167 per 10 000 births (compared with only 3 per 10 000 births in the Pittsburgh series mentioned above). The three leading causes responsible for 73% of the deaths were prolonged labour (mostly uterine rupture), haemorrhage and toxaemia of pregnancy. Puerperal sepsis claimed 65 cases, or 7.6%, of all deaths. It is also important to note that the morbidity rate of rupture of the uterus was high, having been encountered in 786 cases of whom 25% died. Of these uterine rupture cases, 35% occurred in grand multiparas.

Sogbanmu (1979) examined maternal mortality in 2083 deliveries at the General Hospital, Ondo, Nigeria and found a maternal mortality rate of 7.2 per 1000. Major causes of death were anaemia (27%), uterine rupture (20%), and infections (15%). As many as 78.5% of the deaths occurred in multigravida and of these 25% were grand multiparous. In a study at the University Teaching Hospital, Lusaka, Zambia, Hickey & Kasonde (1977) examined 80 maternal mortality cases over a 2-year period and found the mortality rate to be 1.5 per 1000 births. The most common causes were pre-eclampsia and eclampsia, septicaemia, haemorrhage, and ruptured uterus. Mortality was concentrated in two parity groups, the primiparous, representing 26% of the cases (most probably because of young maternal age) and the grand multiparas, representing 22% of the cases. Armon (1977) provided data on a series of women with ruptured uteruses in Malawi and the United Republic of Tanzania based on 22 330 deliveries. Ruptured uterus occurred at a rate of 91 per 10 000 births in Malawi and 40 per 10 000 births in Tanzania. The major cause of ruptured uterus was obstructed labour. Twenty two per cent of the cases were grand multiparous (greater than or equal to 7 pregnancies); the average parity was 4.5 (5 for spontaneous ruptures).

Other reports confirmed the high prevalence of ruptured uterus. An early study in Uganda by Rendle-Short (1960) reported a prevalence rate of 107 per 10 000 births. More recently, Groen (1974) reported a rate of 89 per 10 000 in a rural hospital in Nigeria. Most of the reports relate the incidence of uterine rupture to high parity. This can be partially caused by the build-up of fibrous tissues and thinning of the uterine wall as a result of repeated pregnancies. An additional cause of the observed high rates in hospitals is that many emergency cases are reported to hospitals only after lengthy delays.

Maternal Morbidity

Summary In the developing countries, grand multiparity is still prevalent and is associated with high mortality and morbidity from haemorrhage, sepsis, toxaemia, rupture of the uterus, and anaemia. Some evidence also links high parity with gynaecological problems, such as prolapse, cervicitis, cervical erosion, cancer of the cervix, as well as non-obstetric problems, particularly diabetes and rheumatic conditions. The evidence that hypertension is related to parity is still equivocal, while breast and ovarian cancer may be inversely related to parity.

Maternal morbidity and parity

Morbidity among multiparas does not appear to have been as much reduced by recent improvements in medical care as has mortality. Many authors still report a markedly higher prevalence of maternal morbidity in grand multiparas than in low-parity women.

Maternal morbidity can be conveniently classified into obstetric disorders, gynaecological disorders, and general disease conditions.

Obstetric problems

Several conditions have been reported to increase with parity. Two reports from industrialized countries would illustrate this point. Israel & Blazar (1965) in a collaborative obstetrical survey in 13 hospitals in the USA between 1958 and 1960 reported higher rates of anaemia, pre-eclampsia, chronic hypertension, placental disorders, uterine rupture, and postpartum haemorrhage among women of parity 7 and higher. Vehaskari et al. (1968), reporting on

1567 grand multiparas and 16 432 lower-parity women delivered in a Finnish hospital between 1951 and 1960, show statistically significant higher rates among the grand multiparas for hypertensive disease, abruptio placentae, placenta previa, retained placenta, and breech presentation.

For the developing countries, we return to the multicentre study (Omran, 1978) in Bangladesh, Egypt, Indonesia, Nigeria, Sri Lanka, and Sudan, in which several conditions were found to increase with parity, including anaemia, toxaemia and haemorrhage, malpresentation, and blood disorders. In order to assess the relative medical burden due to high parity, an index of blood transfusion utilization was used. Grand multiparas (of 5 or more births) required twice or three times as many blood transfusions as low-parity women.

Gynaecological problems

A number of gynaecological conditions have been found to be associated with high parity, including cervicitis, cervical erosion, prolapse, and cancer of the cervix.

Prolapse: Prolapse arises from one or more of the following: (*a*) injury or overstretching of the pelvic floor, (*b*) devitalization or damage of tissues during prolonged labour and/or obstetric operations, or failure of the uterosacral ligament to involute after labour, and (*c*) laxity of the cardenal ligaments. These mechanisms are accentuated by repeated pregnancies and labour and/or poor obstetric management resulting, under the stress and strain of active life, in protrusion of the bladder, the rectum, and/or the uterus into the vagina or outside the body. The damage produced by pregnancy and labour may not show in the form of prolapse until later in life. Prolapse may also sometimes occur in multiparas with congenital weakness of the concerned ligaments and other supporting structures.

The prevalence of high parity in developing countries is no doubt a major determinant of the higher incidence of prolapse in these countries as compared with industrialized societies. It has been noted, for example, that the incidence of prolapse is much higher in India than in the USA. Most of the studies relating prolapse and other obstetric and gynaecological conditions to parity and maternal age are based on case reports and hospital records using numerator analysis.

The WHO Family Formation Study (Omran & Standley, 1976) included both inquiries about gynaecological symptoms and general health conditions of the women and gynaecological examinations. The frequency of gynaeco- logical complaints was relatively high in all areas, but only small and inconsistent variations were found by parity. Prolapse, however, was one condition that was reported more frequently by women of higher parity. The gynaecological examinations confirmed this positive relationship between prolapse and parity.

Cancer of the cervix: Several studies suggest a positive association between cervical cancer and parity (Maliphant, 1949; Logan, 1953; Wynder et al., 1954; Lundin et al., 1964; and Wahi et al., 1969). Although Logan (1953)

31

reported a similar association between cervical cancer and marital and childbearing experience, he pointed out that no causal relationship had been established. Some of these articles and others on environmental factors associated with cervical cancer, of which parity is only one, are reviewed by Lundin et al. (1964). In their own study of Memphis women, Lundin and his associates found that age at first pregnancy was highly correlated with cancer of the cervix. They also found a small positive association between high parity and intra-epithelial carcinoma of the cervix in white women, but not in Negro women, and they found no consistent association for squamous cell carcinoma of the cervix.

Breast cancer: An international collaborative study of breast cancer and reproductive experience was undertaken by MacMahon et al. (1970) in hospitals in Brazil, China (Province of Taiwan), Greece, Japan, the USA, Wales, and Yugoslavia. In all, more than 400 women who were hospitalized for a first diagnosis of breast cancer and nearly 13 000 controls (patients in the same hospitals for conditions other than breast cancer) were interviewed. Although the trends were not regular, estimated risks of breast cancer for women of parity 5 or more were between 40% and 60% of the risk for the nulliparous. Furthermore, in all 7 centres, breast cancer increased with increase in the age at which a woman bore her first child, with births after the first having substantially less additional protective influence than that of a first birth at the same age.

General disease conditions

Diabetes: As early as the 1930s, Mosenthal & Bolduan (1933) attributed the higher prevalence of diabetes among women to the possible diabetogenic effects of pregnancy. This report was later supported by Pyke (1956), Fitzgerald et al. (1961), O'Sullivan & Gordon (1966), and Middleton & Caird (1968). The latter study examined the records of 543 women and 413 men between the ages of 40 and 80 years who represented virtually all newly diagnosed cases of diabetes in a population whose age and sex structure were known. For diabetic women, they found an "excess" of those with 4 or more children. They also found that while the likelihood of diabetes increased with age, within each age group the rates also increased " with fair regularity with increasing parity". The results of this study were in close agreement with others and showed that in the postmenopausal years (between the ages of 50 and 80) "the excess risk, above that of a nullipara, is 20% for one child, 45% for two, 100% for three, 200% for four or five, and 400% for six or more children". For men, the risk of diabetes was approximately the same as that for women who had borne two children.

An interesting point about these studies is that they were looking at the onset or at least the existence of diabetes in menopausal or postmenopausal women. Their evidence suggests that there may be certain conditions, such as diabetes, that are associated with multigravidity but do not appear until later in life. It is therefore possible that excessive childbearing may alter women permanently. The same may also be true of other conditions, like prolapse and malignancy.

The United States National Health Examination Survey (O'Sullivan & Gordon, 1966) examined mean blood glucose levels by parity for a wide range of groups. The results indicate that the correlation of parity with blood glucose levels was very low when all parities were considered together. The high parity groups, however, had significantly higher blood glucose levels. Because of the small numbers and a negative finding in a study in Massachusetts, the reporters pointed out that a causal relationship could not be established.

Hypertension and cardiovascular disease: Studies of parity and hypertension are of uneven methodological quality and conclusions are equivocal. The majority of studies, however, have found a negative relationship between hypertension and parity. Miall & Oldham (1958) found that among a sample of 623 persons in two communities in South Wales, age-adjusted scores of blood pressure decreased with parity for all women. The samples were small, however, especially for those of high parity.

The negative associations between parity and hypertension found in the small cross-sectional study in South Wales (Miall & Oldham, 1958) have been substantiated in a follow-up study of one third of the original sample and relatives (Miall, 1959) and in a larger sample in Jamaica (Miall et al., 1962). In the Jamaican study, while mean blood pressure was higher for nulliparous than for parous women, it decreased for parities 2 to 5 and then increased for higher parities. A higher mean blood pressure among primigravidas compared with parous women was also found in a study of 6662 white gravidas by Christianson (1976). Similar results were also found in a Swedish study (Humerfelt & Wedervang, 1957) and in Capetown (Gordon et al., 1970). In the first United States National Examination Survey of 1960–62, although "women of parity 5 or more have higher systolic and diastolic blood pressures" and "the mean for women of parity 6 and over is significantly higher than the means for other women on an age-adjusted basis", the authors concluded on the basis of regression coefficients that neither parity nor gravidity played an independent part in the etiology of cardiovascular hypertension. One of the studies that found a positive relationship between parity and hypertension, as well as cardiovascular disease, was that by Quinlivan (1964) who observed that the incidence of cardiovascular disease was 0.8% in 31 986 women of all parities compared with 8.4% among the 4721 women of parity 6 or more.

II. IMPACT OF MATERNAL AGE

Fetal and Child Mortality

Summary The effect of maternal age is discussed here as a separate entity in order to emphasize the significance of timing in family formation. The close association between age and parity should always be borne in mind. A multitude of studies have revealed a consistent association between maternal age and both morbidity and mortality in mothers and children. These studies uniformly suggest that there is an age-band in the fertility span of a woman during which the reproductive risks are at a minimum; on either side of this relatively safe age-band,

33

the risks progressively increase, describing a J-shaped, a U-shaped, or occasionally a reversed J-shaped curve. These patterns are particularly typical of late fetal deaths, perinatal mortality, and infant mortality.

Child mortality

The noteworthy series of British studies based on record linkage from 1949/1950 to 1980 (Morris & Heady, 1955; Spicer & Lipworth, 1966; Davies, 1980) have generally established the patterns. In the latest report of vital records for 1977 (Davies, 1980), a distinct U-shaped pattern for perinatal mortality by maternal age was observed when parity was controlled. The U-shaped curve was described for parities 1, 2, and 3, while for parities 4 and over the risk was high at all ages. The pattern for infant mortality was a reversed J-shaped curve with the highest mortality for maternal ages under 20. There also was a small increase for ages 35 and over.

National and large community studies in the USA have also corroborated these patterns. For instance, neonatal mortality formed a U- or J-shaped relationship with maternal age for both the 1950 and 1960 cohorts of births (Loeb, 1965; Chase, 1972; Armstrong, 1972). The pattern was observed for both whites and non-whites. Similar patterns have also been observed in several large studies in cities in the USA (Yerushalmy, 1938; Chase, 1961, 1962, 1973; Kessner et al., 1973). Most of the studies reviewed in the section on birth order and parity have also indicated the important role of maternal age.

It is of interest to recognize a rapidly growing body of evidence from developing countries on the relationships between maternal age and child mortality and morbidity. However, the published studies are based mainly on hospital records and have serious limitations as to their representativeness, particularly in those countries where only few deliveries take place in a health facility. It has been encouraging to see that several detailed community-based studies were published during the later part of the 1970s. The influence of maternal age was considered in relationship to parity in the previous sections; studies concerned with other relationships are summarized below.

The WHO Family Formation Study (Omran & Standley, 1976) investigated the relationship between maternal age and pregnancy outcome. In most cultural and residential groups in the five countries, 20–29 seemed to be the maternal age range in which there was least pregnancy wastage (stillbirths and abortions). In most of these groups, pregnancy wastage rates described a J-shaped relationship to maternal age. The exceptions were in Iran and Turkey where abortion rates (including both spontaneous and induced abortion) were lowest at young maternal ages.

Neonatal and infant mortality in relation to maternal age were studied in eight projects of the Inter-American Investigation of Mortality in Childhood (Puffer & Serrano, 1975). For all eight projects, including six in Latin America and two in North America, both neonatal and infant mortality rates were higher for young mothers (under 20 years) than for any of the other four age

34

groups. The lowest rates were for mothers 25–29 years old, indicating that his maternal age span was the most favourable one. Along with the excessive death rates among infants born to young mothers, it was noted that in five of the projects these women accounted for more than 10% of the live births. In a further investigation of immaturity and nutritional deficiency as underlying or associated causes of death, the reversed J-shaped pattern was evident in all six Latin American projects, with greatly increased risk among young mothers (under 20 years), reduced risk for intermediate ages, and somewhat elevated risks for mothers over 35 years.

A recent report from Chile (Cabrera, 1980) corroborates the above' age patterns of risks in a national study of all births and deaths from the civil registry during the five-year period 1969–74. While the infant mortality rate declined over the period from 85.3% per thousand live births in 1969 to 69.4 in 1974, the pattern of mortality with maternal age persisted throughout the period. Thus neonatal, postneonatal, and total infant mortality rates were lowest for maternal ages 20–34 and highest for ages under 20 years and for ages 35 and over.

The WHO Family Formation Study also investigated the relationship between infant mortality and maternal age but found that the typical J-shaped curve was not consistently observed for all cultural and residential groups. For many of the groups in the five-country study the percentage of deaths of children under one year of age described a reversed J-shape with maternal age, with high risks among infants born to mothers under 20 years of age, and with the rates decreasing steeply to a minimum somewhere between ages 20 and 34, then rising again for many groups. The relatively high risk associated with young maternal ages may have been due partly to the higher risks of mortality among births occurring in the early years of the cohort when child mortality was higher than in the more recent years, but part of the risk could be attributed to young maternal age itself.

In two studies in Bangladesh, Swenson & Harper (1979) showed an increase in fetal wastage with increasing maternal age while Stoeckel & Chowdhury (1972) found a distinct reversed J-shaped relationship of neonatal mortality with maternal age and a J-shaped relationship of postneonatal mortality with maternal age. Sullivan (1972) found similar patterns in China (Province of Taiwan).

A large number of recent studies in Africa have investigated the relationships between maternal age and child and maternal health. This is a topic of particular significance in a continent where pregnancy and child-bearing begin so early and continue to a relatively late age, encompassing the two periods of highest reproductive risk. In general, the well-established pattern of increased risks for both very young and older mothers has been confirmed, but with some variation among the various conditions studied.

In a study of national data in Ghana for 1960 and 1971, Tawiah (1979) found that infant mortality rates were highest for mothers in the 15–19 age group, reaching 84.3 per thousand, and in the 45–49 age group, reaching 144.7 per thousand. There was a monotonical rise in the death rates after the 20–24 age group, which had the lowest mortality rate of 74.1 per thousand.

In another community-based study, Voorhoeve et al. (1979) conducted an investigation of factors associated with maternal and child health in Machakos, a rural area in Kenya, covering 2246 births in 1975 and 1976. The perinatal mortality rate was 46.7 per thousand births for all age groups, but higher rates were associated with maternal ages less than 25 years and those over 35 years. A history of previous perinatal death and breech delivery were also associated with high perinatal mortality.

Several reports from African centres have demonstrated similar patterns. Examples include: (a) a study by Arkutu (1978a) among 2791 Tanzanian primiparas revealing an increase in perinatal mortality with age, especially after age 30, and (b) a study by Ayeni & Oduntan (1978) in a rural area in Nigeria, which showed a distinct J-shaped relationship between infant mortality and maternal age, with the lowest infant mortality rate for mothers aged 25–29 (71.7 per 1000 live births), increasing to 115.9 for mothers aged 40–44. In another study in Nigeria, Harrison (1979) found that perinatal mortality was highest for women under 20 and for women over 30. The multicentre study by Omran (1978) also revealed an increase in perinatal mortality with age in the Egyptian and Bangladesh centres and a J-shaped pattern in the Indonesian centres. Another example from Africa is the study by Arkutu (1978b) of 259 Tanzanian primigravidae aged 15 and under showing a higher incidence of low-birth-weight children compared with 377 primigravidae aged 21 to 25, with rates of 30.5 and 12.7%, respectively.

Child Health and Development

Summary   Many studies have shown a consistent relationship between maternal age and child health and development. In regard to birth weight and prematurity, teenage girls and older mothers have been found to be more likely to bear a low-birth-weight baby.

Maternal age (and sometimes paternal age, as well) has been found to be the family formation variable most strongly correlated with congenital malformation and handicapping conditions in children. These conditions, especially Down syndrome, have been shown to increase in incidence with increasing maternal age, especially after age 30.

Prematurity

In regard to birth weight and prematurity, a recent example of the widely found relationships comes from the 1976 United States data analysed by Taffel (1980). As mentioned earlier in this review, teenage girls and older mothers have been shown to be more likely than women of other age groups to bear a low-birth-weight baby. The same pattern was also found by Selvin & Garfinkel (1972) in their study of 1.5 million birth certificates in New York City (see under *Birth Order*).

Congenital malformations

Of the family formation variables, maternal age (and sometimes paternal age as well) is most strongly correlated with congenital malformations and handicapping conditions among children. The relationship of increasing incidence of these conditions with increasing maternal age has been documented in the literature of many conditions, especially for Down syndrome (see, for example, Penrose, 1933, 1962, 1967; Smith & Record, 1955; Stevenson et al., 1966; and Spiers, 1972). More recently, a large study in the USA (Taffel, 1978) has confirmed the relative increase of congenital malformations with age after age 30. The highest incidence, however, was found to occur with unusual age-parity combinations of first births to older mothers.

Newcombe (1964) and Newcombe & Travendale (1964) found a great risk of handicapping conditions for women under 20 years and women over 35 years of age. The risk of handicapping conditions was extremely large for high-order births to young mothers and for first-order births to older mothers.

An international WHO surveillance study of consecutive births in 24 medical centres in 16 countries demonstrated an increase in congenital malformation rates with maternal age, especially after age 30 (Stevenson et al., 1966). In a study of two large cities in the USA, Hay & Barbano (1972) also found an increase in congenital malformations as maternal age increased.

The relationship between maternal age and Down syndrome has been recognized in the literature for many decades. Specific studies are reviewed in the section on child health. In one recent study, Fryers & Mackay (1979) reviewed birth records over the fifteen-year period 1961–1975 in an industrial city in Great Britain. For the whole period, the prevalence of Down syndrome at birth was 0.36 per thousand for mothers under 25, 1.15 per thousand for mothers between 25 and 34, and 5.71 per thousand for mothers aged 35 or more. The authors note that with the recent decline in the birth rate among the higher risk group of mothers aged 35 and over, the prevalence of Down syndrome has been decreasing.

Maternal Mortality

Summary   The risk of maternal mortality describes a parabolic, or J-shaped, curve with maternal age. Minimal risk occurs for maternal ages in the early twenties, with high risk for teenage pregnancies, and higher risk for older mothers over 35. This relationship with maternal age is found for all major causes of mortality, including sepsis, toxaemia, and haemorrhage, and in countries at all levels of maternal mortality.

The parabolic relationship between maternal mortality and maternal age has been found in national data from several countries, with the period of least risk falling typically in the early twenties and with some variation in different countries. This means a high risk of mortality for teenage pregnancy and higher risks for older mothers over 35 years. Nortman (1974) noted the J-shaped relationship for all causes and probably also for the specific major causes of sepsis, toxaemia and haemorrhage in several countries during the 1960s. By 1969, such a relationship had been found under low mortality conditions in 14 countries, under intermediate mortality conditions in 16 countries, and under high mortality conditions in 12 countries. Watson et al. (1979) added 5 more countries from the 1974 and 1976 United Nations Demographic Yearbooks and cited the existence of the pattern in two more countries, bringing the total to an impressive 49 countries displaying the typical pattern.

The J-shaped pattern of maternal mortality with age was also found to persist despite the dramatic decline in maternal mortality in the countries under study. This was demonstrated by Berry (1977) for the USA for the years 1917, 1927, 1937, 1947, 1957, and 1967. Our own analysis has shown that the pattern persists also in 1977.

Maternal Morbidity

Summary   A large number of maternal health conditions have been associated with maternal age. Antenatal complications, disorders of uterine action, diabetes, and hypertension have all been shown to increase at older maternal ages. Teenage pregnancies have increasingly become a major source of concern and have been shown to carry a high risk of toxaemia, prolonged labour, Caesarian section, cervical laceration, and other obstetric complications and maternal health problems.

Most of the studies quoted under maternal health and parity described either a steady increase or a J- or reversed J-shaped relationship with maternal age for several specific disease conditions and health problems. The conditions found to be associated with an increase in maternal age include:

(*a*) antenatal complications, including anaemia, toxaemia, urinary tract infection, blood disorders (Omran, 1978, for centres in Bangladesh, Egypt, and Indonesia),

(b) disorders of uterine action and arrest disorders, increasing with age among 6248 parturients at Beth Israel Hospital in Boston (Cohen et al., 1980),

(*c*) high maternal morbidity and hypertension with and without protein-aemia, hepatogestosis, diabetes, varices, psychic illness in women aged 40 and over in a Helsinki centre over a period of 7 years (Kajanoja & Widholm, 1978),

(*d*) diabetes: the likelihood of diabetes was found to increase both with maternal age and with increasing parity (Middleton & Caird, 1968). Many authors over the last 30 years have drawn attention to the medical, social, and educational problems of pregnant teenagers. For example, a large series of cases of pregnant teenagers in New York City was studied by Pakter et al. (1961) who found a high rate of toxaemia, syphilis, maternal mortality, prematurity, and infant mortality. Increased rates of weight gain, toxaemia, prolonged labour, Caesarian section, and cervical laceration, were also found in pregnant girls aged 12–15. Similar findings were presented by Hassan & Falls (1964) and were also reported in a London series (Obeng, 1969), and in Texas (Duenhoelter et al., 1975) to mention only a few examples. Efiong & Banjoko (1975) demonstrated in a study in Lagos that some of the problems of teenage pregnancy could be diminished with good antenatal care.

38

Finally, the interest in the health aspects of teenage pregnancy has been on the increase, especially in industrialized countries. Many books, monographs and journal articles have been published on the subject. See, for example, the special issue of *Family planning perspectives* (1978) which was devoted to this topic.

III. IMPACT OF BIRTH INTERVAL

Definitions

It is important to note that the term "interval" is often used in published reports without clear definition of what it specifically measures in a particular study. There are several types of interval, including:

(a) *Interbirth interval.* The interval between two successive births, including live and/or stillbirths. This interval will miss an intervening pregnancy ending in abortion or fetal loss; if the second child is born prematurely, the interval is automatically shortened by a number of weeks. Such an effect would introduce bias in the analysis. There is also the possibility of underreporting stillbirths leading to similar bias.

(b) *Inter-live-birth-interval.* The interval between two successive live births. It has the advantages over the *interbirth interval* that it includes only live births, which are usually less underreported than stillbirths in surveys. It still disregards an intervening pregnancy that did not end in a live birth, and is also shortened if the second child is born prematurely.

(c) *Interconception interval* or *onset interpregnancy interval.* The interval between the onset of one pregnancy and the onset of a subsequent one. It has the disadvantage that the exact onset of pregnancy cannot usually be accurately identified in interview surveys. If one or both pregnancies end in abortion, fetal loss, or pre term birth, the interval is automatically shortened.

(d) *End-to-onset interpregnancy interval.* The interval between the end of a pregnancy (whether the outcome was a live birth, stillbirth, or fetal loss) and the onset of a subsequent pregnancy, usually measured as the date of the last menstrual period. This is consonant with the term *pregnancy spacing*. Again, there is a possibility of bias due to underreporting of unsuccessful outcomes or inability to identify accurately the onset of the next pregnancy.

(e) *Pregnancy interval* or *end-to-end interpregnancy interval.* The interval between the end of a pregnancy (whether the outcome was a live birth, stillbirth, or fetal loss) and the end of the subsequent pregnancy (again whether the outcome was a live birth, stillbirth, or fetal loss). This is also used synonomously with the generic term "birth interval", although again bias due to underreporting of unsuccessful outomes is a possibility. Along with interbirth interval, this is the most commonly used term and its is the term used in the present study.

Fetal and Child Mortality

Summary Prevailing medical opinions favour spacing of pregnancies in order to allow restoration of health of mothers, to safeguard the health of the offspring, and to enable mothers to breast feed their children without the added burden of a new pregnancy.

Studies from developed countries and recently from developing countries have shown an association between short birth intervals and higher risks of poor outcome of subsequent pregnancy and of child mortality. The effects are not only associated with the preceding interval, but also with the succeeding interval. It follows that both the displaced child and the displacing child are affected. Birth interval effects are by no means entirely independent of those of age and parity.

Research concerning the influence of birth interval on family health is relatively scanty and fraught with methodological problems. This is an area for further investigation, especially in developing countries where the factors of lactation and nutrition play an important part in these interactions.

The link between short birth intervals and higher risks of infant mortality has been recognized since the early 1920s (Hughes, 1923 and Woodbury, 1925) at a time when infant mortality was high in the USA. For example, in Gary, Indiana, in 1916, Hughes found an infant mortality rate of 169.1 per 1000 for intervals of less than 15 months, compared to 102.8 for intervals of two years or more. Yerushalmy (1945), using an indirect method of estimating the risk, reached similar conclusions in regard to stillbirth rates among the birth cohorts of 1937–41 in the USA. Yerushalmy et al. (1956) investigated this question again in Kauai, Hawaii, by collecting reproductive histories of 6039 women over 12 years of age during 1953. High fetal and childhood mortality were found to be associated with very short intervals (of 4 months or less). The World Health Organization comparative study on perinatal mortality in seven industrialized countries and Cuba indicated that the optimal interval between births in those countries was from 18 months to 3 years (World Health Organization, 1976a, 1978). The risk for those born within 12 months of the completion of a previous pregnancy was 3.5 times greater than for those born during the optimum interval.

The original data from the British Perinatal Mortality Survey (PBMS) (Butler & Bonham, 1963) exhibit an association of high perinatal mortality and short intervals. However, James (1968b) believed that such a relationship is spurious because of the association of low social class with both high perinatal mortality and short interval. He also quoted other authors establishing the relationship between parity (which is inherently associated with birth interval) and perinatal mortality. He obtained and reanalysed the data from the 1958 British Perinatal Mortality Survey using a fixed sibship or a longitudinal approach after making several exclusions from the data set. His conclusions were that, within sibships, stillbirths were associated with long but not with short intervals, while neonatal mortality was associated with short intervals. Such conclusions should be viewed with caution for two reasons: (*a*) selection was introduced in the data set by including in the analysis only "questionnaires in which details were recorded of at least one prior pregnancy and in which the pregnancy immediately preceding the ascertained confinement had yielded a live-born infant ... which had not died before the age of 28 days", and (b) the longitudinal method has since been criticized as introducing its own bias (Mantel, 1979).

Still another reanalysis of the British data set by Fedrick & Adelstein (1973) found neonatal mortality to be greater for short intervals. When social class and outcome of preceding intervals were controlled, the effect of birth interval diminished, except for intervals of 6 months or less where the difference was statistically significant.

A Norwegian study by Erickson & Bjerkedal (1978) failed to find the same effect of short birth interval on child mortality and prematurity. In the study, pairs of first and second births, and pairs of second and third births to the same Norwegian mothers, were studied. There was a fairly marked deficit in average weight at the short intervals and a less pronounced deficit at longer intervals. Higher stillbirth rates were found for longer intervals, while neonatal mortality was higher for short intervals. The authors concluded that "it seems to us highly unlikely that manipulation of the interval between pregnancies will have a marked, direct, beneficial effect on pregnancy outcome". Such a conclusion does not follow from the Norwegian data and is antagonistic to other biological, clinical, and epidemiological evidence (see also the following section).

A more recent longitudinal study by Zimmer (1979) was based on a random sample of 3098 once-married women in Aberdeen, Scotland, who had a pregnancy outcome during the period 1950–55 and whose reproductive behaviour was followed through 1970. They had a total of 10 825 pregnancies which resulted in 285 infant deaths, 173 stillbirths, 712 involuntary terminations, and 200 voluntary terminations. Through longitudinal analysis by pregnancy order (for the pooled data), wastage was found to increase with parity. There was also a two-way interaction between spacing and outcome. Women who had a wastage were more likely to continue on to the next higher pregnancy number (usually at a shorter interval) and those who have a wastage at one pregnancy number were more likely to have a wastage at the next pregnancy outcome also. One of the conclusions relating to spacing and parity was that "spacing between pregnancy events, at any given number, has an impact on outcome. The wastage rate is highest among women who closely space their pregnancies and at higher parity levels".

Evidence from the developing countries points generally in the same direction. High infant mortality was linked at least partly to short birth intervals in several Latin American centres (Puffer & Serrano, 1975). Similarly, in the Punjab, India, infants born less than two years after the previous child were about 50% more likely to die by age one than were infants born 2–4 years after the previous child (Gordon et al., 1967).

The WHO Family Formation Study (Omran & Standley, 1976) found that pregnancy wastage rates (stillbirths and abortions) typically described a reversed J-shape with pregnancy interval, the highest risks being associated with intervals of less than 1 or 2 years, while the lowest risks were associated with intervals of 3–5 years. With the exception of India, the risks increased again for intervals of 6 or more years. The risks of infant mortality were also found to be highest after intervals of less than 1–2 years.

The evidence from Africa and the Middle East is scanty and irregular, being based on hospital studies or small community samples. For example, El-Beheiry et al. (1976) examined birth intervals among 208 children attending the outpatient clinic in a Cairo centre. The average birth interval for 98 children diagnosed as normal was 40.1 months, compared with 34.8 months for the 110 children with health problems (59 cases of underweight, 30 cases of kwashiorkor, 19 cases of marasmas, and 2 cases of marasmic kwashiorkor). The difference of 5.3 months was not statistically significant, but Kamel et al. (1974) found a definite relationship between short birth intervals and high fetal wastage (stillbirth and abortion) especially when the interval was less than 12 months. The sample used was small and included 350 women in a rural community in Egypt.

Sudden infant death syndrome

There is, in Western countries, particularly the USA, a growing interest in investigating the sudden infant death syndrome. One study by Spiers & Wang (1976) linked this syndrome to short birth intervals. In their study, pregnancy intervals were calculated for 54 369 later-born singletons delivered during 1969 in North Carolina. Deaths in this cohort were matched with those in a control group of infants surviving the first year of life. Deaths were categorized as sudden infant death syndrome, deaths due to congenital malformation, and all other deaths. A higher proportion of short intervals was found among cases than among controls. The results were statistically significant only for the sudden infant death syndrome.

Child Health and Development

Summary   Short preceding birth intervals have been linked with higher rates of prematurity, low birth weight, and neonatal mortality, and with lower physical and intellectual development of children. The highest risks of prematurity occur with birth intervals of less than two years. Intervals of two to four years have the least risk of prematurity, while the risk increases for intervals of five or more years. Poorer child health and development may also be associated with the succeeding birth interval, with both the displaced and the displacing child being affected.

Prematurity and preceding birth interval

Higher rates of prematurity were also linked with preceding short intervals in two studies, one in England by Douglas (1950) who studied a nationwide sample of 13 000 births during one week in 1946. The study found that the highest risks of prematurity were associated with intervals of one year or less and the least risks with intervals of 2–4 years. A second but smaller increase in risk was also noted for extra-long intervals of 6 years or more. The second study was reported by Bishop (1964) among 16 000 consecutive deliveries in Philadelphia, which confirmed the increased risks of prematurity with intervals of less than 1 year.

In the multicentre study by Omran (1978), the prematurity risk was higher when the interval since the end of the last pregnancy was less than 21 months than it was for intervals of 30 months and longer. The respective rates of prematurity, for example, were 122 per 1000 and 65 per 1000 in an Indonesian centre, 282 and 175 in a Bangladesh centre, and 65 and 30 in a Swedish centre.

Child development

Physical and mental development also seem to be influenced by the birth interval. In an ongoing longitudinal study by the Perinatal Research branch of the National Institute of Neurological Diseases and Stroke (USA), based on data from 14 collaborating medical centres, Holley et al. (1969) found that "the children with an intersib interval of less than one year had lower birth weight, lower Bayley developmental scores at 8 months of age, lower Binet IQ scores at four years of age, and a greater incidence of neurologically suspicious or abnormal outcome check at one year of age".

Maternal Health

Summary The undermining of a woman's health by repeated pregnancies at short intervals has been an important concern of the medical community. Spacing of pregnancies is regarded as important both for the restoration of the mother's health and to enable the mother to breast feed her child without the added burden of a new pregnancy.

As expected, successive pregnancies deplete the maternal resources and may result in maternal malnutrition, particularly anaemia, the maternal depletion syndrome (Jelliffe, 1966) , and poor quality of breast milk (Kader et al., 1972, in an Egyptian study). This is an important area for further investigation.

Several maternal health problems have previously been discussed in relation to multiparity. It should be pointed out that many of the problems of multiparous and grand multiparous women are also related to age. Likewise, many of the same health problems, including anaemia of pregnancy and maternal malnutrition, may be attributed to too close spacing of pregnancies.

Subsequent Interval Effect

Summary A few studies have examined the impact of the succeeding birth interval on the displaced child. Children whose birth is followed by short birth intervals have been found to have lower survivorship, be less healthy, and have lower physical and intellectual development than those whose birth is followed by a longer interval. This deleterious effect on the earlier child has long been recognized in African and Islamic cultural restrictions on a new pregnancy while a mother is nursing a child.

Scientific literature about the effects of the subsequent birth interval is scanty, although its influence has not escaped notice in folk culture. It is well known that there are cultural restrictions on intercourse by nursing mothers in

Africa. Even in the early Islamic tradition, a new pregnancy while the mother is nursing a child is strongly discouraged, lest the suckling child may incur ill effects that may not appear until adult life. This is known in Islamic tradition as *al-ghail*. Reference may also be made to kwashiorkor, which has been linked in African culture to the close succession of pregnancies interfering with proper feeding of the early child. Cecily Williams (cited in Wray, 1971) has explained that "kwashiorkor" derives from the Ghanian Ga language and means the disease of the baby deposed (from the mother's breast) when the next one is conceived.

A few studies have examined the impact of the succeeding interval on the displaced child. Wray & Aguirre (1969), in their Colombian Study, found that the rate of malnutrition ranged from 40% to 57% with intervals of less than 3 years (succeeding the birth of the index child) compared with about 26% for longer intervals. Although the difference was only of borderline statistical significance, the authors felt that the percentages clearly suggest that an interval of at least 3 years between children in that community "protects" the older child to some extent from malnutrition. Wolfers & Scrimshaw (1974) believed that there is a combined effect of preceding and succeeding intervals. They examined the reproductive histories of 1934 mothers in Guayaquil, Ecuador, and found higher risks of miscarriage and stillbirth rates for very short and for very long interpregnancy intervals (both preceding and succeeding). A minimal risk of postneonatal mortality was found for intervals of about 3 years (both ways).

In a study in a rural area in Bangladesh, Swenson (1978) found that children whose birth was followed by a subsequent pregnancy in less than 12 months have significantly lower survivorship than those followed by longer intervals. The outcome of the second pregnancy (fetal loss or stillbirth as opposed to live birth) and the length of competition from the second pregnancy did not appear to significantly affect the survivorship of the first child in the interval. However, the author suggests that children whose births are followed by short intervals may be less healthy than those whose births are followed by longer intervals, or may have less healthy mothers, and that health conditions that predispose to childhood mortality may be affecting the mortality experience of both children in the interval.

The hypothesis that birth intervals affect the physical and mental development of children as well as infant survival has been investigated in a study in Singapore (Martin, 1979). Five hundred and sixty 9-year old school-children randomly selected from 19 urban schools in 1974 and 1975 were compared on a number of physical and mental measures. It was found that children born after a short birth interval (less than 18 months) scored lower in vocabulary tests than those children born after a longer birth interval. Children born after short intervals consistently had lower scores in perceptual and vocabulary tests, and were smaller in height and weight than those born after longer intervals, with linear improvements in all measures as birth intervals increased from less than 12 months to greater than 24 months. The preceding birth interval was found to be more important. Family size and maternal age by themselves did not seem to affect vocabulary scores; however, income was an important factor, particularly when large family size was combined with poverty to produce a detrimental effect on physical and mental development. The author concluded that a minimum of two years is necessary between births for the best development, and that the linear trend in the tables indicated that a 3-year interval would be even better.

IV. IMPACT OF CHILD LOSS ON FERTILITY BEHAVIOUR

Summary Family formation patterns and objectives (including actual and ideal family size, desired number of male and female children, and regulation of fertility) may be influenced by the child loss experience of individual couples and/or by the fear of child loss based on community experience. The implication of this view is that there will be a major psychological barrier to fertility limitation as long as infant and child mortality remain at high levels. The mechanisms through which infant mortality may affect fertility have been the subject of a number of seminars and reviews (Omran, 1971; Taylor et al., 1976; Friedlander, 1977; Ware, 1977; Preston, 1978; Scrimshaw, 1978).

The four main mechanisms through which child loss or survival is linked to fertility behaviour are:

(*a*) involuntary or biological (physiological) mechanisms, whereby the birth interval following child loss is shorter than that following the birth of a child who survives; among factors to be considered are length of lactation and lactation amenorrhoea, as well as social customs that make for the shunning of a new pregnancy while another child is being nursed;

(*b*) response to loss of own child (replacement motivation);

(*c*) response to fear of child loss (insurance motivation); and

(*d*) societal response whereby social organizations responding to improved child survival may endorse and/or subscribe to fertility regulation.

Although these mechanisms have been widely discussed, existing methodologies have proved inadequate in establishing their independent operation. In particular, it appears that different mechanisms will operate depending on the level of development and the stage of the epidemiological transition. There is, therefore, a need for additional sociodemographic and epidemiological studies of the relationship between child loss and fertility in different cultural and geopolitical settings.

In the previous review (Omran & Standley, 1976), the evidence was classified, for descriptive purposes, into five categories: (1) studies of pre-industrial Europe; (2) studies of national demographic trends; (3) simulation and econometric models; (4) cross-sectional correlation and multivariate analyses; (5) specific family surveys.

The reader is referred to the previous review for details of these categories. Additional discussion can also be found in Preston (1978) and Taylor et al. (1976). In the present report, only a few additional comments will be given for the category of specific family surveys, which represents the most direct method of investigating the impact of infant mortality on the formation of individual families.

Reference has already been made in the previous review to a number of specific family surveys, including: (*a*) Hassan's study in Egypt (1966); (*b*) Adlakha's study in Turkey (1970); (*c*) Harrington's study in West Africa (1971); (*d*) Rutstein's study in China (Province of Taiwan) (1971); (*e*) Heer and Wu's study in China (Province of Taiwan) and Morocco (1975); (*f*) Lery and Vallin's study in France (1975); and (*g*) Chowdhury et al.'s study in Bangladesh (1975).

The WHO Family Formation Study (Omran & Standley, 1976) used a special approach to solve the problem of the time factor by considering women in the 40–44 age group who had experienced 0, 1–2, or 3 losses among their first three live births. In the five collaborating cities, it was found consistently that mean gravidity and mean parity increased progressively with child loss among the first three live births. The ideal family size was not affected, while mean achieved family size decreased with child loss. Contraceptive use was negatively associated with child loss.

Devi (1978) addressed the question of the insurance effect, i.e., whether perception of the level of infant mortality in the community had an influence on fertility. From a study of 1498 currently married women in Kerala, India, grouped according to whether or not they perceived an improvement in infant and child mortality conditions, he concluded that among all age and socio-economic groups, the actual experience of a reduction in infant deaths was the crucial factor leading to a decline in fertility and that the impression of a decline in infant and child deaths had only a negligible influence.

Park et al. (1979) in a recent study in the Republic of Korea investigated the effect of infant deaths on subsequent fertility in a country where both fertility and mortality have undergone recent dramatic declines. They analysed retrospectively 23 635 birth records of 6285 women from the 1971 National Fertility Survey of Korea. Their findings suggest that prior to the introduction of the National Family Planning Program, the influence of infant deaths was limited to the biological effect resulting from a shortened lactational period. Since fertility regulation methods have been made available throughout the country, the effect of motivation to replace the lost child appeared to emerge. Thus, the proportion of excess births attributable to infant deaths was seen to increase in recent years, although because of the lowered infant mortality the overall impact of infant deaths on national fertility appeared to be small.

One indication that the replacement motivation may have been acting independently of a biological effect in some societies is the increased propensity to continue childbearing that has been noted in several societies when the child who died in infancy was a male (Srivastava & Pandey, 1978; Mitra, 1977). For instance, in a study of the effect of infant mortality on subsequent fertility in Uttar Pradesh, India, Srivastava & Pandey (1978) found that the average interval after survival of an infant less than one month old was 15.3 months; if the earlier child lived at least a year, the average interval was 25.3 months. When a male child died after less than a month, the interval was 16.5 months, while when a female child died, the interval was 19.0 months.

A major question in all this research is the direction of causal influence in the relationship between infant mortality and subsequent fertility. Evidence that shortened lactation and close birth spacing result in increased child mortality has been discussed in the section on birth intervals. Evidence for a reverse effect (of child survival on the length of the subsequent interval) also exists, as shown in two recent studies. In a study in Bangladesh, Swenson (1978) has investigated the relationship between child survivorship and the length of the subsequent interpregnancy interval, as well as the outcome of the subsequent pregnancy. Regression analysis showed that children whose birth is followed by another pregnancy in less than 12 months have significantly lower survivorship than those whose birth is followed by longer intervals. (The outcome of the second pregnancy did not appear to have a significant effect on the survivorship of the older child in the interval.)

Zimmer (1979) has noted that analysis of replacement and spacing effects has mostly been limited to live births and infant deaths. In an analysis of birth histories of 3098 once-married women in Aberdeen, Scotland (between 1950 and 1970), he examined all pregnancy outcomes for evidence of replacement and spacing effects. He found that women who experience a stillbirth or involuntary abortion at any given pregnancy number are not only more likely to have another pregnancy, but also do so over a shorter time interval than those whose last pregnancy resulted in a live birth. The wastage rate was found to be highest among women who closely space their pregnancies and at higher parity levels. Since those who experience a loss at one pregnancy are more likely to have a wastage at the next pregnancy outcome, attempts at a further reproduction not only add additional births, but also contribute further to the loss rate.

Finally, it should be emphasized that the crucial question regarding the impact of infant mortality on fertility is the time lag between improvements in infant and childhood survival and the response of the individual families in limiting their fertility and of societal organizations in endorsing and supporting fertility regulation. Multivariate time series of data from communities living under various social and economic conditions are vitally needed for further evaluation of the mechanisms that link mortality to fertility.

V. HEALTH BENEFITS FROM IMPROVED FAMILY FORMATION PATTERNS

Summary Retrospective analysis of trends in the age and parity distribution of births, such as the experience in the USA, reveals measurable reductions in health risks with elimination or modification of certain patterns of family formation. Health risks are shown to be reduced through limiting the number of children, timing pregnancies to occur at maternal ages with minimum risk, and spacing of pregnancies. The decline in certain congenital abnormalities, such as Down syndrome, has been attributed to changes in the maternal age distribution of births.

The preceding sections of this review have concentrated exclusively on characterizing the risks associated with certain patterns of family formation by comparing population groups with varying levels of maternal age, number and

47

rank of pregnancy or birth, and length of birth interval. Collectively, the association between family formation and health has been demonstrated in various social and geographical settings.

A crucial question raised in many countries is whether or not it would be possible, either directly or indirectly, to reduce health risks to children and mothers through family planning, i.e., limiting the number of children, timing pregnancies to occur at maternal ages with minimum risk (20–34 years), and spacing pregnancies. It is difficult to find a direct answer to this question based on experimental design, since such designs would obviously be unethical and extremely complex. But some evidence can be gained from retrospective analysis of trends or from projecting potential changes under certain assumptions. Such evidence is only recent and is still in need of methodological refinement. It nevertheless reveals measurable reductions in health risks with elimination of certain patterns of family formation that are considered potentially hazardous.

Thus, Wright (1972) estimated a 29% reduction in infant mortality (24% in neonatal and 42% in postneonatal mortality) in the USA under optimal assumptions of family size, spacing and timing of first births. Using the US birth cohort of 1960 and the corresponding infant mortality by birth order and maternal age, he found the familiar U-shaped relationship of infant mortality rates with maternal age, while the rates increased steadily with birth order. The stated reductions were estimated under the assumption that within that particular cohort, no birth orders higher than three occurred, with birth order one occurring only to women 20–24 and 25–29, and birth orders two and three to women 25–29 and 30–34, respectively. He also stated that "with 1960 birth order-specific infant mortality rates held constant, the birth order distribution in 1968 on the whole favored a lower overall infant mortality rate than in 1960". He was, however, apprehensive that this effect would be cancelled out by the changing distribution of maternal age toward lower maternal ages between 1960 and 1968.

Morris et al. (1975) used data from the USA for the years 1960–1972 and applied age-birth-order-specific infant mortality rates during 1960 to age-birth-order distribution of births for each of the succeeding years. They found that "whereas shifts in birth order distributions for births since 1960 that would favor lower infant mortality rates were thought previously to be cancelled out by shifts in maternal age distributions that would raise the mortality rate, our data show that the *net* effect actually accounts for about 27 percent of the decline in infant mortality rates".

In an earlier report, Gendell & Hellegers (1973) used special tabulations of matched births and deaths for the city of Baltimore for the years 1960–62 and 1965–67. During this period, births fell by a sixth and perinatal mortality by a quarter. Their calculations indicated that almost one quarter of the 9.3% decline in the perinatal mortality rate for all births between 1961 and 1966 was due to the changes in the maternal-age-birth-order distribution of all births.

Meirik et al. (1979) found that changing age and parity distribution of mothers in Sweden between 1953 and 1975 accounted for only 8.75% of the 16 per 1000 decline in perinatal mortality.

48

In regard to maternal mortality, there is an indication in a study by Berry (1977) of US trends between 1919 and 1969 that "changes in age and parity distributions of births had some influence on maternal mortality trends for the years 1919–1969 in the USA" and that "changes in the age and parity distributions of births for cohorts of U.S. women also influenced crude cohort maternal mortality rates to some extent".

Finally, it is interesting to note that the decline in Down syndrome in certain areas is largely due to the change in distribution of maternal age. This was found by Fryers & Mackay (1979) who analysed comprehensive records of the mentally handicapped over a period of 15 years (1961–1975) in Salford, England. In that city, the prevalence of Down syndrome at birth was shown to have fallen from 17.0 per 10 000 births in the period 1961–65 to 8.4 in 1971–75. Births to mothers aged 35–44 fell by 70% while no births occurred to mothers aged 45 in the period 1963–73. The authors concluded that "the fall in the prevalence can be shown to be largely due to a change in distribution of maternal age".

VI. CROSS-SECTIONAL VERSUS LONGITUDINAL ANALYSIS OF FAMILY FORMATION AND HEALTH: AN ASSESSMENT

Introduction

In recent years, there has been a growing debate on the validity of conclusions based on the traditional cross-sectional analysis of the relationship between health risks and family formation variables. A number of longitudinal and sibship analytical techniques have been proposed that have confirmed the adverse effects of large sibship sizes, but have failed to corroborate an increase in risk with birth order as heretofore universally reported. Instead, the proposed techniques have demonstrated that once the total or "eventual" sibship size or gravidity is controlled, risks decrease with birth order. The increased risk with birth order was, therefore, considered an artifact (James, 1976; Leridon, 1977; Ressiguie, 1977; Roman et al., 1978; Bakketeig & Hoffman, 1979). Similar doubts were cast on the effect of birth interval (James, 1976; Erickson & Bjerkedal, 1978). The new techniques, however, have also been criticized for introducing artifacts of their own (Mantel, 1979; Golding, 1979; Yudkin, 1980);[1] and the validity of cross-sectional analysis has been reaffirmed by studies comparing the two techniques applied to the same data (Naylor, 1974; Phillippe, 1978). Such a debate could have been passed off as an academic exercise, but some of the proponents of the alternative techniques have unwisely concluded that manipulation of the family formation variables would not lead to any direct health benefits. It is necessary, therefore, to make a careful assessment of these issues. Because of space limitations, this discussion will concentrate on two of the most recent papers, one concerning the birth order effect and another the birth interval effect.

---

[1] Also: Gray, R., 1980, personal communication.

The birth order effect

Bakketeig & Hoffman (1979) used data on 294 514 mothers in Norway who gave birth during 1967–1973 to one or more of their first four single babies. The analysis excluded mothers with fifth or higher birth order children and mothers who had multiple births. Thus, 46 981 births were excluded from a total of 464 067 births. Cross-sectional analysis of perinatal mortality (deaths at 16 or more weeks of gestation and during the first week of life) revealed a higher mortality rate (19.4 per 1000 births) for first compared with second order births (14.8 per 1000) and an increasing mortality to 17.0 per 1000 for third- and to 19.5 per 1000 for fourth-order births. Longitudinal analysis, on the other hand, revealed three principal features. First, as the attained sibship size increased from one to four, the perinatal mortality generally increased, a finding in agreement with cross-sectional analysis. Second, within fixed attained sibship sizes, perinatal mortality decreased with birth order. Third, perinatal mortality was higher in babies born to mothers who had had three or four children within a seven-year period than among those born to mothers whose deliveries occurred over a period exceeding seven years.

The findings of the longitudinal analysis confirm the conclusions from cross-sectional studies that perinatal mortality increases with attained sibship size (the first finding of the study). The third finding of the study affirms the health benefit of spacing, although the authors did not explicitly state this obvious conclusion. The controversy remains, therefore, with the birth order effect. Before we address this issue, it is important to emphasize that the policy implications will be the same whether an independent effect of birth order is found or not. In other words, the Norwegian study confirms that *the smaller the sibship size, the lower the perinatal mortality and that the more widely spaced the pregnancies, the lower the perinatal mortality. Hence, no change in policy is warranted.*

Comments on the birth order effect

By resorting to longitudinal analysis in which sibship size was kept fixed, the authors could demonstrate a declining perinatal mortality with birth order, in contrast with the findings of cross-sectional analysis which they claimed were due to an artifact. They concluded that it is the "final" or "eventual" family size, not the birth order, that has the adverse impact. They explained that a first birth to a mother who will eventually attain a family size of four is at a higher risk than a first birth to a mother who will eventually attain a family size of 3 or less. This could imply a retroactive effect of future family size which violates the temporal component of causality. Earlier authors (James, 1968a, 1970; Ressiguie, 1973, 1977) asserted that mothers who are prone to high fertility are also prone to high perinatal mortality among their pregnancies. No convincing biological or epidemiological evidence was given to support such an assertion.

Bakketeig & Hoffman (1979) attempted to explain the relationship on the basis, on the one hand, of increasing birth weight with birth order and on the other hand, of reproductive compensation. Their data suffer, however, from several limitations and the validity of the longitudinal approach itself is impaired by its own bias. In the first place, the restriction of the analysis to only four pregnancies poses severe limitations on the results and precludes generalization to populations where higher parities exist. It is, ironically, higher parities of five or over that sustain the highest risk. In addition to this restriction or selection bias, bias can also arise from inclusion of incomplete families and the inevitability of truncation (Gray, R., personal communication).

Mantel (1979) in a comment on the Norwegian paper, shows that the longitudinal analysis adopted in the paper has introduced its own bias. Bakketeig & Hoffman (1979) argued that their results are consistent with the tendency to become pregnant again after a pregnancy with an early adverse outcome and the higher probability of stopping childbearing after a successful outcome of pregnancy. They go on to relate the phenomenon of declining perinatal mortality to this tendency, but, as Mantel argues, they "show no awareness that their own demonstration would then itself be an artifact". Mantel then gives the following example to demonstrate that artifact:

> Suppose the perinatal mortality rate to be constant at 20 per 1000, and that second pregnancies occur with certainty if the first pregnancy results in mortality, only half the time if the first pregnancy is successful. Accordingly, in 100 000 first pregnancies there would be, on the average, 2000 failures and 98 000 successes. In the 51 000 second pregnancies (2000 + 98 000/2) there would be, on the average, 1020 failures, 40 being repeat failures, 980 first-time failures. If we now compare perinatal mortality rates only for women who have had two pregnancies, we would see $\frac{2000}{51\,000} = 39.2$ per thousand for the first pregnancy, but only $\frac{1020}{51\,000} = 20$ per thousand for the second pregnancy.
>
> By making comparisons fixed on sibship size Bakketeig and Hoffman have only traded one artifact for another. Increasing perinatal mortality with parity (but with no concern for sibship size) could as much reflect that higher parity pregnancies include relatively more high risk mothers as that the risk actually increases with parity.

In another critique, Golding (1979) agrees with Mantel and goes further to emphasize the dilemma that faces clinicians when reading the Norwegian paper. She says "given a group of pregnant women, even the most intuitive clinician is unlikely to be able to determine how many pregnancies the woman will eventually have ... what he will know is how many pregnancies she has already had, and what their outcome was." She closes by saying, "it would be a pity if clinicians and epidemiologists alike were to consider the analysis by Professor Bakketeig and Mr. Hoffman as anything other than an amusing artifact."

Leridon (1977) also used the longitudinal approach but indicated that the method is not applicable beyond the sixth rank because of the complexity of the birth histories when "the number of possible (parity) combinations rapidly exceeds the number of pregnancies observed for the same rank, and the results are no longer valid". This is an inherent limitation of the method making it inapplicable to data from developing countries.

In still another critique of the Norwegian paper, Yudkin (1980) referred to the difficulty in the study of family formation interactions of applying the usual procedure of allowing pregnancy order as a risk factor to vary, while all other relevant variables are held constant. She concludes that if the risk rates are aggregated according to the number of previous outcomes, using a population weighting, "one arrives at the familiar cross-sectional data relating to pregnancy order". We might add that there is also the dilemma that seven years is too short a span for longitudinal observation, while longer periods would, as acknowledged by Bakketeig & Hoffman, introduce a time-trend bias.

Phillippe (1978) has taken issue with the longitudinal approach in a practical way by examining the outcome of both the longitudinal and cross-sectional approaches and finding comparable results. His data were collected from records of married couples distributed over the entire demographic evolution of a rural Quebec population. Cross-sectional analysis indicated that the distribution of infant mortality rates takes the form of a parabola indicating increased risk for first birth, declining until the fourth birth order and undergoing, finally, a constant increase with later birth orders. Longitudinal analysis demonstrated also that, for most family sizes, the risk of infant mortality grows in a parabolic manner with birth order within each family size. The author concludes that the results speak in favour of a genuine increase in risk of infant death with birth order.

In an earlier detailed study, Naylor (1974) looked explicitly for an artifact in the relationship between spontaneous abortion and maternal age and birth order. The material for the study consisted of reproductive histories of women registered in the obstetric services of 13 hospitals during the period 1959–1966. Naylor used various statistical models and techniques to test the artifactual hypothesis and failed to find evidence for such an artifact. The data clearly showed that abortion was greater at higher parity. Although the women sampled tended to be young, an increase of risk with age was demonstrated in the white sample. Such effects were considered by Naylor as genuine. The age effects among Negro women were, however, possibly confounded with other factors.

In commenting on this paper, James (1977) who has been a persistent advocate of the artifact hypothesis since 1963, disagreed with Naylor's conclusions. He most interestingly declared that "I have not suggested that the genuine-effect hypothesis is false, but rather that the artifact hypothesis is true". He also suggested that it is unlikely that this problem will be settled without prospective data on complete obstetric histories.

The birth interval effect

Erickson & Bjerkedal (1978) conducted a paired analysis of the same data set for births in Norway for the period 1967–1973. After making several exclusions, the authors concentrated on pairs of first and second births and pairs of second and third births to the same Norwegian mothers. Most of the pairs were derived from mothers who had only two births during the period. Use of the pair approach, according to the authors, provides one birth which could possibly have been affected by the length of the interval and one birth which could not. The study found that stillbirth rates were higher for long intervals but not for short intervals while neonatal mortality rates were higher for short, but not for long intervals. The report ended with a sweeping conclusion that "it is highly unlikely that manipulation of the interval between pregnancies will have any marked, direct, beneficial effect on pregnancy outcome".

In the first place, such a conclusion is at variance with the stated findings of the study. Nothwithstanding the acceptability of their approach, they found higher risks of stillbirth rates with long intervals and of neonatal mortality rates with short intervals. It is logical to assume that an intermediate interval (one that is not too short or too long) would be associated with a reduction in both mortality risks.

Secondly, the study itself has limitations. In order to get the pairs required for analysis, considerable exclusions were made which rendered the data set unrepresentative of the orginal population of births. Thus, the conclusions of the study cannot be generalized to even the population from which the pairs were drawn. Furthermore, examining the graphs presented in the paper one finds that the pattern of relationships is not sufficiently consistent to allow unequivocal conclusions. Finally, the conclusion about the futility of spacing is in conflict with known physiological and clinical facts, let alone compelling epidemiological evidence. There can be little doubt that a woman needs a period of rest and recuperation before another pregnancy. The least that can be said is that during the intervening period, she will be rebuilding her own resources and will be able to breast-feed her child uninterrupted by a subsequent pregnancy. The epidemiologic evidence regarding the association of short intervals with health risks has been presented earlier and there is no reason to dispute such an evidence.

In closing, we might add that the results of intervention studies would also help to clarify these issues in regard to birth order and birth interval effects. Experimental or quasi-experimental evidence is not easy to come by. An approximation to such evidence is provided by the analysis of the experience of certain countries with a view to examining to what extent the reduction in maternal and child health risks can be attributed to a change in maternal age-parity-birth interval patterns.

REFERENCES

ADLAKHA, A. L. (1970) *A study of infant mortality in Turkey.* Ann Arbor, Michigan, University Microfilms.

ADLAKHA, A. L. & SUCHINDRAN, C. M. (1980) *Differentials of infant mortality in Sri Lanka,* Chapel Hill, University of North Carolina (mimeographed document).

ARKUTU, A. A. (1978a) A clinical study of maternal age and parturition in 2971 Tanzanian primiparae. *International journal of gynaecology and obstetrics,* **16**: 20–23.

ARKUTU, A. A. (1978b) Pregnancy and labor in Tanzanian primigravidae aged 15 years and under. *International journal of gynaecology and obstetrics,* **16**: 128–131.

ARMON, P. J. (1977) Rupture of the uterus in Malawi and Tanzania. *East African medical journal,* **54**: 462–471.

ARMSTRONG, R. J. (1972) A study of infant mortality from linked records: by birth weight, period of gestation and other variables. *Vital and health statistics*, Series 20, Number 12.

AYENI, O. & ODUNTAN, S. O. (1978) The effects of sex, birthweight, birth order and maternal age on infant mortality in a Nigerian community. *Annals of human biology*, 5: 353–358.

BAHR, S. J. & LEIGH, G. K. (1978) Family size, intelligence , and expected education. *Journal of marriage and family*, 40: 331–335.

BAJPAI, P. C. ET AL. (1966) Observations on perinatal mortality. *Indian pediatrics*, 3: 83–98.

BAKKETEIG, L. S. & HOFFMAN, H. J. (1979) Perinatal mortality by birth order within cohorts based on sibship size. *British medical journal*, 2: 693–696.

BAKKETEIG, L. S. ET AL. (1978) Obstetric service and perinatal mortality in Norway. *Acta obstetricia et gynecologica scandinavica*, Suppl. No. 77: 3–19.

BELMONT, L. & MAROLLA, F. A. (1973) Birth order, family size, and intelligence. *Science*, 182: 1096–1101.

BERRY, L. G. (1977) Age and parity influences on maternal mortality: United States, 1919–1969. *Demography*, 14: 297–310.

BISHOP, E. H. (1964) Prematurity: Etiology and management. *Postgraduate medicine*, 35: 185–188.

BLACKER, J. G. C. (1979) The application of indirect techniques for the estimation of fertility and mortality to African data. Paper presented at the Expert Group Meeting on Fertility and Mortality Levels, Patterns and Trends in Africa and their Policy Implications, Monrovia, Liberia, 26 November–1 December 1979.

BONARINI, F. (1979) Preliminary analysis on the dynamics of the birth weight in sibs. *Genus*, 35, 7–52.

BRELAND, H. M. (1974) Birth order, family configuration, and verbal achievement. *Child development*, 45: 1011–1019.

BUTLER, N. R. & ALBERMAN, E. D. (1969) *Perinatal problems: The second report of the 1958 perinatal mortality survey*, Edinburgh, Livingstone.

BUTLER, N. R. & BONHAM, D. G. (1963) *Perinatal mortality: The first report of the 1958 British perinatal mortality survey*, Edinburgh, Livingstone.

CABRERA, RENE (1980) The influence of maternal age, birth order and socioeconomic status on infant mortality in Chile. *American journal of public health*, 70: 174–177.

CANTRELLE, P. & LERIDON, H. (1971) Breast feeding, mortality in childhood and fertility in a rural zone of Senegal. *Population studies*, 25: 505–533.

CHAMBERLAIN, R. ET AL. (1975) *British births 1970, Vol. 1: The first week of life*, London, Heinemann medical.

CHASE, H. C. (1961) *The relationship of certain biologic and socio-economic factors to fetal, infant and early childhood mortality—I. Father's occupation, parental age, and infant's birth rank*, Albany, New York State Department of Health (mimeographed document).

CHASE, H. C. (1962) *The relationship of certain biologic and socio-economic factors to fetal, infant and early childhood mortality—II. Father's occupation, infant's birth weight and mother's age*, Albany, New York State Department of Health (mimeographed document).

CHASE, H. C. (1972) A study of infant mortality from linked records: Comparison of neonatal mortality from two cohort studies. *Vital and health statistics*, Series 20, Number 13.

CHASE, H. C. (1973) A study of risks, medical care and infant mortality. *American journal of public health*, 63, Suppl.

CHOWDHURY, A. K. A. ET AL. (1975) The effect of child mortality experience on subsequent fertility: An empirical analysis of Pakistan and Bangladesh data. Paper presented at a Seminar on Infant Mortality in Relation to the Level of Fertility, Bangkok, Thailand, 6–12 May 1975.

CHRISTIANSON, R. (1976) Studies on blood pressure during pregnancy: Influence of parity and age. *American journal of obstetrics and gynecology*, 125: 509–513.

COHEN, W. R. ET AL. (1980)   Risk of labor abnormalities with advancing maternal age. *Obstetrics and gynecology*, **55**: 414–416.

DAVIES, I. M. (1980)   Perinatal and infant deaths: Social and biological factors. *Population trends*, **19**: 19–21.

DEVI, V. S. (1978)   Effect of perception of infant mortality on actual family size. *Journal of family welfare*, **24**: 26–33.

DINGLE, J. H. ET AL. (1964)   *Illness in the home: A study of 25,000 illnesses in a group of Cleveland families*, Cleveland, Press of Western Reserve University.

DOUGLAS, J. W. B. (1950)   Some factors associated with prematurity: The results of a national survey. *Journal of obstetrics and gynaecology of the British Empire*, **57**: 143–170.

DOUGLAS, J. W. B. & BLOMFIELD, J. M. (1958)   *Children under five: The results of a national survey*, London, Allen & Unwin.

DOUGLAS, J. W. B. & SIMPSON, H. R. (1964)   Height in relation to puberty, family size and social class: A longitudinal study. *Milbank Memorial Fund quarterly*, **42**: 20–35.

DUENHOELTER, J. H. ET AL. (1975)   Pregnancy performance of patients under 15 years of age. *Obstetrics and gynecology*, **46**: 49–52.

EFIONG, E. I. & BANJOKO, M. O. (1975)   The obstetric performance of Nigerian primigravidae aged 16 and under. *British journal of obstetrics and gynaecology*, **82**: 228–233.

EL-BEHAIRY, F. ET AL. (1976)   The nutritionally at risk child: Part 2: Study of factors pertinent to the child, siblings, or mother. *Gazette of the Egyptian paediatric association*, **24**: 31–41.

ERICKSON, J. D. & BJERKEDAL, T. (1978)   Interpregnancy interval: Association with birth weight, stillbirth, and neonatal death. *Journal of epidemiology and community health*, **32**: 124–130.

Family planning perspectives (1978)   A special issue on teenage pregnancy, Vol. 10, No. 4.

FAN, K. Y. & OMRAN, A. R. (1981)   *Family formation patterns and health in Taiwan*, Taichung, Taiwan, Maternal and Child Health Institute, in press.

FEDRICK, J. & ADELSTEIN, P. (1973)   Influence of pregnancy spacing on outcome of pregnancy. *British medical journal*, **4**: 753–756.

FITZGERALD, M. G. ET AL. (1961)   The effect of sex and parity on the incidence of diabetes mellitus. *Quarterly journal of medicine*, **30**: 57–70.

FRACCARO, M. (1956)   A contribution to the study of birth weight based on an Italian sample. *Annals of human genetics*, **20**: 282–298.

FRIEDLANDER, D. (1977)   The effect of child mortality on fertility: theoretical framework of the relationship.   *Proceedings of the International Population Conference, Mexico*, Liège, Belgium, IUSSP.

FRYERS, T. & MACKAY, R. I. (1979)   Down syndrome: Prevalence at birth, mortality and survival. A 17-year study. *Early human development*, **3**: 29–41.

GEBRE-MEDHIN, M. ET AL. (1976) Association of maternal age and parity with birth weight, sex ratio, stillbirths and multiple births. *Journal of tropical pediatrics*, **22**: 99–102.

GENDELL, M. & HELLEGERS, A. E. (1973)   The influence of the changes in maternal age, birth order and color on the changing perinatal mortality, Baltimore, 1961–66. *Health services reports*, **88**: 733–742.

GOLDING, J. (1979) Perinatal epidemiology in wonderland. *British medical journal*, **2**: 1436.

GOPALAN, C. (1968) Nutrition and family planning. *Population review*, **12**: 33–38.

GORDON, H. ET AL. (1970)   Genetic and interracial aspects of hypertensive toxemia of pregnancy—A prospective study. *American journal of obstetrics and gynecology*, **107**: 254–262.

GORDON, J. E. ET AL. (1967) The second year death rate in less developed countries. *American journal of medical science*, **254**: 357–380.

GRANT, M. W. (1964) Rate of growth in relation to birth rank and family size. *British journal of preventive and social medicine*, **18**: 35–42.

GROEN, G. P. (1974) Uterine rupture in rural Nigeria: Review of 144 cases. *Obstetrics and gynecology*, **44**: 682–687.

GUHA-RAY, D. K. (1976) Maternal mortality in an urban hospital. A 15-year survey. *Obstetrics and gynecology*, **47**: 430–433.

HARRINGTON, J. (1971) The effect of high infant and childhood mortality on fertility: The West African case. *Concerned demography*, **3**: 22–35.

HARRISON, K. A. (1979) Nigeria. *Lancet*, **2**: 1229–1232.

HASSAN, S. (1966) *Influence of child mortality on population growth*, Ann Arbor, Michigan, University Microfilms.

HASSAN, H. M. & FALLS, F. Y. (1964) The young primipara. *American journal of obstetrics and gynecology*, **8**: 256–269.

HAY, S. & BARBANO, H. (1972) Independent effects of maternal age and birth order on the incidence of selected congenital malformations. *Teratology*, **6**: 271–279.

HEADY, J. A. & MORRIS, J. N. (1955) Social and biologic factors in infant mortality III: The effect of mother's age and parity on social-class differences in infant mortality. *Lancet*, **1**: 445–448.

HEER, D. M. & WU, H. Y. (1975) The separate effects of individual child loss, perception of child survival and community mortality level upon fertility and family-planning in rural Taiwan with comparison data from urban Morocco. Paper presented at a Seminar on Infant Mortality in Relation to the Level of Fertility, Bangkok, Thailand, 6–12 May 1975.

HEFNAWI, F. ET AL. (1972) Lactation patterns in Egyptian women: Milk yield during the first year of lactation. *Journal of biosocial science*, **4**: 397–401.

HICKEY, M. J. & KASONDE, M. (1977) Maternal mortality at University Teaching Hospital, Lusaka. *Medical journal of Zambia*, **11**: 74–78.

HOLLEY, W. L. ET AL. (1969) Effect of rapid succession of pregnancy. In: *Perinatal factors affecting human development*, Washington, Pan American Health Organization (Scientific Publication No. 185), pp. 41–44.

HUGHES, E. (1923) Infant mortality: Results of a field study in Gary, Indiana, based on births in one year. *Children's Bureau Publication*, No. 12: 44–45.

HUMERFELT, S. & WEDERVANG, F. (1957) A study of the influence upon blood pressure of marital status, number of children, and occupation, *Acta medica scandinavica*, **159**: 489–497.

ISRAEL, S. L. & BLAZAR, A. S. (1965) Obstetric behavior of the grand multipara. *American journal of obstetrics and gynecology*, **91**: 326–332.

JAFFE, F. & POLGAR, S. (1964) *Epidemiological indications for fertility control*, New York, Planned Parenthood-World Population.

JAMES, W. H. (1968a) Stillbirth and birth order. *Annals of human genetics*, **32**: 151–162.

JAMES, W. H. (1968b) Stillbirth, neonatal death and birth interval. *Annals of human genetics*, **32**: 163–172.

JAMES, W. H. (1969) Birth weight and birth order. *Annals of human genetics*, **32**: 411–413.

JAMES, W. H. (1970) Neonatal death and birth order. *Annals of human genetics*, **33**: 385–394.

JAMES, W. H. (1976) Birth order, maternal age and birth interval in epidemiology. *International journal of epidemiology*, **5**: 131–132.

JAMES, W. H. (1977) Observations on the artifact hypothesis and Naylor's "Sequential aspects of spontaneous abortion: Maternal age, parity and pregnancy compensation artifact". *Social biology*, **24**: 86–89.

JELLIFFE, D. B. (1966) *The assessment of nutritional status of the community*, Geneva, World Health Organization (Monograph Series No. 53).

56

KADER, M. M. ET AL. (1973) Lactation patterns in Egyptian women: Chemical composition of milk during the first year of lactation. *Journal of biosocial science*, **4**: 403–409.

KAJANOJA, P. & WIDHOLM, O. (1978) Pregnancy and delivery in women aged 40 and over. *Obstetrics and gynecology*, **51**: 47–51.

KAMEL, W. H. ET AL. (1974) Pregnancy wastage in a rural community in Egypt. *Egyptian population and family planning review*, **7**: 11–20.

KARN, M. N. & PENROSE, L. S. (1951) Birth weight and gestation time in relation to maternal age, parity and infant survival. *Annals of eugenics*, **16**: 147–164.

KESSNER, D. M. ET AL. (1973) *Infant death: an analysis by maternal risk and health care*, Washington, Institute of Medicine, National Academy of Sciences.

KHAN, A. A. & GUPTA, B. M. (1979) A study of malnourished children in Children's Hospital, Lusaka (Zambia). *Tropical pediatrics and environmental child health*, **25**: 42–45.

LERIDON, H. (1977) *Human fertility: The basic components*, Chicago, University of Chicago Press.

LERY, A. & VALLIN, J. (1975) Attempt to estimate the over-fertility consecutive to the death of a young child. Paper presented at a Seminar on Infant Mortality in Relation to the Level of Fertility, Bangkok, Thailand, 6–12 May 1975.

LESINSKI, J. (1976) Family size: Its influence on family's health, economic status and social welfare. *Obstetrical and gynecological survey*, **31**: 421–452.

LEWIS, J. R. (1974) The birth weights of babies in the Cameroon Grasslands. *Journal of tropical pediatrics and environmental child health*, **20**: 300–301.

LOEB, J. (1965) Weight at birth and survival of newborn, by age of mother and total birth order: United States, early 1950. *Vital and health statistics*, Series 21, Number 5.

LOGAN, W. P. D. (1953) Marriage and childbearing in relation to cancer of the breast and uterus. *Lancet*, **265**: 1199–1202.

LUNDIN, F. E. ET AL. (1964) *Socio-economic distribution of cervical cancer*, Washington, Goverment Printing Office (Public Health Monograph No. 73).

MACMAHON, B. ET AL. (1970) Age at first birth and breast cancer risk. *Bulletin of the World Health Organization*, **43**: 209–221.

MALIPHANT, R. G. (1949) The incidence of cancer of the uterine cervix. *British medical journal*, **1**: 978–982.

MANTEL, N. (1979) Perinatal mortality by birth order. *British medical journal*, **2**: 1147.

MARTIN, E. C. (1979) A study of the effect of birth interval on the development of 9-year old school children in Singapore. *Journal of tropical pediatrics and environmental child health*, **25**: 46–76.

MBISE, R. L. & BOERSMA, E. R. (1979) Factors associated with low birth weight in the population of Dar es Salaam, Tanzania. *Tropical and geographical medicine*, **31**: 21–32.

MEHDI, Z. ET AL. (1961) Incidence and causes of perinatal mortality in Hyderabad, Andhra Pradesh, India. *Indian journal of medical research*, **49**: 897–946.

MEIRIK, O. ET AL. (1979) Impact of changing age and parity distributions of mothers on perinatal mortality in Sweden, 1953–1975. *International journal of epidemiology*, **8**: 361–364.

MEME, J. S. (1978) A prospective study of neonatal deaths in Nairobi, Kenya. *East African medical journal*, **55**: 262–267.

MIALL, W. E. (1959) Follow-up study of arterial pressure in the population of a Welsh mining valley. *British medical journal*, **2**: 1204–1210.

MIALL, W. E. ET AL. (1962) Factors influencing arterial pressure in the general population in Jamaica. *British medical journal*, **2**: 497–506.

MIALL, W. E. & OLDHAM, P. D. (1958) Factors influencing arterial blood pressure in the general population. *Clinical science*, **17**: 407–444.

MIDDLETON, G. D. & CAIRD, F. I. (1968) Parity and diabetes mellitus. *British journal of preventive and social medicine*, **22**: 100–104.

MILLIS, J. & SENG, Y. P. (1954) The effect of age and parity of the mother on birth weight of the offspring. *Annals of human genetics*, **19**: 58–73.

MITRA, A. (1977) National population policy in relation to national planning in India. *Population and development review*, **3**: 297–306.

MORLEY, K. ET AL. (1968) Factors influencing the growth and nutritional status of infants and young children in a Nigerian village. *Transactions of the Royal Society of Tropical Medicine and Hygiene*, **62**: 164–199.

MORRIS, J. N. & HEADY, J. A. (1955) Social and biological factors in infant mortality. I. Objects and methods. *Lancet*, **1**: 343–349.

MORRIS, N. M. ET AL. (1975) Shifting age-parity distribution of births and the decrease in infant mortality. *American journal of public health*, **65**: 359–362.

MOSENTHAL, H. O. & BOLDUAN, C. (1933) Diabetes mellitus: Problems of present day treatment. *American journal of the medical sciences*, **186**: 605–621.

NAMBOODIRI, N. K. & BALAKRISHNAN, V. (1959) On the effect of maternal age and parity on the birth weight of the offspring (Indian infants). *Annals of human genetics*, **23**: 189–203.

NAYLOR, A. F. (1974) Sequential aspects of spontaneous abortion: maternal age, parity and pregnancy compensation artifact. *Social biology*, **21**: 195–204.

NEWCOMBE, H. B. (1964) Screening for effects of maternal age and birth order in a register of handicapped children. *Annals of human genetics*, **27**: 367–382.

NEWCOMBE, H. B. & TRAVENDALE, O. G. (1964) Maternal age and birth order correlations: Problems of distinguishing mutational from environmental components. *Mutation research*, **1**: 446–467.

NORTMAN, D. (1974) Parental age as a factor in pregnancy outcome and child development. In: *Reports on population/family planning*, New York, The Population Council.

OBENG, B. B. (1969) Pregnancy in girls under 16 years. *Journal of obstetrics and gynaecology of the British Commonwealth*, **76**: 640–644.

OMRAN, A. R. (1971) *The health theme in family planning*, Chapel Hill, Carolina Population Center (Monograph No. 16).

OMRAN, A. R. (1975) Health rationale for family planning. In: Block, L. S., ed. *Population Change: A Strategy for Physicians. Proceedings of the International Conference on the Physician and Population Change, September 4–6 1974, Stockholm, Sweden*, Bethesda, Maryland, World Federation for Medical Education.

OMRAN, A. R. (1978) Health consequences of high risk pregnancies in Muslim women: A cross-national maternity center study. Paper presented at the Pan-Islamic Conference on Motherhood, Cairo, Egypt.

OMRAN, A. R. (1980) *Population in the Arab World: Problems and prospects*, New York, United Nations Fund for Population Activities.

OMRAN, A. R. & STANDLEY, C. C., ED. (1976) *Family formation patterns and health*, Geneva, World Health Organization.

O'SULLIVAN, J. B. & GORDON, T. (1966) Childbearing and diabetes mellitus. *Vital and health statistics*, Series 11, No. 21.

PAKTER, J. ET AL. (1961) Out of wedlock births in New York City. I. Sociologic aspects. *American journal of public health*, **51**: 683–696.

PARK, C. B. ET AL. (1979) The effect of infant death on subsequent fertility in Korea and the role of family planning. *American journal of public health*, **69**: 557–565.

PATHAK, S. K. B. (1978) Infant mortality, birth order and contraception in India. *Journal of family welfare*, **25**: 12–21.

PENROSE, L. S. (1933) The relative effects of paternal and maternal age in mongolism. *Journal of genetics*, **27**: 219–224.

PENROSE, L. S. (1962) Paternal age in mongolism. *Lancet*, **1**: 1101.

PENROSE, L. S. (1967) The effects of change in maternal age distribution upon the incidence of mongolism. *Journal of mental deficiency research*, **11**: 54–47.

PHILLIPPE, P. (1978) Analyse transversale et longitudinale du risque de mortalité infantile en fonction du rang de naissance et de la dimension finale de la famille. *Canadian journal of public health*, **69**: 109–112.

PHILLIPS, O. C. ET AL. (1965) Obstetric mortality: A 26-year survey. *Obstetrics and gynecology*, **25**: 217–222.

PRESTON, S. H., ED. (1978) *The effects of infant and child mortality on fertility*, New York, Academic Press.

PUFFER, R. R. & SERRANO, C. V. (1975) *Birthweight, maternal age, and birth order: Three important determinants in infant mortality*, Washington, DC, Pan American Health Organization (Publication No. 294).

PYKE, D. A. (1956) Parity and the incidence of diabetes. *Lancet*, **1**: 818–821.

QUINILIVAN, W. L. G. (1964) Maternal death rates and incidence of abnormalities in women of parity 6 or more. *Obstetrics and gynecology*, **23**: 451–456.

RADOVIČ, P. (1966) Frequent and high parity as a medical and social problem. *American journal of obstetrics and gynecology*, **94**: 583–585.

RAO, K. B. (1975) Maternal mortality in a teaching hospital in southern India: A 13-year study. *Obstetrics and gynecology*, **46**: 397–400.

RECORD, R. G. ET AL. (1969) The relation of measured intelligence to birth order and maternal age. *Annals of human genetics*, **33**: 61–69.

REHAN, N. E. & TAFIDA, D. S. (1979) Birth weight of Hausa infants in northern Nigeria. *British journal of obstetrics and gynaecology*, **86**: 443–449.

REINHARDT, M. C. ET AL. (1978) A year of deliveries at the Adjamé Maternity Hospital in Abidjan (Ivory Coast). *Helvetica paediatrica acta* Suppl. No. 41: 7–20.

RENDLE-SHORT, C. (1960) Rupture of the gravid uterus in Uganda. *American journal of obstetrics and gynecology*, **79**: 1115–1120.

RESSIGUIE, L. J. (1973) Influence of age, birth order and reproductive compensation on stillbirth ratios. *Journal of biosocial science*, **5**: 443–452.

RESSIGUIE, L. J. (1977) The artifactual nature of effects of maternal age on risk of stillbirth. *Journal of biosocial science*, **9**: 191–200.

ROBERTS, D. F. & TANNER, R. E. S. (1963) Effects of parity on birth weight and other variables in a Tanganyika Bantu sample. *British journal of preventive and social medicine*, **17**: 209–215.

ROMAN, E. ET AL. (1978) Fetal loss, gravidity, and pregnancy order. *Early human development*, **2**: 131–138.

RUTSTEIN, S. O. (1971) *The influence of child mortality on fertility in Taiwan: Study based on sample surveys conducted in 1967 and 1969*. Ann Arbor, Michigan, University Microfilms.

SCOTT, J. A. (1962) Intelligence, physique, and family size. *British journal of preventive and social medicine*, **16**: 165–173.

SCRIMSHAW, S. C. M. (1978) Infant mortality and behavior in the regulation of family size. *Population and development review*, **4**: 383–404.

SELVIN, S. & GARFINKEL, J. (1972) The relationship between parental age and birth order with the percentage of low birth-weight infants. *Human biology*, **44**: 501–509.

SHAH, F. K. & ABBEY, H. (1971) Effects of some factors on neonatal and post-neonatal mortality. *Milbank Memorial Fund quarterly*, **49**: 33–57.

SHAPIRO, S. (1954) Influence of birth weight, sex and plurality on neonatal loss in the U.S. *American journal of public health*, **44**: 1142–1153.

SHAPIRO, S. ET AL. (1968) *Infant, perinatal, maternal and childhood mortality in the U.S.*, Cambridge, Massachusetts, Harvard University Press.

SHAPIRO, S. ET AL. (1970) Factors associated with early and late fetal loss. In: *Proceedings of the 8th Annual Meeting of the AAPPP, 9–10 April 1970, Boston, Massachusetts*, Excerpta Medica International Congress, Series No. 224.

SIMPKISS, M. J. (1968) Birth weight, maternal age and parity among the African population of Uganda. *British journal of preventive and social medicine*, **22**: 234–237.

SMITH, A. & RECORD, R. G. (1955) Maternal age and birth rank in the aetiology of mongolism. *British journal of preventive and social medicine*, **9**: 51–55.

SOGBANMU, M. O. (1979) Perinatal mortality and maternal mortality in General Hospital, Ondo, Nigeria. Use of high-risk pregnancy predictive scoring index. *Nigerian medical journal*, **9**: 123–127.

SPENCE, J. ET AL. (1954) *A thousand families in Newcastle upon Tyne: An approach to the study of health and illness in children*, London, Oxford University Press.

SPICER, C. C. & LIPWORTH, L. (1966) Regional and social factors in infant mortality. In: *Studies on medical and population subjects*, No. 19, London, Her Majesty's Stationery Office.

SPIERS, P. S. (1972) Father's age and infant mortality. *Social biology*, **19**: 275–284.

SPIERS, P. S. & WANG, L. (1976) Short pregnancy interval, low birthweight, and the sudden infant death syndrome. *American journal of epidemiology*, **104**: 15–21.

SRIVASTAVA, S. V. K. & PANDEY, G. D. (1978) Infant mortality and fertility: An empirical investigation. *Journal of family welfare*, **25**: 57–63.

STEVENSON, A. C. ET AL. (1966) Congenital malformations. *Bulletin of the World Health Organization*, **34** (Suppl.): 5–127.

STOECKEL, J. & CHOWDHURY. A. K. A. (1972) Neonatal and post-neonatal mortality in a rural area of Bangladesh. *Population studies*, **26**: 113–120.

STUKOVSKY, R. ET AL. (1967) Family size and menarcheal age in Constanza, Roumania. *Human biology*, **39**: 277–283.

SULLIVAN, J. (1972) The influence of demographic and socio-economic factors on infant mortality rates in Taiwan, 1966–1969. New York, The Population Council (unpublished manuscript).

SWENSON, I. (1978) Early childhood survivorship related to the subsequent interpregnancy interval and outcome of the subsequent pregnancy. *Journal of tropical pediatrics and environmental child health*, **24**: 103–106.

SWENSON, I. & HARPER, P. A. (1979) High risk maternal factors related to fetal wastage in rural Bangladesh. *Journal of biosocial science*, **11**: 465–471.

TAFFEL, S. (1978) Congenital anomalies and birth injuries among live births: United States, 1973–1974. *Vital and health statistics*, Series 21, No. 31.

TAFFEL, S. (1980) Factors associated with low birthweight. *Vital and health statistics*, Series 21, No. 37.

TANNER, J. M. (1968) Earlier maturation in man. *Scientific American*, **218**: 21–27.

TAWIAH, E. (1979) *Levels, patterns, trends and differentials in infant and early childhood mortality, Ghana, 1960 and 1971*, Ann Arbor, Michigan, University Microfilms.

TAYLOR, C. E. ET AL. (1976) The child survival hypothesis. *Population studies*, **30**: 263–278.

VEHASKARI, A. ET AL. (1968) Hazards of grand multiparity. *Annales chirurgiae et gynaecologiae Fenniae*, **57**: 476–484.

VELANDIA, W. ET AL. (1978) Family size, birth order, and intelligence in a large South American sample. *American education research journal*, **15**: 399–416.

VOORHOEVE, A. M. ET AL. (1979) Agents affecting health of mother and child in a rural area of Kenya: XVI. The outcome of pregnancy. *Tropical and geographical medicine*, **31**, 607–627.

WAGNER, M. E. & SCHUBERT, H. J. P. (1979) Sibship-constellation effects on psychosocial development, creativity and health. *Advances in child development behavior*, **14**: 57–148.

WAHI, P. N. ET AL. (1969) Factors influencing cancer of the uterine cervix in North India. *Cancer*, **23**: 1221–1232.

WARE, H. (1977) The relationship between infant mortality and fertility: Replacement and insurance effects. *Proceedings of the International Population Conference, Mexico, 1977*, Liège, Belgium, IUSSP.

WATSON, W. ET AL. (1979) Health, population and nutrition: Interrelations, problems and possible solutions. In: Hauser, P., ed. *World population and development, challenges and prospects*, New York, United Nations Fund for Population Activities.

WOLFERS, D. & SCRIMSHAW, S. (1974) Child survival and interval between births in Guayaquil, Ecuador (mimeographed document).

WOODBURY, R. M. (1925) Causal factors in infant mortality, a statistical study based on investigations in eight cities. *Children's Bureau Publication*, No. 142, pp. 60–67.

WORLD HEALTH ORGANIZATION (1976) Comparative study of social and biological effects on perinatal mortality. *World health statistics report*, **29**: 228–234.

WORLD HEALTH ORGANIZATION (1978) Main findings of the comparative study of social and biological effects on perinatal mortality. *World Health Organization statistical quarterly*, **31**: 74–83.

WRAY, J. D. (1971) Population pressure on families: Family size and child spacing. In: *Rapid population growth, Vol. II*, prepared by a study committee of the Office of the Foreign Secretary, National Academy of Sciences, Baltimore, Johns Hopkins Press, pp. 403–461.

WRAY, J. D. & AGUIRRE, A. (1969) Protein-calorie malnutrition in Candelaria, Colombia: I. Prevalence; social and demographic causal factors. *Journal of tropical pediatrics*, **15**: 76–98.

WRIGHT, N. H. (1972) Some estimates of the potential reduction in the United States infant mortality rate by family planning. *American journal of public health*, **62**: 1130–1134.

WYNDER, E. L. ET AL. (1954) A study of environmental factors in carcinoma of the cervix. *American journal of obstetrics and gynecology*, **68**: 1016–1052.

WYON, J. B. & GORDON, J. E. (1962) A long-term prospective-type field study of population dynamics in the Punjab, India. In: Kiser, C. V., ed. *Research in family planning*, Princeton, Princeton University Press, pp. 17–32.

YERUSHALMY, J. (1938) Neonatal mortality by order of birth and age of parents. *American journal of hygiene*, **28**: 244–270.

YERUSHALMY, J. (1945) On the interval between successive births and its effect on survival of infant—I. An indirect method of study. *Human biology*, **17**: 65–106.

YERUSHALMY, J. ET AL. (1956) Longitudinal studies of pregnancy on the island of Kauai, Territory of Hawaii—I. Analysis of previous reproductive history. *American journal of obstetrics and gynecology*, **71**: 80–96.

YUDKIN, P. (1980) Pregnancy order and reproductive loss. *British medical journal*, **280**: 715–716.

ZAJONC, R. B. (1976) Family configuration and intelligence. *Science*, **192**: 227–236.

ZAJONC, R. B. & MARKUS, G. B. (1975) Birth order and intellectual development. *Psychological review*, **82**: 74–88.

ZAJONC, R. B. ET AL. (1979) The birth order puzzle. *Journal of personality and social psychology*, **37**: 1325–1341.

ZIMMER, B. G. (1979) Consequences of the number and spacing of pregnancies on outcome and of pregnancy outcome on spacing. *Social biology*, **26**: 161–178.

Chapter Two

RESEARCH DESIGN
FOR THE COLLABORATIVE STUDIES

A. R. Omran, C. C. Standley & A. Kessler

THE RESEARCH PROBLEM AND OBJECTIVES

The Research Problem

When these collaborative studies were first considered in 1970, several studies had already indicated that the health of mothers and children might be affected by certain components of family formation, particularly the age of the mother at pregnancy, pregnancy intervals, parity, and family size. However, most of the evidence for these relationships came from Europe, the USA, and other developed countries. The question remained whether the same relationships were to be found in the developing countries, where the environment was more hostile, the social and economic conditions poorer, and health care less adequate.

Because of the close association between unfavourable socioenvironmental conditions and poor health, it seemed likely that the relationships between factors determining family formation and health would be different in developing countries. It was possible, for example, that when social and environmental conditions were bad, family formation effects might be obscured.

It was also of interest to examine in developing communities the possible impact that child loss early in the reproductive span of a woman might have on her subsequent fertility. This was of particular significance to the debated question of whether the level of fertility was closely associated with the level of childhood mortality, especially in infancy.

Specific Questions and Objectives of the Study

More specifically, the questions that required answers were:

1. Will high parity, large family size, and close spacing of pregnancies in the less developed countries be associated with:

(a) poor pregnancy outcome;

(b) high infant and childhood mortality and morbidity, especially from infectious diseases and undernutrition;

(c) poor physical development and lower intellectual achievement of children;

(d) poor maternal health, especially in regard to gynaecological and obstetrical problems?

2. Do pregnancies at an early or late maternal age have poorer pregnancy outcomes? Are they also associated with adverse effects on maternal and child health?

3. Does high child loss in the early stages of a woman's reproductive life lead to higher subsequent fertility?

4. Are the health effects of family formation the same among different socioeconomic groups? Are they the same among rural and urban groups and among various cultural subgroups under similar socioeconomic conditions?

Under the auspices of the World Health Organization, a collaborative study was therefore organized among research centres in several countries to investigate the above questions in different cultural settings. Each centre tested the study hypotheses in its own context; the findings cannot be extrapolated to a national context. The study was intended as a first step, possibly to be followed by more detailed investigations. These were in fact carried out by the centres in India, Lebanon, and the Philippines.

It was hoped, however, that it would, through the collection of local data, answer some questions of interest to those involved in policy formulation and implementation in both health and family planning programmes. Moreover, if different patterns of family formation were shown to affect significantly the health of mothers and children, this would prove a powerful argument for family planning for both the medical profession and for the public at large.

Some operational questions were also considered. The main ones were (a) whether it would be possible to use cross-culturally a unified research design and instruments, and (b) whether it would be possible to carry out, in some settings, physical and other examinations on samples of women and children or to obtain reliable answers to questions relating to many "personal" matters, such as family formation, health, and fertility behaviour.

Finally, another fundamental objective was institutional development, since WHO was interested in developing a network of research teams with competence in epidemiological studies in human reproduction.

ORGANIZATION OF THE STUDY

Collaborating Centres

At the outset of the study, only the following six centres were involved:

China (Province of Taiwan)	Maternal and Child Health Institute, Taichung
India	Gandhigram Institute of Rural Health and Family Planning, Madurai District, Tamil Nadu
Iran	School of Public Health, Teheran University
Lebanon	School of Public Health, American University in Beirut
Philippines	Institute of Public Health, University of the Philippines, Manila
Turkey	Department of Community Medicine, Hacettepe University, Ankara

The findings from these centres were published in 1976,[1] with the exception of those from the Chinese centre, which withdrew from the study in 1972 and is publishing its findings separately.

While these studies were in progress, the governments of Egypt, Pakistan, and the Syrian Arab Republic, as well as an institution in Colombia, expressed interest in joining them. As a result, the following four centres were added to the collaborative study:

Colombia	School of Public Health, Medellin
Egypt	Institute of Public Health, Alexandria; Department of Preventive Medicine, Assiut University
Pakistan	National Research Institute of Fertility Control, Karachi
Syrian Arab Republic	Central Bureau of Statistics, Damascus

Coordination

The responsibility for planning, coordination and follow-up of the study was shared between the WHO Special Programme of Research, Development and Research Training in Human Reproduction and the WHO Collaborating Centre for Epidemiological Studies of Human Reproduction in Chapel Hill. Frequent site visits and consultations by Dr Omran, who acted as coordinator of the studies, were supplemented by several meetings of investigators.

Study Organization in Each Centre

The head of the collaborating institution or agency selected a team of investigators and consultants and was officially responsible for the administration of the study on behalf of the institution. A field director was also named and became responsible for the field operation, record keeping, local analysis, etc. The composition of the research teams was multidisciplinary, including specialists in public health, biostatistics, obstetrics and gynaecology, paediatrics, and social sciences.

Writing of the Reports

The format for the reports was discussed and adopted at a meeting of investigators in 1972 and has been maintained for this second series of reports.

---

[1] OMRAN, A. R. & STANDLEY, C. C., ED. (1976) *Family formation patterns and health*, Geneva, World Health Organization.

65

Drafts of the different chapters were prepared by the investigators, discussed at common meetings, and edited by the WHO Special Programme and the WHO Collaborating Centre in Chapel Hill.

Timetable

The data were collected by the centres in Colombia, Egypt, Pakistan and the Syrian Arab Republic in the years between 1972 and 1976. Data verification and analysis took place between 1976 and 1978, and the centres prepared draft reports in 1978–1979.

RESEARCH HYPOTHESES *

Selection of Study Variables and Indices

The variables selected for study can be classified into 4 categories: (1) sociocultural variables, (2) family formation variables, (3) health variables, and (4) family planning behaviour variables. The variables are shown in Table 1.

---

* A glossary of key terms used in the study is provided on page 71.

TABLE 1. STUDY VARIABLES

I. SOCIOCULTURAL VARIABLES	II. FAMILY FORMATION VARIABLES	III. HEALTH VARIABLES	IV. FAMILY PLANNING BEHAVIOUR VARIABLES
Social class		A. *Pregnancy outcome*	
Education of husband	Family size	Abortion	Family planning practices
Education of wife	Age of mother	Stillbirth	Ideal family size
Occupation of husband	Parity	Livebirth	Attitudes toward contraception
Occupation of wife	Gravidity		abortion
Residence	Birth order	B. *Child health and development*	sterilization
	Pregnancy order	Neonatal mortality	Pregnancy interval preference
	Birth interval	Postneonatal mortality	Ideal age for boys or girls to marry
	Age at marriage	Child mortality, 1–4 years	Eligible women's opinions on health & family formation
	Interval between marriage and first pregnancy	Morbidity in children under 5 years: percentage with fever/diarrhoea in preceding month	Timing failure of last pregnancy
	Duration of marriage	Health examination of children under 5 years: weight height haemoglobin infection	
	Family type: nuclear/extended	IQ of children	
	Ideal family size		
		C. *Maternal health*	
		Weight/height	
		Haemoglobin	
		Blood pressure	
		Gynaecological: complaints findings	
		Lactation practices	

Statement of the Research Hypotheses

Two overall hypotheses were considered:

1. Health risks for mothers and children increase with high frequency of pregnancies, large family size, short birth intervals, and too young or too old age of mother at the time of pregnancy.

2. Experience of child loss raises subsequent fertility.

RESEARCH SETTING

Study population

Family formation patterns and health in two or more different population subgroups were compared, each collaborating centre choosing its subgroups (see sampling below) from different residential areas, e.g., from urban or rural districts.

Sampling

Sampling technique

The choice of subgroups was decided upon by the collaborating centre, and the chosen samples were not intended to represent the national population.

In most centres, the sampling frame was based on local area maps or on a baseline census of households. Some variation in sampling occurred between centres. The details of each centre's sample are found in the individual country reports. In each case, sampling was done by or in consultation with the team's statistician.

Determination of sample size

In determining sample size, one usually considers the frequencies of the most pertinent variables in the study. In this case, because of the multiplicity of variables and because of varying frequencies, infant mortality was chosen (a) because it was a very important variable in the study, and (b) because its frequency was relatively lower than that of many other indices in the study.

Calculations indicated that a sample size of 2000 women in each subgroup would be adequate and would allow 4 subclassifications (e.g., subclassification by urban/rural residence and simultaneously by middle and low social status could be made). For the populations considered in the study, an estimate of 130 infant deaths per 1000 live births was used in calculating sample size. While allowing for a relative error $\pm 25\%$ (or ± 32.5 per 1000 births), the sample size (with $\alpha = 0.05$ and $1-\beta = 0.80$)[1] is approximately

$$N = \frac{11.68 \times (0.0975 \times 0.9025 + 0.13 \times 0.87)}{(0.0325)^2}$$

---

[1] "α" represents the probability of finding a significant difference when there is actually none, while "β" represents the probability that even when there is a significant difference the sampling procedure will fail to detect it.

which gives 2224 births. Assuming a conservative average of 4 births per ever-married female, then 556 ever-married females are required per sub-classification, or 2224 ever-married females for each cultural or religious group comprising 4 subclassifications. With a sample size of 2000 females, any observed difference more than ± 26.2 per 1000 births between any two subclassifications can be considered statistically significant at the 1% level (ignoring the multiple-comparison problem).

Controls

In this study, the groups (and classes within each group) for each centre acted as controls for one another.

Study Components

The material for the collaborative study was obtained through: (a) household surveys; (b) structured interviews with married women under 45 years of age (referred to as eligible women or EWs; (c) medical examination of these women; (d) paediatric examination of their children under 5 years of age; and (e) IQ testing of children 8–14 years old.

Household survey

A household survey was done in each of the chosen areas according to the sampling design. A standardized household questionnaire was administered in order to obtain identification data for the household and information on its composition as well as demographic and social data.

Eligible woman interview

Each eligible woman in the study sample was interviewed according to the standardized EW questionnaire, which takes approximately 45 minutes to one hour to administer. Some of the main areas covered by the EW questionnaire are: (a) demographic and social characteristics; (b) pregnancy history with additional details for last pregnancy; (c) mortality particulars, if applicable, for her dead children; (d) selected morbidity particulars for children and mothers in the preceding month; (e) health service utilization by family; (f) perception of mortality and fertility and consciousness of change in each; (g) concepts of "ideal family sizes", best age at marriage, sex preference, etc.; (h) knowledge, attitudes, and practice of contraception (KAP), (i) attitudes towards abortion, sterilization, lactation, and family formation; (j) fertility of EW's parents; (k) attitudinal questions regarding childhood mortality and whether improvement in childhood survival would be taken into consideration in decision-making regarding family planning.

Paediatric examination of children under five

A physical examination was done on all children under 5 years of age belonging to the eligible women, or on samples of such children. The examination included: (*a*) weight and height; (*b*) physical abnormalities and diseases; (*c*) history of illness and use of medical care in the preceding month; and (*d*) haemoglobin level and stool examination for parasites.

Medical examination of the eligible women

The following information was collected for all or samples of the EW population: (*a*) weight and height; (*b*) blood pressure; (*c*) gynaecological examination; (*d*) obstetric history; and (*e*) haemoglobin level.

Intelligence quotient of children

The Cattell & Cattell Culture-Fair Test designed for children 8–14 years of age was used in all centres except for the Egyptian centre which employed the Goodenough Test, and applied it to children aged 6–11 years. The raw scores from these tests were converted into standardized scores by using a conversion table, which allowed for the age of the child. The results were expressed as standardized IQ norms, with mean = 100.

Research Instruments

The household and eligible woman's questionnaires were developed by Dr Omran in consultation with the WHO Special Programme. These instruments were revised by teams of investigators from India, Iran, Lebanon, and Turkey during a conference held in Gandhigram, India, 1970. At the same meeting, the medical and other examination procedures were also standardized. The questionnaire, shown in the Annex to the previous volume, was slightly modified for this study.

Training of interviewers and other personnel

Training of interviewers and other personnel was a crucial part of the preparation for the investigation and was conducted with the utmost care. Every effort was made to avoid creating interviewer bias, either by not discussing the hypotheses with the interviewers or, if the hypotheses were already known, by strongly emphasizing that the purpose of the study was to *test* rather than to verify these hypotheses. The interviewers were made completely familiar with the instruments (in the local language) and with the technique they were to use. Demonstration interviews, role-playing by interviewers and observations of interviews in a field situation were used as steps to train a new interviewer. Also, the first ten or so interviews of a new trainee were carefully scrutinized by a supervisor and errors in recording were pointed out and discussed.

Reliability checks

Because of the importance of the EW interviews in the whole study, reliability checks were introduced in order to test the recall consistency of the interviewees. This was done in two ways. Some questions concerning certain items in the pregnancy history chart were also included in other parts of the questionnaire and served as built-in reliability checks. Discrepancies were used for further probing until consistent responses were obtained. Secondly, each team was requested to re-interview at least 5% of the women as the study progressed; for this purpose, factual items in the questionnaire rather than opinion questions were asked. The results were used to correct interviewing techniques. Thirdly, a very detailed list of consistency checks developed at the WHO Collaborating Centre for Epidemiological Studies in Human Reproduction at Chapel Hill was applied in each centre for cleaning the data decks or tapes.

Pretesting the instruments

The study instruments were carefully translated into the local language and dialect. Some of the items were independently retranslated into English as a test of accuracy, and necessary modifications were made. Pretesting of the translated instruments was carried out locally; several women (about 10 in each cultural or residential group) were interviewed. These women had characteristics comparable to the study population but were not included in the actual study. Any ambiguity was eliminated from the instruments and culturally objectionable or easily misunderstood wording was altered.

Data Processing and Analysis

The questionnaires and other forms

Editing and coding of questionnaires and other data collection forms, subsequent transfer of data to punch cards and verification were done by the research team in each centre. The data were then transferred from the cards to computer tapes, either in Geneva or at the centre. Analysis was carried out in Geneva, in collaboration with the Chapel Hill centre, except for the data from the centres in Egypt, where data processing and analysis were carried out locally.[1]

Tabulation scheme

A tabulation scheme was developed when the study was designed. Volumes of dummy tables were prepared; these were of 3 kinds: (a) descriptive tables; (b) correlation tables; and (c) tables designed to test the specific hypotheses.

---

[1] Although the WHO computer program for data analysis was made available to the Egyptian investigators, only a partial analysis was made of the Egyptian data.

Statistical analysis

The statistical methods used included: (*a*) descriptive statistics applied to frequency distribution, (*b*) the control or frequency table technique, widely used in epidemiology, where the relation of each of two independent variables to a dependent variable was examined in a simple fashion, and (*c*) tests of association.

GLOSSARY
Definitions of Terms as used in the Study

Abortion (fetal loss)—loss of the fetus or termination of pregnancy under seven months (28 weeks), including both induced and spontaneous abortions

Actual or achieved family size—number of children born to each eligible woman who are still living at the time of the survey

Age at marriage—in this study the term "age at marriage" is used synonymously with "age at consummation"

Birth order—the rank of an index live birth among other live births for each woman

Child loss—number of children born alive who died under 5 years of age

Childhood mortality—death of children (under 1 month, 1–11 months, under 1 year, under 5 years) per hundred reported live births per eligible woman

Eligible woman—woman under 45 years of age who was married at the time of the survey

Extended family—household including, in addition to nuclear family, relatives of husband or wife

Family size—see "actual or achieved family size"

Family structure—classification of family according to nuclear or extended family

Gravidity—number of pregnancies per woman

Household—those people living together in one dwelling (house, apartment, or room) sharing food and/or economically interdependent, including at least one eligible woman

Household head—person recognized by the members of a household as leader or economic provider based on economic, seniority, or other cultural considerations

Ideal family size—number of children considered by an interviewee to be desirable under circumstances similar to her own

Interval between marriage and conception—duration in months between the date of marriage and the beginning of the first pregnancy within the specified marriage

Maternal age—age of the eligible woman at termination of a given pregnancy (birth, abortion, stillbirth)

Nuclear family—family composed of husband, wife, and their unmarried offspring

Parity—number of children ever born alive or number of live births per woman

Ponderal index—an index of body bulk incorporating both height and weight

$$\text{ponderal index} = \frac{\text{height in inches}}{\sqrt[3]{\text{weight in pounds}}}$$

Preceding pregnancy interval—the interval (in months) between the termination of the preceding pregnancy and the termination of the given pregnancy (this definition automatically excludes the first pregnancy as a given pregnancy)

Pregnancy order—rank of index pregnancy among total pregnancies per woman

71

Pregnancy outcome—the result of a pregnancy including live birth, stillbirth, and abortion, whether induced or spontaneous

Pregnancy wastage—abortions and stillbirths combined

Social status—a composite score based on education and occupation of household head, family income, and average number of persons per room. The rating was done according to local standards and was relative within each area. Households were divided into high status, middle status, and low status according to a scheme attached to the questionnaire.

PART II. REPORTS FROM COLLABORATING CENTRES

Chapter One

STUDY AREAS AND
POPULATION CHARACTERISTICS

INTRODUCTION

A. R. Omran

In this chapter, each of the collaborating centres describes the physical features of the area covered by its study, the transporation, medical, and other service facilities of the region, and the social and demographic characteristics of the study population. The general procedure of each centre was to select two or more residential groups that might differ in their patterns of family formation, but the method of selection varied from centre to centre. It was not possible to select areas that would necessarily be representative of the total population of a country, of a region within a country, or of a residential group.

To be eligible for inclusion in the study, a woman had to be under 45 years of age and married, with a husband present at the time of the study. This made it possible to cover nearly the full fertility span, except for the few women aged 45 or more who might yet be found to be fecund.

The social classification is a composite index based on the education and occupation of the head of the household (usually the spouse of the woman interviewed), the income of the family, and the number of individuals per room (an indication of the quality of housing). Because this index is "culture bound", i.e., heavily influenced by local norms, an inter-country comparison of social status groups should not be attempted. Furthermore, as the classification index is only relative, it may not be representative of the general social status conditions of the country from which the specific area of study was chosen. So few high status households were included in the study that in all areas they were added to the middle status group.

A. COLOMBIA

A. Gil, G. Ochoa & L. F. Duque

Introduction

This study was carried out by the National School of Public Health of the University of Antioquia in Medellín, Colombia. Its purpose is to examine the interactions between health and reproductive behaviour in two geographic zones of the city of Medellín.

Study Areas

Each of the research centres participating in the collaborative study had been asked to select for comparison two or more population groups differing in culture or religion and from different social backgrounds. As the population of Colombia is predominantly Catholic, it was not possible to make such a selection on the basis of religious differences. Moreover, it was not practicable to compare an urban with a thoroughly rural area because of the inaccessibility of Colombia's rural populations. It was therefore decided to restrict the study to the city of Medellín and to compare two residential zones within the city, differing in degree of urbanization and probably in their migratory history.

The city of Medellín is located in one of the more mountainous regions of Colombia in a narrow valley 1538 metres above sea level and with an average daily temperature of 22°C. The unvarying weather conditions and the consistently temperate climate have earned the city the name "City of eternal spring". It is the principal industrial city of the country, specializing in textiles. The 1973 population census revealed a total of 1 100 082 inhabitants. In the same year, the crude birth rate was 36.7 births per 1000 population and the crude death rate was 7.2 per 1000 population (*Annual Statistics of Medellín*, 1974).

Selection of the two zones was based on a rigorous analysis of their population characteristics, such as origin, degree of urbanization, and fertility patterns. The first zone comprised mainly migrant farm workers (actually daily labourers) who had been established in marginal areas of the city for some time and were then relocated as a result of government housing projects. This zone will be referred to as the *newly settled zone*. In contrast, the other zone was one of the old districts of the town and had a population that had almost always resided in this city. This zone will be referred to as the *old urban zone*.

The newly settled zone (NSZ). We chose the barrios (neighbourhoods) Tejelo, Florencia, Girardot, and 12 de Octubre. These barrios were constructed by a governmental agency, the Territorial Credit Agency, after 1968. They are located to the northwest of the city, and were classified by a government study as of low socioeconomic status. This classification was based on external characteristics relative to living units and dwellings, energy consumption, transportation, etc.

The old urban zone (OUZ). Selection of the OUZ was based on the same government study, which classified it as of middle socioeconomic status; it was internally homogeneous and large enough to yield the desired sample size.

The following neighbourhoods, located in the southwestern sector of the city, were selected: San Javier, La Floresta, El Danubio, Santa Monica, and Campo Alegre.

76

It is of interest to note that under a four-year health plan carried out from 1969 to 1972 the city of Medellín was divided into 5 areas. The NSZ was located in the area with the highest infant mortality rate (63.8 per 1000 live births). It also had the highest mortality rate from infectious intestinal diseases and tuberculosis. There are 6 public elementary (primary) schools in this zone and one high school (secondary school). However, there are no private schools. There is a public health centre but there are no private health services. The monthly earnings for the average worker in this zone ranged from US$50 to US$100.

The OUZ had a lower infant mortality rate than the NSZ. It enjoys the lowest mortality rate in Medellín, especially from intestinal infections. There are 4 official public schools and numerous private ones. It has one official health centre and numerous private medical services. The monthly earnings range from US$120 to US$240.

Sampling

Sampling technique

The general procedure was to use area sampling (on the basis of predetermined quotas) for the interview survey followed by probability systematic sampling for additional examinations.

Urban plans were obtained and a preliminary list of all dwellings in the area was made. In order to find out the proportion of all dwelling units with women eligible for the study and to be able to delimit exactly the number of blocks necessary to achieve the target population, a pilot study was run. The objectives of the pilot study were (a) to refine the test instruments (questionnaire, interview, etc., including back-translation), (b) to secure community acceptance of the project, (c) to ascertain how long each interview would take, and (d) to assess the numbers of eligible women (EW) and children under 5.

In the NSZ, it was found that there were 75 eligible women per 100 dwelling units, which meant that an area with 3825 dwellings was required to obtain the target population of 2500 for interviewing. In the OUZ, it was found that there were 35 eligible women per 100 dwelling units, making it necessary to cover an area with 5032 dwellings to complete the desired number of interviews.

Applying a systematic (probability) sampling procedure, and using a constant sampling interval for all the dwelling units, a sample was selected to undergo a gynaecological examination, cervical cytology, and haemoglobin test, and to fill out a Cornell Medical Index (CMI). All children under 5 years of age belonging to the eligible women who were selected for a medical examination were submitted to a paediatric examination and a haemoglobin test and their heights and weights were measured. Children aged 8–14 years, who were sons and daughters of the eligible women in the subsample chosen for medical examination, were selected for intelligence testing, using the Cattell & Cattell Culture-Fair Test.

Data Collection Procedures

A group of 17 students of sociology, social work, and auxiliary nursing were selected to carry out the data collection. They received a 3-week training course covering the methodology of social investigation, human reproduction, sickness and health, and family planning. An interview manual was prepared that described general methodological considerations and gave specific advice about questionnaires to be used as text material during the course of training. Finally, 10 interviewers, 3 supervisors, and a general coordinator (a professional nurse) were selected to work 8 hours a day during the 6 months that the field work lasted (June to December, 1975). In each study area a health centre was used as headquarters for the interviewers, supervisors, and medical examiners.

Clinical evaluations

Forms for the physical (including gynaecological) examinations of the eligible women chosen for this study and for the paediatric evaluation of the children under 5 were designed separately, and all procedures were standardized for both areas.

Both the paediatric examination of the children under 5 and the medical examination of the eligible women included measurement of weight and height and determination of the haemoglobin level. In addition, for all the eligible women examined information was collected regarding blood pressure, obstetric history, and gynaecological complaints.

The clinical evaluations were carried out in parallel with the household interviews. Four doctors (two general practitioners, a gynaecologist, and a paediatrician) worked in collaboration with three auxiliary nurses and two recorders to collect the medical information and research data.

Interviewing

At the end of each interview, a record card was made out showing the names of the woman's children under 5 years of age, those between 8 and 14 years of age, the schools they were currently attending, and the grades they had reached, and spaces were left for checking the completeness of the examination or test. The interviewer made the appointments for the eligible women and their sons and daughters. If an appointment was broken, the woman was given a second appointment. If a woman refused medical examination, the health coordinator tried to obtain her cooperation. Three broken appointments were considered to constitute a rejection.

A Spanish version of the Cornell Medical Index (CMI) was applied as a health questionnaire. It was administered in a self-response format to 2000 women in the old residential area of the project, the OUZ, and was completed by them while they were waiting to be examined. It is to be noted that 94% of the women were literate.

78

IQ testing

The Cattell & Cattell test, which is designed to ensure freedom from cultural influences, was administered to all schoolchildren aged 8 to 14 years belonging to the women who had undergone the gynaecological examination. Details of the test and the way in which it was administered are given in chapter 5.

Coverage

The coverage reached substantially high levels, especially in the interviewing stage of the study (97.9% coverage; see Table 1.A.1). This can be attributed to the intense period of preparation (3 months) and the motivating influences that were brought to bear on individual community organizations, such as parent meetings, religious organizations, school programmes, and community action organizations. Even the gynaecological examination was accepted by over 80% of eligible women. Details of each type of examination are given in chapters 5 and 6.

In the NSZ, the coverage was higher than in the OUZ. This zone seems to have better community organization and places great priority on health.

To satisfy the health needs of the families that were interviewed, a total of 403 medical examinations were made, mainly on children. This definitely contributed to the acceptance of the study by the community. These examinations were excluded from the analysis.

Characteristics of the Study Population

Social status, education, occupation, and the woman's age were the indices selected for comparing eligible women and their husbands in the NSZ and the OUZ (Table 1.A.2).

Social status

A social status scale was constructed based on education and occupation of the household head, the annual family income, and the average number of persons living in a room. The women were classified according to social status as upper, middle, and low social status. Very few women could be classified as of upper social status. This group was therefore merged with the middle social status group. There was some difference in social status distribution for the two residential groups.

In the OUZ 94.31% were classified as of middle social status while in the NSZ 62.0% were classified as of low social status. Social status is the variable that was found to have the most influence on family formation patterns and it will therefore be taken into consideration whenever possible.

TABLE 1.A.1. POPULATION AND COVERAGE

Type of sample	Old urban zone			Newly settled zone			Totals in both zones combined		
	Population sample (No.)	Coverage		Registered population (No.)	Coverage		Total registered population (No.)	Coverage	
		No.	%		No.	%		No.	%
Eligible women:									
(a) Interviewed	2747	2678	97.5	2663	2601	97.7	5380	5270	97.9
(b) Subsample for physical and gynaecological examination	1306	1063	81.4	1275	1147	90.0	2581	2210	85.6
Children under 5: Physical examination	1141	943	82.6	1351	1234	91.3	2492	2177	87.3
Children aged 8–14: IQ test	1283	1074	83.7	1154	1025	88.8	2437	2099	86.1

TABLE 1.A.2. CHARACTERISTICS OF STUDY POPULATION BY RESIDENCE AND SOCIAL STATUS (PERCENTAGE DISTRIBUTION)

Characteristic	Old urban zone			Newly settled zone		
	Middle	Low	Total	Middle	Low	Total
	N = 2516[a]	N = 153	N = 2669	N = 966	N = 1635	N = 2601
Education of EW						
Illiterate + no school	4.3	34.6	6.0	21.9	49.2	39.1
Primary	67.8	62.7	67.6	69.5	49.9	57.2
Secondary	22.7	2.6	21.6	8.1	0.9	3.5
College or graduate	5.1	0.0	4.8	0.5	0.1	0.2
Education of EW's husband						
Illiterate + no school	3.3	30.1	4.5	19.9	45.2	35.8
Primary	42.6	66.0	43.9	57.6	52.5	54.4
Secondary	28.2	3.3	26.8	18.5	1.8	8.0
College or graduate	26.0	0.7	24.5	4.0	0.5	1.8
Occupation of EW						
Housewife	86.7	94.8	87.2	86.1	94.6	91.3
Clerical/professional	7.6	0.7	7.2	3.2	0.4	1.4
Agricultural/industrial	4.9	3.3	4.8	10.1	5.0	7.1
Janitorial/other	0.8	1.3	0.8	0.2	0.1	0.2
Occupation of EW's husband						
Unskilled worker	16.3	92.5	19.9	56.0	92.5	79.0
Skilled worker	4.5	0.4	4.3	9.4	0.4	3.8
Landowner	19.5	2.6	19.2	6.2	2.6	4.0
Clerical/professional	58.5	1.7	55.2	27.7	1.7	11.3
Supported by family	1.3	2.7	1.4	0.6	2.7	1.9
Family structure						
Nuclear	74.0	67.3	73.6	67.2	67.5	67.4
Extended	26.0	32.7	26.4	32.8	32.5	32.6
Age of EW						
<20	2.5	2.0	2.5	4.3	3.4	3.8
20–24	15.0	13.7	14.9	19.4	14.5	16.3
25–29	25.3	19.0	25.0	26.3	22.0	23.6
30–34	22.1	22.9	22.1	22.8	23.4	23.1
35–39	19.5	25.5	19.8	14.7	20.9	18.6
40–44	15.7	17.0	15.1	12.5	15.8	14.6
Mean ages of EW	31.4	32.5	31.5	30.2	31.6	31.1

[a] N = total number of eligible women in group.

Age structure

There was almost no difference in the mean ages of the eligible women in the two zones of residence (31.5 years in the OUZ and 31.1 years in the NSZ). Women in the middle social status group were just one year younger than those of low social status. It is noteworthy that in a national survey on fertility in Colombia (1976), the mean age of the women was 31.8 years in the urban area.

Formal education

The percentage of eligible women and their husbands without any education in the NSZ was high. Thus, 39.1% of the women and 35.8% of their husbands were illiterate and had no schooling. In the OUZ, the figures were much lower: 6.0% and 4.5%, respectively.

In the latter zone, the education of the husbands reached a higher level than that of their wives: 51.3% finished secondary school or college while only 26.4% of the wives reached the same level. In the NSZ, educational levels were similar for the husbands and wives except in the middle social status group where 22.5% of the husbands and only 8.6% of the wives finished secondary school or college.

The differences in educational level according to social status showed a similar tendency in the two zones. The low social status group had a high percentage of women in the "illiterate and no school" category in both zones.

Occupation

In regard to the occupation of the husband, there were marked differences between the two zones. The NSZ had a much higher percentage of unskilled workers than the OUZ—79.0% as against 19.9%. The low social status groups had a high percentage of unskilled labourers (92.5%) in both zones. In the OUZ, 55.2% of the husbands were employed in clerical or professional positions, compared with only11.3% in the NSZ. The great majority of the women (87.2% in the OUZ and 91.3% in the NSZ) were housewives. However, in the OUZ a larger percentage of the women (7.2%) were employed in clerical and professional jobs.

B. EGYPT

A. Bindari, M. H. El-Sammaa, A. Z. Zaghloul,
H. M. Hammam & A. F. El-Sherbini

Introduction

This investigation was carried out by the Department of Epidemiology and Public Health, Faculty of Medicine, Assiut University, Egypt (the rural and urban areas); and the High Institute of Public Health, Alexandria University (the industrial area).

The data were collected and analysed locally in Egypt. Not all the needed statistical tables were available, owing to technical problems; therefore Egypt studies include less information than the other studies reported in this volume.

Study Areas

The study covered a rural and an urban area in Upper Egypt and an industrial area in Lower Egypt. The areas that were studied in Upper Egypt are as follows:

1. *Rural area.* Abnub district in Assiut governorate, Upper Egypt, was selected as a typical rural area. During the past decade, the Faculty of Medicine at Assiut University has conducted extensive field studies in the area east of the Nile. Hundreds of medical students, interns, residents and postgraduate students from Assiut University have been trained in primary health care and field research.

The main characteristic of this area is that it has to a large extent retained the tribal pattern of rural Upper Egypt, with extensive feudal relationships and a low level of socioeconomic development. The main current of civilization and technological development, including the provision of education and health services, transportation, and electricity as well as industrialization, has passed on the west side of the Nile, while the east side has for a long time been largely deprived of such services. There is only one bridge by which civilization could be transmitted to this side, namely, the Assiut barrage. Moreover, few boats come to this area. Only in the last 10 years have serious efforts been made to reach this area to improve services and bring about socioeconomic development.

The homogeneity of this area allowed the research group to select Beni Muhammadeyat village for the main bulk of the rural sample, supplemented by Abnub, which is also rural. The estimated population of Beni Muhammadeyat was 20 000.

2. *Urban area.* To obtain a contrast between rural and urban communities an area on the opposite (west) bank of the Nile was selected. This included Walideya, where a large group of infrastructure and lower echelon University workers and employees live; it is actually semi-urban and is still influenced by the rural culture of Upper Egypt. The estimated population of Walideya was 27 000.

3. *Industrial area.* This area was selected from Kafr El Dawar industrial complex which lies 30 kilometres southeast of Alexandria. One of the three textile plants sited there, El Beida Dyeing company, was chosen for this study. It consists of a residential colony beside the plant building for the workers and their families. The medical services are provided by specialists in a polyclinic. Social services are also available to these families.

Sampling

A sample size of 2000 women in each study area was determined to be adequate to allow the study of the 6 categories classified according to urban, rural, or industrial residence and to middle or low social status.

The target was to cover approximately 2000 potentially reproductive married women under 45 years of age in each of the urban and rural areas. These are referred to as "eligible women" or EW.

1. *Rural area.* Households with an eligible woman in Beni Muhammadeyat were included in this study. The number of eligible women registered in the 1973 census was 1800 but only 1600 were available for study. To complete the required number, 600 eligible women were added from Abnub through systematic random sampling.

2. *Urban area.* Among households in Walideya, the total number of eligible women in the 1973 census was 2200, of whom 2097 were available for interview.

In both the rural and the urban areas, the target population for the physical examination included all women interviewed and their children under 5 years of age. However, for the Goodenough Intelligence Test a representative sample of schoolchildren aged 6–11 years were asked to take the test. Gynaecological examinations were conducted only when necessary; hence, the results are excluded from this report.

3. *Industrial area.* According to the original design for the industrial sample all eligible women in the families of El Beida were to be included. Out of 1232 eligible women living in the residential colony, 619 or 50.2% agreed to be interviewed (Table 1.B.1).

Data Collection Procedure

To pretest the questionnaire a pilot study was conducted on 100 eligible women in Beni Mohammadeyat. It was found necessary to rephrase certain questions and to add others; also the approximate time required to fill out and complete each question was determined. As a result of this pilot study, the final form of the questionnaire was developed.

In selected urban and rural areas, mapping, numbering of houses, and a complete census were carried out. Family folders were developed.

Each eligible woman in the study was interviewed according to the standardized questionnaire. Each day a list of households with eligible women was prepared from family folders kept in the health centre, and a list of 5 households was given to each of the interviewers. They visited the houses, interviewed the women, and made appointments for later visits if the women were absent. They scheduled appointments for eligible women and their children aged up to 5 years to visit the clinic in the health centre. On the chosen day, the eligible women and their children were brought to the clinic by the assistant midwife from the health centre. She was usually a local person who knew them.

In the rural and urban areas, 3 physicians and 2 paediatricians from the Departments of Epidemiology and Paediatrics of Assiut Medical School conducted physical examinations and measurements of weight and height. Two laboratory technicians carried out blood and stool specimen examinations. Interviews were conducted by 9 trained female medical students and 1 female agriculture student. Those who failed to attend the clinic were visited at home, given stool boxes, and advised to report to the clinic. Intelligence tests were carried out by two psychologists.

In the industrial area, the physical examination was carried out in the polyclinic by the staff of the Family Health Department of the High Institute of Public Health, Alexandria.

Coverage

Table 1.B.1. shows the percentages covered by the interview and the physical examination and the numbers taking the intelligence tests in 3 areas.

TABLE 1.B.1. POPULATION COVERAGE

Stage of study	Rural			Urban			Industrial		
	Registered population = 100%	Persons interviewed or examined		Registered population − 100%	Persons interviewed or examined		Registered population = 100%	Persons interviewed or examined	
		No.	%		No.	%		No.	%
Interview	2400	2145	89.4	2200	2097	95.3	1232	619	50.2
Physical examination									
Women	2145	1504	70.1	2097	1868	89.1	619	338	54.6
Children under 5	2187	1678	76.7	2195	1631	74.3			
IQ test									
Schoolchildren aged 6–11		548			1172			1330	

Characteristics of the Study Population

Table 1.B.2 shows the indices that were selected for comparison among the rural, urban, and industrial groups in the categories of education, occupation, family structure, and age distribution by social classes.

Social status. Social status was determined by a social status scoring system, which included the education and occupation of the household head, annual family income, and average number of persons per room. On this basis, women were classified as of high, middle, or low social status. Since there were very few women in the high social status category, this was merged with the middle status category.

Table 1.B.2 shows that of 4861 eligible women, 47.9% were of middle social status and 52.1% were of low social status. The middle social status category was larger in the urban and industrial areas than in the rural area, the proportions being 59.0%, 58.8%, and 33.8%, respectively.

Age structure. The rural and urban groups had a similar age structure. For rural women the percentages were 27.5%, 39.5%, and 33.0%, respectively, in the age groups under 25 years, 25–34 years, and 35 years and older. This can be compared with 29.8%, 40.3%, and 29.9%, respectively, in those age groups for urban women. On the other hand, in the industrial area, there were

TABLE 1.B.2. CHARACTERISTICS OF STUDY POPULATION BY RESIDENCE AND SOCIAL STATUS (PERCENTAGE DISTRIBUTION)

Characteristic	Rural			Urban			Industrial		
	Middle	Low	Total	Middle	Low	Total	Middle	Low	Total
	N = 724[a]	N = 1421	N = 2145	N = 1238	N = 859	N = 2097	N = 364	N = 255	N = 619
Education of EW									
Illiterate + no school	90.7	96.9	94.8	67.5	80.2	72.7	66.2	78.2	71.1
Primary	8.5	3.0	4.8	30.6	13.9	23.8	32.7	21.3	27.9
Secondary	0.8	0.1	0.4	1.6	5.6	3.2	1.1	0.5	1.0
College +	—	—	—	0.3	0.3	0.3	—	—	—
Education of EW's husband									
Illiterate + no school	57.3	87.9	77.6	14.2	49.5	28.6	11.8	13.5	12.4
Primary	29.8	12.1	18.1	55.3	42.9	50.2	75.0	73.7	74.5
Secondary	11.9	—	4.0	26.4	3.5	17.0	13.2	12.8	13.1
College +	1.0	—	0.3	4.1	4.1	4.2	—	—	—
Occupation of EW									
Housewife	98.1	99.7	99.1	95.6	97.4	96.4	98.6	98.9	98.7
Clerical/professional	1.1	0.0	0.4	4.0	2.2	3.2	1.4	0.7	1.1
Agricultural/industrial	0.8	0.3	0.5	0.4	0.2	0.3	—	0.4	0.2
Others	—	—	—	—	0.2	0.1	—	—	—

TABLE 1.B.2. (continued)

Characteristic	Rural			Urban			Industrial		
	Middle	Low	Total	Middle	Low	Total	Middle	Low	Total
	N = 724[a]	N = 1421	N = 2145	N = 1238	N = 859	N 2097	N = 364	N = 255	N = 619
Occupation of EW's husband									
Unskilled worker	—	1.0	1.0	0.5	0.1	0.4	—	—	—
Skilled worker	42.9	95.9	76.7	43.1	72.7	55.2	87.9	92.7	89.8
Landowner	28.6	2.0	10.8	9.5	9.8	9.6	0.9	0.4	0.7
Clerical/professional	22.4	2.0	8.8	40.2	11.1	28.2	9.6	5.0	7.8
Supported by family	2.0	0.0	0.7	3.4	3.5	3.4	0.9	0.9	0.9
Unknown	4.1	.1	2.0	3.3	2.8	3.2	0.7	1.0	0.8
Family structure									
Nuclear	87.8	96.0	93.2	84.9	84.0	84.5	76.9	82.3	79.1
Extended	12.2	4.0	6.8	15.1	16.0	15.5	23.1	17.7	20.9
Age of EW									
<20	6.9	7.2	7.0	12.8	8.8	10.2	6.3	5.1	5.8
20–24	22.6	17.7	20.5	22.0	18.3	19.6	26.4	12.9	20.8
25–29	21.1	19.9	20.8	22.4	21.5	21.6	16.8	18.8	17.6
30–34	19.3	18.0	18.7	16.2	20.0	18.7	10.4	16.9	13.1
35–39	16.7	20.8	18.3	15.0	19.1	17.7	17.9	27.5	21.9
40–44	13.4	16.4	14.7	11.6	12.3	12.2	22.2	18.8	20.8

[a] N = total number of eligible women in group.

87

relatively fewer women in the two lower age groups, while there were 42.7% aged 35 years and older, a proportion one and half times as large as that in the rural or urban groups.

Among women of middle social status, there was a higher percentage in the young age group of less than 25 years than among women of low social status. This pattern was reversed for 35 years of age and older in each of the rural, urban and industrial groups. The 2 social classes did not show consistent patterns in the other age groups.

Education. Rural women had the highest proportion of illiteracy (94.8% illiterate), followed by urban women (72.7%) and industrial women (71.7%). Secondary education was attained by very few women: 0.4% in the rural, 3.2% in the urban, and 1.0% in the industrial area. College level education was attained only in the urban group (0.3%).

Many more men than women received formal education. The literacy level of respondent's husbands was higher in urban and industrial areas than in the rural area. The proportions of husbands with secondary education were 17.0% urban, 13.1% industrial, and 4.0% rural. College level education was attained by 4.2% in the urban group, compared with 0.3% in the rural and 0.0% in the industrial group. With regard to social status, the literacy level was always higher among middle, than among low social status groups. In general, the rural and low social status groups of eligible women and husbands received less formal schooling than those in the other groups.

Occupation. Over 95% of the eligible women were housewives. Only 0.4% of women in the rural area, 3.2% in the urban area, and 1.1% in the industrial area had clerical or professional jobs. They belonged to the middle rather than the low social status category.

Among the husbands, skilled workers led all occupations and were most prevalent in the industrial area (89.8%). In the rural area they totalled 76.7% and in the urban area, 52.2%. There were more skilled workers in the middle social status groups. The proportion of clerical and professional workers was high (as expected) in the urban area, being 28.2% compared with 8.8% in the rural and 7.8% in the industrial area. Landowners accounted for 10.8% of the rural, 9.6% of the urban, and 0.7% of the industrial groups. Unskilled workers were lowest in number (1.0% rural, 0.4% urban, and 0.0% industrial).

C. PAKISTAN

Batul Raza

Introduction

The study was carried out by the National Research Institute of Fertility Control (NRIFC).

The National Research Institute of Fertility Control is the technical arm of the Pakistan Population Planning Organization and has been responsible for population research for the last 15 years. Besides conducting clinical trials of new contraceptives, it has participated in several collaborative studies with population planning organizations and agencies abroad. The National Research Institute of Fertility Control has also been designated as one of the Collaborating Centres for Clinical Research in Human Reproduction of the World Health Organization.

The study aroused great interest not only at the National Research Institute of Fertility Control, but also amongst teachers and researchers at other academic institutions, who considered that the findings of this study would be useful as baseline information for planning and developing similar research studies and for undertaking future comparisons.

Study Area

Two areas of the city of Karachi, representing different socioeconomic and cultural backgrounds, were selected. The two areas, Malir/Saudabad and Nazimabad, were selected for practical reasons, such as acceptability of interviewers and the fact that complete registration of eligible women had already been effected under the Health and Family Welfare Project in Malir/Saudabad and the Continuous Motivation System (CSM) in Nazim-abad/Paposhnagar. Moreover, no research studies had been conducted in these two areas in the past, whereas in other areas of the city several research studies had been undertaken by various organizations and institutions. It is emphasized that the purpose of the study was not to present findings on the national level, but to investigate differences in family formation and health patterns in two groups living under contrasting economic and social conditions.

A brief description of the two areas is given below:

Malir/Saudabad is a low-income, semi-urban area situated about 17 miles east of Karachi. Approximately 12 817 households with a population of about 90 000 were registered in the year 1973. It is worth noting that a considerable proportion of the population consists of immigrants from India as well as from other parts of Pakistan. The migration from India occurred some 30 years ago. This area has been considered semi-urban because of its proximity to Karachi, although at the time of the collection of the data it had most of the characteristics of a rural community. Most of the houses had no water supply, no electricity, and no roads. The hygienic conditions were poor. Most of the people belonged to the low-income group. At the time of the launching of the study, the population of the area suffered from inadequate transportation and lack of health personnel. The main occupations are agriculture, fishing, carpet making, factory work (skilled and unskilled labour), clerical jobs, and other related services. These are representative of the usual occupations of the country. There were two dispensaries in the study area, which were administered by the local municipality, but with insufficient numbers of staff. Many apothecaries (hakeems) and homeopaths were also serving the area. The houses were small and made of concrete. They were systematically planned and numbered. Thus they could be easily located by the field workers.

Nazimabad/Paposhnagar is an urban area located to the north of the city. The sample area consisted of approximately 35 800 households with a population of about 209 000. The residents of this area are migrants from up-country as well as other parts of the city. The population of the area have low to middle incomes and represent different cultures and traditions. Most of the people work in clerical and professional jobs, others are land owners and a smaller number skilled and unskilled workers. Comparatively better health facilities are available in this area than in Malir/Saudabad. Two government hospitals and a number of private health centres are located in the area. The houses provide better accommodation than those in Malir. Here, too, the field workers had no problem in locating the addresses.

Sample Design

As stated earlier, the registration of all the houses in Malir/Saudabad had previously been completed for the Health and Family Welfare Project. The listing was used as the sampling frame for the study. For the purposes of sampling, the area was divided into 60 wards of varying size in terms of both number of households and population. According to the study protocol, 2500 eligible women aged 15–44 years were to be interviewed and medically examined, and their children were also to be medically examined and subjected to an intelligence test. On the basis of a preliminary enquiry conducted in this area, there were about 80 eligible women per 100 households; the remaining 20 were women who failed to respond, or were aged over 45, or were widows. Thus 2500 women could be found for the study by covering 3100 households in the area. With a view to selecting the required number of households in such a way as to be representative of the Project Area, the technique of cluster sampling was used as the population was homogeneous. Two adjoining registration wards were grouped to form one cluster. Thus, in all, 30 clusters were constructed. Out of these, 8 were randomly selected for undertaking intensive work. About 380 households from each cluster were selected randomly to obtain the desired size of sample, i.e., 2500 eligible women.

In Nazimabad/Paposhnagar the household lists and registers prepared by Family Planning Workers under the Continuous Motivation System (CMS), which aimed to maintain a complete record of all households and of all the eligible women in the community, were used to select the sample cases. The data obtained from the registers provided the basis for drawing the sample of currently married women aged 15–44 years. Since the population occupied a wide area, two blocks out of five were selected. Out of these two, about 3000 households were selected randomly to provide 2500 eligible women for the study.

The study ultimately included 2473 eligible women from the urban area and 2383 eligible women in the semi-urban area, thus achieving a response of 98.9% and 95.6% respectively, in the two areas.

Data Collection Procedures

The standardized proforma, i.e., the household and eligible woman questionnaires developed by WHO to be used in several countries were translated into Urdu. To check the validity, the questionnaires were back-translated into English. After pretesting, the questionnaires were finalized.

The interviewers were selected from candidates who replied to a formal advertisement placed in a daily paper, the choice being made by a selection board consisting of experts in medicine, demography and social science research.

Each of the investigators and interviewers engaged for the project had an M.A. in Social Science, Social Work, Sociology, or Psychology. The candidates selected were well versed in the techniques of interviewing and establishing rapport, and had the ability to win the confidence of the respondents. Some of them had previous experience in working with social welfare organizations and some were involved in research work in university projects.

For this specific study, interviewers were trained through lectures on new techniques of interviewing. Instructions were also given in solving field problems, etc. Besides this, information on population dynamics and family planning methods was also provided.

Each interviewer was responsible for interviewing 5–6 eligible women per day and also for editing and coding the completed questionnaire. Two supervisors checked the completeness of the recorded information by re-interviewing 10% of the interviewed eligible women.

In each sample area, a central place was hired for a temporary office to interview those eligible women who did not prefer home surroundings for the interview and/or medical examination of themselves and their children. A team consisting of interviewers, medical doctors, family welfare visitors, laboratory technicians, IQ test administrators, and health educators was responsible for collection of data, medical check-up, and IQ tests. From the sample areas, the eligible women and their children under 5 years of age were physically examined. Their children aged 8–14 years were selected for intelligence testing.

The medical examination of the eligible women included: general physical examination, recording of blood pressure, recording of height and weight, determination of haemoglobin, taking of a cervical smear for cytological examination, and testing of a cervical smear for infections.

The paediatric examination of children of the eligible women under 5 years of age included: general physical examination, examination of urine for albumin and sugar, and stool examination for parasites.

The intelligence quotient of children of the eligible women in the age group 8–14 years was determined using the Cattell and Cattell Culture-Fair Test.

Coverage

To ensure good working relations before starting the project a team of social workers was sent to the communities (research areas) to explain the objectives of the study and its value to the family and to the country. The coverage for the different study components was better in the urban area than in the semi-urban area. Table 1.C.1 describes the details of coverage for each study component.

TABLE 1.C.1. POPULATION COVERAGE

| Stage of study | Semi-urban | | | Urban | | |
| | Number in sample | Persons interviewed or examined | | Number in sample | Person interviewed or examined | |
		No.	%		No.	%
Interview	2500	2389	95.6	2500	2473	98.9
Physical examination						
Women	2388	1753	73.0	2473	2050	83.0
Children under 5	2558	1397	54.6	2367	1690	71.4
IQ test						
Children aged 8–14	3463	1325	38.3	2947	2069	70.2

Interview of eligible women

In the semi-urban, low-income area, 95.6% of the eligible women were interviewed whereas in the urban area, with incomes in the low-to-middle range, the coverage was 98.9%.

Of the women interviewed, 73% in the semi-urban area and 83% in the urban area were given a physical examination. There was some resistance to the gynaecological examination, particularly when it was attempted at the eligible woman's residence. The resistance was atrributable to cultural values, lack of privacy, and objections from in-laws and other members of the family. Overall, about 80% of the women accepted physical examination and 40% accepted the gynaecological examination. Of those women who had undergone the gynaecological examination, a cytological test was performed on 43.1% of the semi-urban women and 51.2% of the urban women.

The coverage for haemoglobin testing in the semi-urban area was 83.0% of those women who were physically examined; in the urban area, the correspondingly figure was 88.0%.

The field workers encountered problems in collecting samples for the urine examination. The women could not comprehend the value of testing urine, so they did not bother to collect samples even when containers were provided for them. This lack of interest resulted in a coverage of 50.8% of the semi-urban women and 63.4% of the urban women.

Physical examination of children under 5 years of age

The physical examination of children under 5 years of age could be carried out on 54.6% of the children of this age group in the semi-urban area and on 71.4% in the urban area.

Blood samples for the haemoglobin test were drawn from about 41.9% of the children who were physically examined in the semi-urban area and from about 57.5% of those in the urban area.

The urine test for albumin and sugar was performed on 23.2% of the children in the semi-urban area and on 28.5% of those in the urban area. The low percentage was due to ignorance and failure of the mothers to realize the importance of the test.

IQ testing

Among the children 8–14 years of age, 38.3% in the semi-urban area and 70.2% in the urban area were subjected to IQ tests. The low coverage in the semi-urban area indicates a lower proportion of school-going children in the semi-urban area than in the urban area. The Professor of Psychology and Dean of the Arts Faculty, Karachi University, was responsible for organizing the IQ testing.

Characteristics of the Study Population

Some selected characteristics of the sample population are presented in Table 1.C.2. The information includes education and occupation of eligible women and their husbands, composition of the family, age composition of the eligible women, mean age of the eligible women, and mean age at marriage of the eligible women in both sample areas. These characteristics are further classified according to socioeconomic status. The main findings are summarized below.

Socioeconomic status. The socioeconomic status (SES) was determined on the basis of the scores for education and occupation of the household head, the annual family income, and the average number of persons living per room. On this basis the respondents were classified into high, middle, or low SES groups.

Very few respondents qualified for inclusion in the high SES group; this is in accordance with the objective of the survey which was to investigate the low and low middle income groups of society.

As expected, in the urban area 92.8% of the respondents belonged to the middle SES group, compared with 49.8% in the semi urban sample. The population of respondents in low SES groups was considerably lower in the urban area than in the semi-urban area.

Educational status of respondents and their husbands. Both the literacy rate and formal educational attainment were higher in the middle SES group than in the low SES group in both the areas. The proportion of women who were illiterate and had no schooling was considerably higher in the semi-urban (70%) than in the urban area (33%). The educational attainment level, particularly the secondary and college level, was considerably higher for urban women.

The literacy level of respondent's husbands was considerably higher in the urban than in the semi-urban area. The educational attainments of husbands,

93

TABLE 1.C.2.   CHARACTERISTICS OF STUDY POPULATION BY RESIDENCE AND SOCIAL STATUS (PERCENTAGE DISTRIBUTION)

Characteristic	Semi-urban			Urban		
	Middle	Low	Total	Middle	Low	Total
	N = 1189[a]	N = 1199	N = 2388	N = 2294	N = 179	N = 2473
Education of EW						
Illiterate + no school	54.7	85.8	70.4	29.7	81.0	33.4
Primary	30.2	12.8	21.5	29.3	18.4	28.5
Secondary	10.8	1.2	5.9	22.4	0.6	20.9
College +	4.3	0.2	2.2	18.6	—	17.2
Education of EW's husband						
Illiterate + no school	6.9	63.9	35.5	4.0	62.0	8.2
Primary	25.7	22.6	24.2	10.5	19.6	11.2
Secondary	37.1	11.3	24.1	30.2	13.4	28.9
College +	30.3	2.2	16.2	55.3	5.0	51.7
Occupation of EW						
Housewife	95.6	95.2	95.4	96.0	92.2	95.7
Clerical/professional	2.6	0.6	1.6	3.4	2.8	3.4
Agricultural/industrial	1.0	2.7	1.8	0.3	2.2	0.5
Janitorial/other	0.8	1.5	1.2	0.3	2.8	0.4
Occupation of EW's husband						
Unskilled worker	3.8	35.4	19.6	1.5	39.7	4.3
Skilled worker	14.9	18.3	16.6	3.7	7.8	4.0
Landowner	9.2	18.8	14.0	30.5	34.7	30.8
Clerical/professional	68.7	21.4	45.0	59.5	6.1	55.6
Supported by family	3.4	6.1	4.8	4.8	11.7	5.3
Family structure						
Nuclear	68.1	74.5	71.3	55.1	70.4	56.2
Extended	31.9	25.5	28.7	44.9	29.6	43.8
Age of EW						
<20	6.0	3.9	4.9	4.0	1.7	3.9
20–24	20.5	12.6	16.5	17.3	15.1	17.1
25–29	21.9	22.3	22.1	26.9	24.6	26.8
30–34	18.6	25.2	22.0	18.5	23.5	18.8
35–39	16.4	19.6	18.0	15.5	16.7	15.6
40–44	16.6	16.4	16.5	17.8	18.4	17.8
Mean age of EW	29.7	31.2	30.7	30.4	31.4	30.7
Mean age of EW at marriage			16.7			18.3

[a] N = total number of eligible women (EW) in group.

particularly at the college level, was considerably higher in the urban (52%) than in the semi-urban area (16%).

Occupation of respondents and their husbands. Most of the respondents (96%) reported that they were housewives. Only 1.6% of the respondents in semi-urban areas and 3.4% in urban areas reported that they were working in clerical and professional jobs. This proportion was higher among the middle SES than among the low SES group in both the areas. About 3.0% of women in the semi-urban area and 0.9% in the urban area reported that they were engaged in agricultural, industrial and janitorial work.

As regards the respondent's husbands, nearly 20% were unskilled workers in the semi-urban area compared with 4.3% in the urban area. The proportion of skilled workers was considerably higher in the semi-urban area (16·6%) than in the urban area (4%). The proportion of land owners was higher in the urban area (30.8%) than in the semi-urban area (14%). The proportion of clerical and professional workers was lower in the semi-urban area (45.0%) than in the urban area (55.6%). The proportion of unskilled workers in both the sample areas was higher in the low SES groups, whereas the proportions of clerical and professional workers in both areas were higher in the middle SES group than in the low SES group. In the urban area, the proportion of clerical and professional workers was considerably higher in middle SES group (59.5%) than in the low SES group (6.1%). In both areas, more of the husbands belonging to the low SES group were supported by their family members than in the middle SES group. The proportion supported by family members was particularly high (11.7%) in the low SES group in the urban area.

Age structure. The age composition of eligible women was almost the same in each of the two sample areas. The proportion of younger women below 25 years of age was 21% in both areas. However, in the middle SES group, it was higher in the semi-urban area (26.5%) than in the urban area (21.3%). The proportion of women in the age group 25–34 was 44.1% in the semi-urban area and 45.6% in the urban area. Older women, i.e., those in the age group 35–44, comprised 34.5% of all eligible women in the semi-urban area and 33.4% of those in the urban area.

In both the sample areas, the mean age of respondents at the time of interview was 30.7 years. It was found that mean age at interview in both the sample areas was higher in the low SES group than in the middle SES group. However, there was little difference by residence between the two social status groups.

Mean age at marriage. The mean age at marriage was slightly higher for urban women than for semi-urban women, the figures being 18.3 years and 16.7 years, respectively.

D. SYRIAN ARAB REPUBLIC

F. El-Boustani

Introduction

The Central Bureau of Statistics, which is affiliated to the Prime Minister's Cabinet, carried out this study in 1973 in collaboration with the Ministry of Health.

The Central Bureau of Statistics, which is located in Damascus, is the country's leading statistical institution.

Study Areas

The areas covered by the study were: the large city of Damascus (urban area), the small towns of Sweida, Salkhad, and Shahba, making up the urban area of Al-Sweida Mohafaza (administrative division), and the rural area of Aleppo Mohafaza.

According to the 1970 Census, the population of the Damascus City was 836 668, of whom 45.8% were under 15 years of age and only 3.5% were above 65 years of age. The annual rate of growth of Damascus was 45.6% during the period 1960–1970, which is one of the highest rates in the country; this is due partly to migration from the rural to the urban area. The illiteracy rate was 28.5% for those aged 10 years and above; 53.7% had a primary level education, 15.3% had an intermediate or secondary (general and vocational) level of education, and only 2.5% had an advanced level of education. There were 734 primary schools, both public and private, and 214 intermediate and secondary schools. The health facilities included 8 state hospitals with 2225 beds and 17 private hospitals with 395 beds; in addition, there were 2 sanatoriums with 435 beds. The occupational structure in 1970 was as follows: 46%, production and related workers; 14%, sales workers; 13%, clerical and related workers; 10% professional, technical, and related workers; and 17%, other occupations.

The population of the urban area of Sweida Mohafaza (1970 Census) was 38 706, of whom 47% were under 15 years of age and only 3.7% were above 65 years of age. The illiteracy rate was 47% for those aged 10 years and above; 45% had a primary level of education, 7% had an intermediate or secondary (general and vocational) level of education, and only 2% had an advanced level of education. There were 196 primary schools, both public and private, and 27 intermediate and secondary schools. There was one state hospital with 197 beds.

The population of the rural area of Aleppo Mohafaza (1970 Census) was 608 367, of whom 51% were under 15 years of age and only 4.5% were above 65 years of age. The illiteracy rate of the two Nahia (districts) covered by the study was 73%; 24% had a primary level of education and only 3% had an intermediate or higher level of education. Sixty-nine percent of the active population were working in agricultural sectors while the others were distributed equally between construction, trade, transport and services. These areas had been chosen to reflect the impact on family health of the differences between rural areas, urban areas, and large cities. At the same time, Damascus City, the urban area of Sweida Mohafaza, and the rural area of Aleppo Mohafaza were considered to be representative samples of the large cities, urban areas, and rural areas of Syria.

Sample Design

The basis of the sample frame was the 1970 housing census. The census figures were updated in the three areas chosen in 1973. Since the target population was 2000 women of reproductive age, a representative sample was taken from the sampling frame. The ratios in the three areas were as follows: Damascus, 2.03%; Rural Aleppo, 3.86%; Sweida, 11.65%.

The representativeness of the sample was tested by comparing the literacy rates in the chosen sample and in the reference population (as revealed in the 1978 census).

The results were as follows:

Area	Illiteracy rate in sample (%)	Illiteracy rate in reference population (%)
Damascus	29.7	28.5
Rural Aleppo	74.9	76.0
Sweida	48.0	53.4

Data Collection Procedures

The questionnaire forms for households and eligible women were discussed and approved by the advisory committee. The survey was undertaken in two stages: The first stage started at the beginning of July 1973 and aimed to provide the Syrian Central Bureau of Statistics with a complete listing of households in the areas chosen in the sample so that a roster of the married women aged between 15 and 45 and their living children could be obtained. The second stage started at the end of July 1973 and included formulating a comprehensive system for instructing the interviewers, training the interviewers, preparing centres for medical examinations and IQ tests, and visiting the households to collect the statistical data. The medical examinations and IQ tests were conducted in the health centres. There were over 80 persons engaged in the survey: 60 interviewers and 21 physicians, of whom 8 were gynaecologists and 8 were paediatricians. The period of the study (survey design, field work, medical examinations, data processing, data tabulation, and final report) was from 1973 to 1978.

It is important to note that all the gynaecologists were women, in the hope that this would increase the acceptability of a gynaecological examination in this traditional society.

Population Coverage

Table 1.D.1 shows that out of the target of 2000 eligible women in Damascus, 1975 were interviewed, making a response rate of 98.9%. In Sweida, the number of interviewed women was 1711, giving a response rate of 86%, while in rural Aleppo the response rate was 96.8%. This was considered a very good achievement. For the gynaecological examination, for which the target for each area was 1500 eligible women, the response rates were 80.93% in Damascus, 74.4% in Sweida, and 93% in rural Aleppo. Again, this was considered quite an achievement for a traditional society; the success was attributed to the good rapport with the project staff and the use of female gynaecologists.

For the paediatric examination of children under 5 years, 67% of the target sample size (1000) were achieved in Damascus, 60.1% in Sweida, and 95.3% in rural Aleppo. These figures do not, however, reflect the level of refusal or achievement, because the numbers of children registered for examination were much higher than the target figure. On the basis of the numbers of registered children, the rates of coverage become 26.7%, 28.3%, and 33.6% for Damascus, Sweida, and rural Aleppo, respectively.

With regard to the IQ test, Table 1.D.1 shows that out of 2954 registered children in Damascus, 1541 had taken the test, an achievement rate of 52.2%. In Sweida and rural Aleppo; the coverage rates were 51.9% and 27.4%, respectively.

TABLE 1.D.1. POPULATION COVERAGE

Stages of study	Damascus			Sweida			Rural Aleppo		
	Registered population = 100%	Persons interviewed or examined		Registered population = 100%	Persons interviewed or examined		Registered population = 100%	Persons Interviewed or examined	
		No.	%		No.	%		No.	%
Interview	2000	1975	98.8	2000	1711	86.0	2000	1935	96.8
Physical examination									
Women	1975	1214	61.5	1711	1116	65.2	1935	1394	72.0
Children under 5	2511	671	26.7	2124	601	28.3	2840	953	33.6
IQ test									
Children aged 8–14	2954	1541	52.2	2395	1244	51.9	2492	683	27.4

The high refusal rate for the gynaceological examination was due to the fact that Syrian women are unwilling to submit to such an examination by a strange doctor, especially when they see no medical purpose for it. More urban than rural women refused the examination, because urban women are more prosperous and more likely to have their own physician. The same reason accounted for the low coverage of the paediatric examinations. For the IQ test the rate of refusal varied from 47.8% in Damascus to 72.6% in rural Aleppo. This high rate of refusal was due to many factors, such as the considerable refusal rate for the women's physical examinations, the widely scattered distribution of children in the schools of the three areas under study and the refusal of the family to allow their children to be submitted to an IQ test.

Despite these shortcomings, however, it is believed that the sample coverage achieved can be taken to be representative of the main characteristics of the eligible women.

Characteristics of the Study Population

Social status, age structure, education, and occupation were selected as indicators to compare women and their husbands within each of the 3 study areas (Damascus, Sweida, and rural Aleppo) and between these areas.

TABLE 1.D.2 CHARACTERISTICS OF THE STUDY POPULATION BY RESIDENCE AND SOCIAL STATUS (PERCENTAGE DISTRIBUTION)

	Damascus			Sweida			Rural Aleppo		
	Middle	Low	Total	Middle	Low	Total	Middle	Low	Total
	N = 1590[a]	N = 335	N = 1975	N = 1314	N = 397	N = 1711	N = 668	N = 1267	N = 1935
Education of EW									
Illiterate + no school	66.0	91.5	71.0	76.3	97.3	81.2	97.6	99.8	99.0
Primary	23.2	7.8	20.0	17.8	2.8	14.3	2.4	0.2	1.0
Secondary	8.8	0.8	7.2	5.5	0	4.2	—	—	—
College or graduate	1.9	0	1.5	0.4	0	0.4	—	—	—
Education of EW's husband									
Illiterate + no school	33.2	93.6	44.9	38.7	96.2	52.1	59.1	96.4	83.6
Primary	33.4	4.4	27.7	37.4	3.5	29.6	24.1	2.4	9.9
Secondary	20.6	1.8	17.0	17.3	0.3	13.3	12.9	1.1	5.2
College or graduate	12.8	0.3	10.3	6.5	0	5.0	3.9	0.1	1.4
Occupation of EW									
Housewife	93.9	97.4	94.6	93.5	98.5	94.7	95.1	95.5	95.3
Clerical/professional	5.3	1.3	4.5	5.0	0	4.0	0.6	1.0	1.5
Agricultural/industrial	0.6	0.6	0.6	0.6	1.3	0.8	3.1	2.9	3.0
Janitorial/other	0.2	0.6	0.2	0.5	0.3	0.4	0.2	0.3	0.3
Occupation of EW's husband									
Unskilled worker	17.8	67.5	27.5	23.0	72.3	34.4	21.1	53.4	42.2
Skilled worker	11.8	2.6	16.3	23.2	2.8	18.5	27.2	9.6	15.7
Landowner	45.9	21.8	13.8	11.6	15.4	12.5	15.9	29.5	24.8
Clerical/professional	19.6	1.0	37.2	37.2	1.3	28.8	31.6	2.0	12.2
Supported by family	4.9	6.8	5.3	5.1	8.3	5.8	4.2	5.5	5.1
Family structure									
Nuclear	79.4	73.5	78.3	83.6	83.6	83.1	65.1	60.9	62.4
Extended	20.6	26.5	21.7	16.4	16.4	16.4	34.9	39.1	37.6
Age of EW									
<20	6.5	8.6	6.9	4.6	1.5	3.9	10.9	7.7	8.8
20–24	18.8	14.0	17.6	17.0	6.8	14.6	24.0	17.7	19.8
25–29	20.8	14.3	19.6	24.3	15.1	22.2	21.6	16.5	18.2
30–34	22.3	19.7	21.8	22.1	20.4	21.7	14.8	19.8	18.1
35–39	16.9	22.3	18.1	14.5	22.4	16.4	14.8	18.5	17.2
40–44	14.8	20.5	15.9	17.5	33.8	21.3	13.9	19.9	17.8
Mean age of EW	30.5	32.0	30.9	30.8	34.8	31.7	28.8	30.9	30.2

[a] N = total number of eligible women in group.

99

Social status. Social status was determined by a scoring system that included the education and occupation of the household head, the annual income of the family, and the habitation. Initially, the population was classified into three different categories, high, middle, and low, but as only a small number of eligible women fell into the high category, this was combined with the middle category; thus, the women were classified into middle and low social status groups.

Age structure. Although the mean age of the women of Sweida was a little higher than the mean age of the women in Damascus and in rural Aleppo, it is worthy of mention that the difference in mean ages between Damascus and Sweida was not large, while there was a large mean age difference between Sweida and rural Aleppo; this could be the result of the younger age at marriage for the rural women. The difference in age structure is more significant; 28.6% of the eligible rural women were under 24, compared with 24.5% and 18.5% of the eligible women of Damascus and Sweida, respectively. The percentage of the eligible women aged between 25 and 29 was 22.2% in Sweida, 19.6% in Damascus, and 18.2% in rural Aleppo. Within each residential category, there was a difference in mean age by social status. Generally, the eligible women of middle social status were younger than the eligible women of low social status.

Education. Of the eligible women in Damascus, 71% were illiterate or had received no formal schooling; 81.2% in Sweida and 99% in rural Aleppo were illiterate. The proportion having no education was much greater among those classified as of low social status than among those who were classified as of middle social status. The husbands were better educated than their wives. This was noticed in the middle social class where the illiterates and those with no formal schooling comprised 33.2% of the eligible women's husbands in Damascus, 38.7% in Sweida, and 59.1% in rural Aleppo.

Occupation. At least 94% of the women in all 3 areas studied, whether of middle or low social status, were housewives. Among the husbands of the eligible women, rural Aleppo had a higher proportion of unskilled workers and a lower proportion of skilled and professional workers than Damascus and Sweida. This reflects the better educational opportunities in Damascus and Sweida.

Chapter Two

FAMILY FORMATION
AND SOCIAL CHARACTERISTICS

INTRODUCTION

A. R. Omran, C. C. Standley & M. R. Bone

Patterns of family formation differ from culture to culture and from place to place. The aim of this chapter is to identify those social variables that are strongly associated with patterns of family formation, so that they can be taken into account when health patterns are examined in subsequent chapters.

Six characteristics of family formation are discussed here in the context of the cultural (or residential) situation and social status.

(a) *Family structure.* A nuclear family consists of a father and mother and their children who are unmarried at the time of the survey. If in-laws, married children and/or other blood relatives live in the same family unit, then the family is described as an extended one.

Although information was gathered in the study on whether families were nuclear or extended, this was not found on the whole to be analytically meaningful. This does not imply that the structure of a family fails to influence family formation. Such an influence may have been present but may have been masked by the fact that the main criterion for classifying a family was the physical situation. Thus, an interfering mother-in-law who lived round the corner would have been excluded from consideration because the family was defined as physically nuclear, though socially extended. The survey was not, however, designed for an in-depth sociological inquiry into family network influences, and hence, this variable is rarely used in the analysis.

(b) *Age at marriage.* There is known to be a pronounced negative association between age at marriage and fertility; this makes it important to consider intergroup variations and variations over time. Within each group, the age at marriage is examined in terms of education, occupation, and social status.

(c) *Gravidity.* This denotes the number of pregnancies per woman up to the time of the survey. In a comparative study such as this, age-specific figures must be used. The number of pregnancies in the age group 40 to 44 years comes close to being a measure of the completed fertility of a woman and is frequently used as such in this report.

Though the gravidity figures are based upon a detailed pregnancy history obtained from each woman, the possibility of underreporting cannot be excluded, since the reproductive history of an older woman covers some 30 years. Also, some pregnancies ending in abortion, stillbirth, or even the death of a young child, may have been suppressed for psychological reasons.

(d) *Parity.* This is defined as the number of live births per woman until the time of the survey. In the present study, age-specific parity is used. Like gravidity, parity in the age group 40 to 44 years is often taken as an approximation to completed parity, even though children might occasionally be born to older women. While parity is definitely more reliable than gravidity, the possibility of underreporting cannot be excluded.

(e) *Family size.* This indicates the number of living children a woman had at the time of the survey.

(f) *Ideal family size.* This indicates a woman's estimate of the optimal family size for a family with economic and social traits similar to her own. Though it is a theoretical index and is therefore liable to inaccuracies related to the education and other social situations of the eligible woman, it is nevertheless valuable as a reflection of cultural and social variations in the different groups.

A. COLOMBIA

A. Gil & G. Ochoa

Family Structure

Family structure can be either nuclear or extended. A nuclear family is defined as consisting of a father and mother and their children. If any in-laws, married children, or blood relatives live in the same family unit, this constitutes an extended family.

The majority of the families who lived in the OUZ were nuclear (73.6%); among those of middle social status, 74.1% of the families were nuclear in structure. In the NSZ, around 67% of the families were nuclear in both social status groups. Because several of the nuclear families were socially extended. family structure was not a meaningful variable in this study; it is not therefore included in the subsequent analysis.

102

Age at Marriage

The average age at marriage for women in the study was just over 20 years. In the OUZ the average age at marriage was 20.7 years, while in the NSZ it was 19.7 years. This difference is statistically significant at the 0.01 level.[1] In

[1] For many of the following tables a large number of statistical tests were performed. Only a few of the more important results are mentioned in the text. Where a test is statistically significant at a probability level of 0.01 or 0.05 this is indicated in parentheses following the summary of the data (e.g., $P < 0.01$).

TABLE 2.A.1 PERCENTAGE DISTRIBUTION OF ELIGIBLE WOMEN BY AGE AT MARRIAGE AND SOCIAL CHARACTERISTICS

Characteristic	Percentage of eligible women who married at age:						Number (all ages)
	12–14	15–19	20–24	25–29	30–34	35–44	
Residence and social status							
Old urban zone							
Middle	2.5	38.8	43.5	12.1	2.7	0.4	2516
Low	5.2	49.0	30.7	10.5	1.3	3.3	153
All OUZ	2.7	39.3	42.8	12.0	2.6	0.6	2669
Newly settled zone							
Middle	3.5	46.6	38.8	8.8	2.1	0.2	966
Low	4.3	52.5	33.3	8.0	1.8	0.1	1635
All NSZ	4.0	50.3	35.3	8.3	1.9	0.2	2601
Education of EW							
Old urban zone							
Illiterate + no schooling	8.1	42.9	33.5	11.8	3.7	0.0	161
Primary	2.8	43.9	40.0	10.5	2.2	0.6	1803
Secondary	1.2	28.6	50.5	15.3	3.6	0.5	576
College + college graduate	0.0	19.4	58.1	19.4	3.1	0.0	129
Newly settled zone							
Illiterate + no schooling	5.6	51.5	32.3	9.2	1.3	0.2	1016
Primary	3.2	51.0	36.0	7.3	2.3	0.0	1487
Secondary	0.0	26.1	56.5	15.2	2.2	0.0	92
College + college graduate	16.7	33.3	50.0	0.0	0.0	0.0	6
Occupation of EW							
Old urban zone							
Housewife	2.7	41.8	41.6	10.9	2.4	0.6	2327
Clerical/professional	0.5	17.6	56.0	21.8	3.1	1.0	193
Agricult./janit./ industrial	3.9	25.8	45.3	18.8	5.5	0.7	128
Others	9.5	47.6	28.6	9.5	4.8	0.0	21
Newly settled zone							
Housewife	4.0	51.6	34.8	7.7	1.8	0.1	2376
Clerical/professional	2.7	13.5	56.8	24.3	2.7	0.0	37
Agricult./janit./ industrial	4.3	39.7	39.1	13.0	3.3	0.6	184
Others	0.0	100.0	0.0	0.0	0.0	0.0	4

both the OUZ and the NSZ, the percentage of women marrying before the age of 20 was higher in the lower social status group than in the middle social status group ($P < 0.10$) (Table 2.A.1 and Fig. 2.A.1). Even larger variations in the age at marriage were evident when education was considered. The age at marriage increased with higher education of the women in both residential areas. In the OUZ, 51.0% of the illiterates were married before age 20, compared with 29.8% of those with secondary school education. In the NSZ, the respective percentages were 57.1% and 26.1% (Table 2.A.1). In both zones

FIG. 2.A.1. FAMILY FORMATION BY SOCIAL CHARACTERISTICS

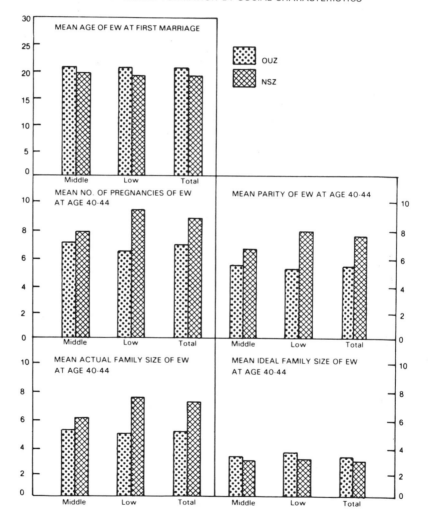

SOCIAL STATUS

these educational differentials are significant at the 0.01 level. With regard to occupation, housewives married at a younger age than working women in both the OUZ and the NSZ. It can be seen that 44.5% and 55.6% of the housewives were married before 20 years of age in the OUZ and NSZ, respectively, in contrast with 18.1% and 16.2% of those employed in clerical/professional work (Table 2.A.1).

Gravidity

Gravidity increased steadily with age. A clear difference was observed in the mean gravidity by residence; it was higher in the NSZ than in the OUZ. For women under 20, the mean gravidity was 0.45 in the OUZ and 0.90 in the NSZ. By age group 40–44 years, it was found that in the NSZ women had approximately three more pregnancies than women in the OUZ. The gravidity was higher in the low social status group in each zone for nearly all age groups (Table 2.A.2 and Fig. 2.A.1 and 2.A.2).

TABLE 2.A.2. MEAN GRAVIDITY BY AGE OF ELIGIBLE WOMEN, RESIDENCE AND SOCIAL STATUS*

Residence and social status	Mean gravidity at age:						Number (all ages)
	< 20	20–24	25–29	30–34	35–39	40–44	
Old urban zone							
Middle	0.44	1.24	2.16	3.61	5.23	6.83	2516
Low	(0.67)	(1.90)	3.72	4.71	7.08	6.23	153
All OUZ	0.45	1.28	2.23	3.67	5.37	6.79	2669
Newly settled zone							
Middle	0.01	1.42	2.71	4.11	6.40	8.00	966
Low	1.98	2.08	4.03	6.06	7.92	9.75	1635
All NSZ	0.90	1.79	3.48	5.35	7.48	9.19	2601

* Figures in parentheses refer to fewer than 25 eligible women.

Parity

A pattern similar to that for gravidity was found for parity. Women in the NSZ had more live births than women in the OUZ in all age groups and in both social status groups. At age 40–44 years, women in the NSZ had two more live births than women in the OUZ ($P < 0.01$). (Table 2.A.3 and Fig. 2.A.1 and 2.A.2.)

The average mean parity declined with increase in educational level for almost all ages in both zones. In the NSZ, the number of women who reached an educational level of at least secondary school was so small that this relationship could not be observed in most age groups. A similar inverse association was observed between mean parity and the husband's education.

105

FIG. 2.A.2. FERTILITY VARIABLES SPECIFIC FOR AGE, BY RESIDENCE AND SOCIAL STATUS

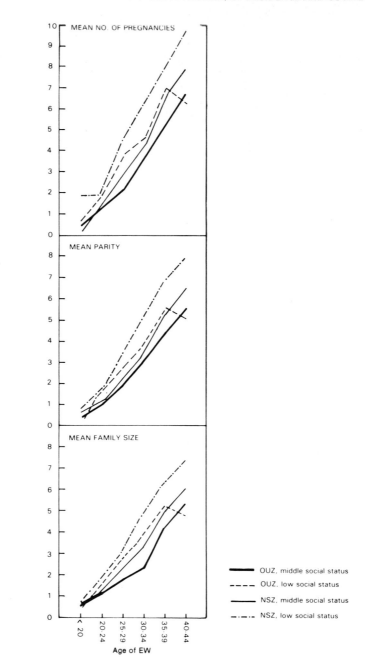

106

TABLE 2.A.3.   MEAN PARITY BY AGE OF ELIGIBLE WOMEN, RESIDENCE, AND SOCIAL CHARACTERISTICS*

Social characteristic and residence	Mean parity at age:						Number (all ages)
	< 20	20–24	25–29	30–34	35–39	40–44	
Social status							
Old urban zone							
Middle	0.40	1.08	1.90	3.,11	4.43	5.66	2516
Low	(0.33)	(1.71)	2.86	4.06	5.67	5.12	153
All OUZ	0.39	1.11	1.94	3.17	4.52	5.63	2669
Newly settled zone							
Middle	0.76	1.23	2.37	3.59	5.37	6.58	966
Low	0.80	1.84	3.43	5.26	6.85	8.15	1635
All NSZ	0.79	1.57	2.99	4.65	6.41	7.65	2601
Education of EW							
Old urban zone							
Illiterate + no schooling	(1.00)	(1.64)	2.70	3.63	5.68	6.02	161
Primary	0.36	1.22	2.16	3.36	4.62	5.75	1803
Secondary	(0.50)	1.00	1.59	2.54	3.78	4.77	576
College + college graduate	(0.00)	0.58	1.18	(2.04)	(3.50)	(4.50)	129
Newly settled zone							
Illiterate + no schooling	1.50	1.89	3.49	5.14	6.65	8.33	1016
Primary	0.71	1.47	2.77	4.40	6.30	7.01	1487
Secondary	(0.50)	(1.00)	3.37	(2.52)	(4.18)	(7.00)	92
College + college graduate	—	(0.50)	(0.40)	—	—	—	6
Education of husband							
Old urban zone							
Illiterate + no schooling	(0.00)	(1.36)	(3.60)	3.92	5.85	5.82	128
Primary	(0.27)	1.26	2.04	3.29	4.83	5.72	1172
Secondary	0.52	1.15	2.08	3.06	4.01	5.45	714
College + college graduate	(0.44)	0.93	1.64	2.93	3.77	5.38	655
Newly settled zone							
Illiterate + no schooling	(1.00)	1.98	3.50	5.19	6.68	8.19	931
Primary	0.80	1.47	2.80	4.38	6.16	7.29	1415
Secondary	(0.38)	1.41	2.61	4.05	(6.31)	(6.50)	208
College + college graduate	(1.00)	(1.27)	(2.47)	(3.13)	(8.00)	(5.00)	47
Occupation of EW							
Old urban zone							
Housewife	0.43	1.23	2.12	3.25	4.56	5.75	2327
Clerical/professional	(0.00)	0.42	0.96	2.23	3.83	(2.84)	193
Agricultural/industrial	—	(0.56)	1.03	2.89	4.44	(5.35)	128
Janitorial/others	(0.00)	(0.73)	(2.00)	(8.00)	(7.50)	(2.00)	20
Newly settled zone							
Housewife	0.80	1.61	3.09	4.82	6.56	7.72	2376
Clerical/professional	—	(1.40)	(1.93)	(2.70)	(3.50)	(4.33)	37
Agricultural/industrial	(0.67)	1.10	1.55	3.07	4.86	6.96	184
Janitorial/others	(0.00)	—	(4.00)	—	(10.00)	—	4

* Figures in parentheses refer to fewer than 25 eligible women.

107

Housewives in all age groups experienced higher parity than working women in both residential zones. However, the small numbers of women in the other working categories made comparisons of parity between these groups less reliable (Table 2.A.3).

TABLE 2.A.4. MEAN FAMILY SIZE BY AGE OF ELIGIBLE WOMEN, RESIDENCE, AND SOCIAL CHARACTERISTICS*

Social characteristic and residence	Mean family size at age:						Number (all ages)
	< 20	20–24	25–29	30–34	35–39	40–44	
Social status							
Old urban zone							
Middle	0.40	1.05	1.86	2.31	4.22	5.35	2516
Low	(0.33)	(1.67)	2.76	3.89	5.36	4.77	153
All OUZ	(0.39)	1.08	1.90	3.08	4.30	5.32	2669
Newly settled zone							
Middle	0.69	1.19	2.27	3.37	4.94	6.07	966
Low	0.77	1.77	3.29	4.98	6.45	7.46	1635
All NSZ	0.73	1.52	2.87	4.39	6.00	7.02	2601
Education of EW							
Old urban zone							
Illiterate + no schooling	(1.00)	(1.45)	2.56	3.39	5.38	5.49	161
Primary	0.36	1.20	2.12	3.28	4.41	5.44	1803
Secondary	(0.50)	0.96	1.56	2.51	3.54	4.61	576
College + college graduate	(0.00)	0.58	1.16	(1.91)	(3.40)	(4.33)	129
Newly settled zone							
Illiterate + no schooling	0.93	1.81	3.31	4.86	6.18	7.52	1016
Primary	0.66	1.43	2.67	4.15	5.94	6.53	1487
Secondary	(0.50)	(1.00)	2.30	(2.48)	(4.00)	(6.83)	92
College + college graduate	—	(0.50)	(3.75)	—	—	—	6
Occupation of EW							
Old urban zone							
Housewife	0.43	1.20	2.08	3.16	4.35	5.42	2327
Clerical/professional	(0.00)	0.42	0.94	2.23	3.72	(2.85)	193
Agricultural/industrial	—	(0.53)	1.00	2.79	3.78	(5.10)	128
Janitorial/others	(0.00)	(0.73)	(1.50)	(6.00)	(7.50)	(2.00)	20
Newly settled zone							
Housewife	0.74	1.56	2.97	4.54	6.14	7.10	2376
Clerical/professional	—	(1.20)	(1.79)	(2.70)	(3.50)	(4.33)	37
Agricultural/industrial	(0.67)	1.07	1.81	2.98	4.57	5.14	184
Janitorial/others	(0.00)	—	(3.50)	—	(6.00)	—	4

* Figures in parentheses refer to fewer than 25 eligible women.

Family Size

The difference between parity and family size is a result of child loss. The values for family size were just smaller than those for parity in each zone. The important difference was in the low social status group, which experienced a higher child loss than the middle social status group. The pattern of association between family size and age was similar to that of gravidity and parity. (Table 2.A.4 and Fig. 2.A.1 and 2.A.2.) Mean family size varied inversely with the women's level of education.

In relation to occupation, housewives had an average family size greater than women employed in other occupational categories (Table 2.A.4).

The NSZ had an average family size that was greater than that of the OUZ for almost all age categories (Table 2.A.5). In both zones, there was an inverse association between average family size and age at marriage for women in each age group. The younger a woman married, the more children she was likely to have.

TABLE 2.A.5. MEAN FAMILY SIZE BY AGE OF ELIGIBLE WOMEN, RESIDENCE, AND AGE AT MARRIAGE*

Residence and age at marriage	Moan family size at age:						Number (all ages)
	<20	20–24	25–29	30–34	35–39	40–44	
Old urban zone							
<15	—	(2.00)	(3.85)	(5.43)	(5.67)	(7.40)	71
15–19	0.39	1.44	2.73	4.08	5.36	6.43	1050
20–24	—	0.65	1.59	2.89	4.19	5.25	1141
25–44	—	—	0.64	1.54	2.22	3.42	407
Newly settled zone							
<15	(1.67)	2.92	(5.04)	(6.59)	(7.76)	(6.84)	105
15–19	0.67	1.81	3.55	5.37	6.89	8.57	1308
20–24	—	0.82	2.12	3.86	5.73	6.94	919
25–44	—	—	0.74	1.86	3.36	4.39	269

* Figures in parentheses refer to fewer than 25 eligible women.

Ideal Family Size

Each woman was asked what she considered to be the ideal number of children for a family in circumstances similar to her own. The average ideal family size was 3.2 in both zones (Table 2.A.6) with only small differences between social status groups. There was a slight tendency for ideal family size to be positively associated with the woman's parity and age. There was no clear association between the parity of the woman and that of her mother.

TABLE 2.A.6. MEAN IDEAL FAMILY SIZE BY POPULATION CHARACTERISTICS*

Characteristic	Mean family size by social status					
	Old urban zone			Newly settled zone		
	Middle	Low	Both categories	Middle	Low	Both categories
All characteristics combined	3.21	3.20	3.22	3.23	3.21	3.22
Parity						
0	2.91	(2.10)	2.89	3.22	2.77	3.04
1	2.84	(2.32)	2.82	2.88	2.73	2.82
2	2.99	3.14	3.00	3.23	3.08	3.15
3	3.39	(3.45)	3.39	3.18	3.37	3.29
4	3.51	(4.18)	3.55	3.26	3.37	3.33
5	3.59	(3.93)	3.56	3.64	3.26	3.38
6 and over	3.68	3.16	3.63	3.48	3.29	3.39
Parity of EW's mother						
1	3.04	—	3.04	(2.31)	(3.00)	2.71
2	2.89	(3.57)	2.93	3.04	2.82	2.91
3	3.24	(2.75)	3.23	3.09	3.08	3.08
4	3.07	(4.43)	3.13	3.22	2.95	3.07
5	3.08	(3.22)	3.08	3.53	3.01	3.19
6	2.97	(3.23)	2.99	3.80	3.28	3.48
7	3.23	(3.00)	3.22	2.99	3.14	3.09
8	3.30	(3.25)	3.30	3.04	3.24	3.17
9	3.24	(2.76)	3.19	3.03	3.16	3.11
10 and over	3.32	(3.11)	3.30	3.43	3.29	3.33
Education of EW's husband						
Illiterate + no schooling	3.50	3.35	3.45	3.49	3.16	3.22
Primary	3.24	3.12	3.23	3.25	3.26	3.26
Secondary	3.19	(3.40)	3.19	3.18	2.79	3.13
College + college graduate	3.17	(4.00)	3.17	3.10	(3.00)	3.92
Education of EW						
Illiterate + no schooling	3.32	3.02	3.22	3.45	3.22	3.27
Primary	3.26	3.32	3.27	3.22	3.19	3.20
Secondary	3.12	(2.75)	3.12	3.37	(3.43)	3.30
College + college graduate	2.95	—	2.95	(3.20)	(4.00)	(3.33)
Occupation of EW						
Housewife	3.25	3.21	3.24	3.30	3.23	3.26
Clerical/professional	3.04	(2.00)	3.03	3.16	1.33	2.86
Agricultural/industrial	3.07	(2.80)	3.05	3.15	(2.95)	3.06
Janitorial/others	(3.00)	(4.50)	(3.14)	(2.50)	—	(1.25)
Age of EW						
<20	2.75	(2.67)	2.74	4.19	2.75	3.37
20–24	2.90	(2.38)	2.87	3.05	2.95	3.00
25–29	3.11	3.07	3.11	3.17	3.20	3.19
30–34	3.21	3.40	3.22	3.34	3.41	3.38
35–39	3.44	3.18	3.43	3.48	3.21	3.29
40–44	3.50	3.85	3.52	3.19	3.24	3.23

* Figures in parentheses refer to fewer than 25 eligible women.

TABLE 2.A.7. PERCENTAGE DISTRIBUTION OF IDEAL FAMILY SIZE BY ACTUAL
FAMILY SIZE

Actual family size	Percentage of EW choosing ideal family size of:				Number of women
	0–3	4	5	6 and over	
Old urban zone					
0	71.4	24.1	2.7	1.7	294
1	75.0	20.6	2.8	1.6	500
2	63.9	31.2	3.6	1.4	587
3	54.9	36.8	5.7	2.6	386
4	36.3	53.0	3.6	7.1	281
5	48.8	23.7	19.9	7.6	211
6 and over	46.3	37.3	4.2	12.2	410
All OUZ	58.7	31.9	5.0	4.4	2669
Newly settled zone					
0	65.8	26.2	3.7	4.3	187
1	74.0	20.9	3.5	1.5	339
2	56.7	35.8	3.5	4.0	427
3	59.1	31.0	4.9	4.9	345
4	42.4	44.4	4.9	8.2	304
5	56.9	22.0	15.0	6.1	246
6 and over	51.8	33.1	4.6	10.5	753
All NSZ	56.9	31.4	5.3	6.4	2601

In the OUZ, an inverse association existed between ideal family size and the
education of the eligible women and their husbands. The pattern was not clear
in the NSZ. Women in clerical and professional occupations preferred a
smaller ideal family size than the housewives (Table 2.A.6).

The actual size of the family was compared with ideal family size and the
data are presented in Table 2.A.7. A direct positive association was observed
between a woman's opinion about ideal family size and the actual size of her
family (r – 0.205). However, more than 80% of the women with 6 or more
children in both the OUZ and the NSZ selected 4 or fewer children as the ideal
size of the family.

B. EGYPT

H. M. Hammam, A. H. A. Zaraour, M. El-Amine, & A. F. El-Sherbini

Family Structure

Table 1.B.2 shows that 93.2%, 84.5%, and 79.1% of families within the rural, urban, and industrial groups, respectively were nuclear. Nuclear families were found more often among the low than among the middle social status groups in the rural and industrial areas, while both social status groups were equally represented in the urban area. It is possible that families of low social status tend to disintegrate as a result of the economic pressures involved in maintaining a large family. Also, it should be noted that an entire village like Beni-Muhammadeyat could be formed from 3 large extended families, even though couples with children live separately. In other words, although some families live separately from others and seem to be physically nuclear, they are in fact socially extended and behave likewise. Hence, this type of family will not be considered as a separate variable in this report.

Age at Marriage

The mean age of women at marriage was 17 years in the rural area, 17.6 years in the urban area, and 18 years in the industrial area. In all areas the majority of women were married by or shortly after the age of 20. Table 2.B.1 shows that the proportion of women whose age at marriage was under 20 years was 85.8%, 83.1%, and 85.3% in the rural, urban, and industrial areas, respectively. However, the rural area had a much higher proportion of women (27.6%) marrying under 15 years of age. The comparable rates for the urban and industrial women were 18.9% and 7%, respectively. This is attributable to the highly traditional society in Upper Egypt, especially in villages where rich and poor folk alike tend to marry their daughters off as early in their reproductive lives as possible. Only slight social status differences were revealed in the percentages of women married before the age of 20. In the urban area, the middle social status group had a slightly higher percentage of marriage at this early age than the low social status group (84.0% and 81.6%, respectively). Industrial groups had nearly equal percentages for both social classes.

Primary education of eligible women as opposed to illiteracy or no schooling was associated with a lower proportion marrying under 15 years of age in all 3 study areas, as shown in the following figures: 28.2% for illiterate and 18.4%

for primary education in the rural area, 21.5% and 13.9%, respectively, in the urban area, and 7.2% and 5.8%, respectively, in the industrial area. Regarding secondary education, the numbers of women with this level of education in the rural and industrial areas were too small to make meaningful comparisons. Out of 68 women in the urban area with secondary education, only 33.9% were married before 20 years of age. This shows that secondary education could have played a remarkable role in raising the age of marriage.

With regard to occupation, women in the housewife category married at a younger age than those with clerical or professional occupations in the urban

TABLE 2.B.1.   PERCENTAGE DISTRIBUTION OF ELIGIBLE WOMEN BY RESIDENCE, AGE AT MARRIAGE AND SOCIAL CHARACTERISTICS*

Social characteristic and residence	Percentage of eligible women who married at age:						Number (all ages)
	10-14	15–19	20–24	25–29	30–34	35–44	
Social status							
Rural							
Low	27.0	58.8	11.6	2.0	0.4	0.2	1412
Middle	28.8	57.0	11.3	1.8	0.7	0.4	718
Both categories	27.6	58.2	11.4	1.9	0.6	0.3	2130
Unknown							15
Urban							
Low	20.3	61.3	15.5	1.9	0.6	0.4	858
Middle	18.1	65.9	13.7	1.6	0.5	0.2	1235
Both categories	18.9	64.2	14.4	1.7	0.5	0.3	2093
Unknown							4
Industrial							
Low	8.6	76.1	13.7	1.2	—	0.4	255
Middle	5.5	79.9	12.9	1.4	—	0.3	364
Both categories	7.0	78.3	13.2	1.2	—	0.3	619
Education of EW							
Rural							
Illiterate + no schooling	28.2	58.1	11.1	1.9	0.4	0.3	2020
Primary	18.4	60.3	18.4	1.9	1.0	—	103
Secondary	—	(50.0)	(33.4)	(16.6)	—	—	6
Unknown							16
Urban							
Illiterate + no schooling	21.5	64.0	12.3	1.3	0.5	0.4	1522
Primary	13.9	69.2	15.3	1.2	0.4	—	497
Secondary	1.5	32.4	51.5	11.8	2.8	—	68
College	—	—	(50.0)	(33.4)	(16.6)	—	6
Unknown							4
Industrial							
Illiterate + no schooling	7.2	79.8	11.8	0.7	—	0.5	440
Primary	5.8	76.9	15.0	2.3	—	—	173
Secondary	0.0	(16.6)	(66.7)	(16.7)	—	—	6

113

TABLE 2.B.1 (continued)

Social characteristic and residence	Percentage of eligible women who married at age:						Number (all ages)
	10–14	15–19	20–24	25–29	30–34	35–44	
Occupation of EW							
Rural							
Housewife	27.6	58.4	11.4	1.9	0.5	0.2	2113
Clerical/professional	(12.5)	(50.0)	(25.0)	(12.5)	—	—	8
Agricult./janit./ industrial	(44.4)	(11.1)	(22.2)	—	—	(22.2)	9
Unknown							15
Urban							
Housewife	19.6	65.4	13.3	1.2	0.4	0.1	2018
Clerical/professional	1.6	25.0	50.0	15.6	4.7	3.1	64
Agricultural/industrial	(11.2)	(33.3)	(22.2)	(11.1)	(11.1)	(11.1)	9
Others	—	(100.0)	—	—	—	—	2
Unknown							4
Industrial							
Housewife	6.8	79.0	13.1	1.1	—	—	610
Clerical/professional	(14.2)	(28.6)	(28.6)	(14.3)	—	(14.3)	7
Agricultural/industrial	—	(100.0)	—	—	—	—	1
Others	—	—	—	—	—	(100.0)	1

* Figures in parentheses refer to fewer than 25 eligible women.

area where 85.0% of housewives were married before the age of 20 years, compared with 26.6% in the clerical or professional occupations. No such comparison was possible for the other two areas because of the small numbers of women in the clerical and professional categories.

Gravidity

The 4861 women in the study had 24 979 pregnancies, giving a mean gravidity of 5.1 per woman; for the 3 areas separately, the figures were: 5.6 among urban, 5.3 among rural, and 4.6 among industrial women.

Table 2.B.2 shows that, as expected, mean gravidity increased with age for the 3 groups. Rural women had higher gravidity than urban women for age groups 20–34, whereas urban women beyond 35 years of age had higher gravidity than rural women. This does not necessarily mean an early onset of menopause in rural women, but on the whole it reveals that the reproductive life of rural women started earlier than that of urban women and that they reproduced faster than urban women up to 35 years of age, after which the pace of reproduction of rural women slowed down compared to that of urban women. Another factor is that the maternal mortality rate, especially among women with high gravidity, was higher in the rural than in the urban area.

At 40–44 years of age, when it is assumed that women have completed their reproductive span, urban women had the greatest number of pregnancies

TABLE 2.B.2. MEAN GRAVIDITY BY AGE OF ELIGIBLE WOMEN, RESIDENCE, AND SOCIAL STATUS

Residence and social status	Mean gravidity at age:						Number (all ages)
	< 20	20–24	25–29	30–34	35–39	40–44	
Rural							
Middle	0.8	2.4	4.5	6.8	7.8	9.7	723
Low	0.9	2.9	4.4	6.7	7.7	8.7	1414
Both categories	0.9	2.7	4.4	6.7	7.7	9.1	2137
Unknown							8
Urban							
Middle	1.0	2.3	4.3	5.9	8.1	10.1	1238
Low	2.1	2.2	4.2	6.4	8.6	10.5	858
Both categories	1.5	2.2	4.2	6.1	8.2	10.2	2096
Unknown							1
Industrial							
Middle	0.6	1.6	2.7	4.7	6.5	8.8	364
Low	0.9	2.0	3.3	5.6	8.1	8.8	255
Both categories	0.7	1.7	3.0	5.2	7.3	8.8	619

FIG. 2.B.1. FAMILY FORMATION BY SOCIAL CHARACTERISTICS

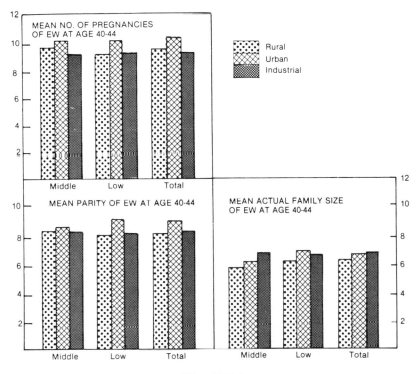

(10.2), followed by rural women (9.1), and industrial women (8.8) (Table 2.B.2 and Fig. 2.B.1 and 2.B.2). There was no appreciable difference in mean gravidity at age 40–44 by social status for either urban or industrial women. Rural women of middle social status, however, had on the average one more pregnancy than those of low social status.

FIG. 2.B.2. FERTILITY VARIABLES SPECIFIC FOR AGE, BY RESIDENCE AND SOCIAL STATUS

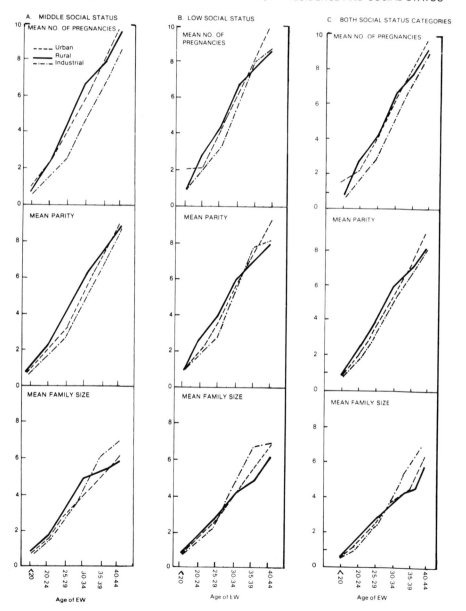

Parity

Table 2.B.3 shows that mean parity increased with age; at 40–44 years mean parities were 8.2, 9.1, and 8.4 for rural, urban, and industrial women, respectively.

In the urban and industrial areas, women of low social status had higher mean live births than did women of middle social status, in most age groups. Rural women showed a reversal of this pattern at age 40–44, where mean

TABLE 2.B.3. MEAN PARITY BY AGE OF ELIGIBLE WOMEN, RESIDENCE, AND SOCIAL CHARACTERISTICS*

Social characteristic and residence	Mean parity at age:						Number (all ages)
	< 20	20–24	25–29	30–34	35–39	40–44	
Social status							
Rural							
Middle	0.8	2.1	4.1	5.9	7.2	8.8	723
Low	0.9	2.6	3.9	5.9	7.0	8.0	1414
Both categories	0.9	2.4	4.0	5.9	7.0	8.2	2137
Unknown							8
Urban							
Middle	0.8	1.9	3.1	5.2	7.1	9.0	1238
Low	0.9	1.9	3.5	5.6	7.5	9.3	858
Both categories	0.9	1.9	3.6	5.3	7.3	9.1	2096
Unknown							1
Industrial							
Middle	0.5	1.5	2.6	4.7	6.4	8.6	364
Low	0.8	1.8	2.8	5.4	7.7	8.1	255
Both categories	0.6	1.5	3.0	5.1	7.0	8.4	619
Education of EW							
Rural							
Illiterate + no schooling	1.3	2.4	4.1	5.9	7.0	8.3	2034
Primary	1.0	2.4	3.7	5.3	6.8	7.6	104
Secondary	—	—	(2.8)	—	(6.0)	—	6
Unknown							1
Urban							
Illiterate + no schooling	1.3	2.0	3.7	5.5	7.5	9.3	1525
Primary	0.5	2.0	3.9	5.3	6.6	8.6	497
Secondary	—	0.8	2.1	3.5	6.7	—	68
College	—	(1.0)	(3.0)	(4.5)	—	(10.0)	7
Unknown							1
Industrial							
Illiterate + no schooling	0.6	1.8	3.1	5.0	7.0	8.4	440
Primary	0.6	1.4	2.8	5.4	6.8	8.2	173
Secondary	—	(0.3)	(1.0)	(2.5)	—	—	6

117

TABLE 2.B.3 (continued)

Social characteristic and residence	Mean parity at age:						Number (all ages)
	< 20	20–24	25–29	30–34	35–39	40–44	
Education of husband							
Rural							
Illiterate + no schooling	1.0	2.1	4.0	6.0	7.0	8.3	1664
Primary	1.1	3.0	4.3	5.7	7.6	7.9	387
Secondary	0.4	1.9	3.2	4.5	5.8	7.8	86
College	—	—	—	—	(7.0)	(11.0)	7
Unknown							1
Urban							
Illiterate + no schooling	1.3	2.0	3.4	5.7	7.5	8.8	601
Primary	1.6	2.1	3.9	5.4	7.4	9.1	1053
Secondary	0.5	1.6	3.2	4.9	7.9	11.5	357
College	0.5	1.5	3.6	5.0	6.2	10.0	86
Industrial							
Illiterate + no schooling	0.8	2.0	4.0	5.6	7.8	8.9	77
Primary	0.4	1.8	2.9	5.0	7.0	8.5	461
Secondary	1.4	1.1	2.6	5.0	4.5	5.8	78
Unknown							3
Occupation of EW							
Rural							
Housewife	0.9	2.4	4.1	5.9	7.1	8.2	2126
Clerical/professional	(—)	(1.0)	(2.8)	(—)	(—)	(5.0)	8
Agricultural/industrial	(5.0)	(1.0)	(3.0)	(—)	(3.0)	(11.4)	10
Unknown							1
Urban							
Housewife	1.3	1.9	3.8	5.4	7.4	8.7	2020
Clerical/professional	—	0.9	1.8	4.1	4.8	—	65
Agricultural/industrial	(1.0)	(2.3)	—	—	(13.7)	—	7
Others	—	—	(5.0)	—	—	—	2
Unknown							3
Industrial							
Housewife	0.5	1.6	3.0	5.1	7.0	8.0	611
Clerical/professional	(2.0)	(2.0)	(1.0)	(2.0)	—	(7.0)	7
Agricultural/industrial	—	(3.0)	—	—	—	—	1

* Figures in parentheses refer to fewer than 25 eligible women.

parity was 0.8 live births higher for middle than for low social status women.[1] (Fig. 2.B.1 and 2.B.2.)

Table 2.B.3 shows the presence of an inverse relationship between the educational level of the women and mean parity in most age groups in the three

[1] The fact that both mean gravidity and mean parity were higher in urban than in rural areas and for richer than for poorer women in rural areas is interesting, since the reverse was expected according to Western experience. But unlike European women, these communities practise little contraception so that the better health of the urban women means higher fertility; similarly, among rural women higher incomes are associated with greater fertility.

areas. Women aged 40–44 years with primary education in the rural, urban, and industrial areas had lower mean parities (7.6, 8.6, and 8.2, respectively) than did illiterate women (8.3, 9.3, and 8.4, respectively). Women with secondary education had the lowest mean parity, but the numbers were too small to permit valid conclusions to be drawn.

With regard to the education of the husbands, the following relationships were observed:

1. In the urban area, a direct relationship existed between parity and educational level. Thus, the mean parity of women aged 40–44 whose husbands were illiterate was only 8.8, compared with 11.5 for women whose husbands had had secondary education.

2. Among rural women, there was a weak but consistent inverse relationship between the educational level of the husbands and mean parity.

3. In the industrial area, the inverse relationship between the education of the husbands and mean parity was well marked. While mean parity at age 40–44 was 8.9 for women married to illiterate husbands, it was only 5.8 for women married to husbands with secondary education.

As for the effect of occupation on parity, the number of professional women was too small to permit valid conclusions.

Family Size

Family size (number of living children) is a function of parity and child loss. Table 2.B.4 shows that at 40–44 years the highest mean family size was 6.9 among women in the industrial area, compared with 6.6 and 6.0 for urban and rural women, respectively.

TABLE 2.B.4. MEAN FAMILY SIZE BY AGE OF ELIGIBLE WOMEN, RESIDENCE, AND SOCIAL CHARACTERISTICS*

Social characteristic and residence	Mean family size at age:						Number (all ages)
	< 20	20–24	25–29	30–34	35–39	40–44	
Social status							
Rural							
Middle	0.7	1.6	3.0	4.8	5.2	5.8	723
Low	0.8	1.8	2.7	4.0	4.7	6.1	1414
Both categories	0.8	1.7	2.8	4.3	5.1	6.0	2137
Unknown							8
Urban							
Middle	0.7	1.6	3.0	4.0	5.0	6.2	1238
Low	0.8	1.5	2.7	3.9	5.3	7.0	858
Both categories	0.7	1.6	2.8	4.0	5.1	6.6	2096
Unknown							1
Industrial							
Middle	0.5	1.4	2.7	4.1	6.2	6.9	364
Low	0.7	1.5	2.5	4.8	6.6	6.9	255
Both categories	0.6	1.4	2.6	4.6	6.4	6.9	619

TABLE 2.B.4 (*continued*)

Social characteristic and residence	Mean family size at age:						Number (all ages)
	< 20	20–24	25–29	30–34	35–39	40–44	
Education of EW							
Rural							
Illiterate + no schooling	0.9	1.7	2.7	4.9	4.9	6.0	2034
Primary	0.8	1.8	3.2	4.7	4.8	6.3	104
Secondary	—	—	(2.2)	—	(4.0)	—	6
Unknown							1
Urban							
Illiterate + no schooling	0.9	1.6	2.8	3.8	5.1	6.5	1525
Primary	0.5	1.6	3.2	4.4	5.3	6.3	497
Secondary	—	0.7	1.6	3.1	6.0	—	68
College	—	(1.0)	(1.0)	(2.0)	—	—	4
Unknown							3
Industrial							
Illiterate + no schooling	0.5	1.6	2.8	4.5	6.6	7.0	440
Primary	0.9	1.2	2.4	4.7	5.5	6.4	173
Secondary	—	(0.3)	(1.0)	(2.5)	—	—	6
Occupation of EW							
Rural							
Housewife	0.6	1.7	2.8	4.0	4.8	6.0	2126
Clerical/professional	—	(1.0)	(2.2)	—	—	(5.0)	7
Agricultural/industrial	—	(1.0)	(2.5)	—	(3.0)	(7.6)	9
Unknown							3
Urban							
Housewife	1.2	1.6	2.9	4.0	5.2	5.9	2020
Clerical/professional	—	0.9	1.5	3.4	3.4	—	65
Agricultural/industrial	(1.0)	(2.3)	—	—	(13.7)	—	9
Others	—	—	(4.0)	—	—	—	2
Unknown							1
Industrial							
Housewife	0.7	1.4	2.6	4.5	6.4	6.9	611
Clerical/professional	(2.0)	(1.0)	(1.0)	(2.0)	—	(3.0)	7
Agricultural/industrial	—	(3.0)	—	—	—	—	1

* Figures in parentheses refer to fewer than 25 eligible women.

With regard to social status, at age group 40–44 mean family size was higher among low than among middle social status women in both the rural and the urban areas. In the rural area the figures were 6.1 and 5.8, respectively, while in the urban area they were 7.0 and 6.2, respectively. Industrial women had the same mean family size of 6.9 for both social status categories (Table 2.B.4 and Fig. 2.B.1 and 2.B.2). Different age groups showed no consistent pattern.

Differences between mean parity and mean family size result from child loss. A comparison of Tables 2.B.3 and 2.B.4 shows that women aged 40–44 years had on the average experienced 2.2 child losses in the rural area, 2.5 in the urban area and 1.5 in the industrial area. Thus, child loss was higher among rural and urban women than among women in the industrial area.

Table 2.B.4 shows that the relationship between primary education and family size was not as consistent as that between parity and education. In the urban and industrial areas, women with primary education had a lower mean family size at 40–44 years than illiterate women, the figures being 6.3 for women with primary education compared with 6.5 for illiterate women in the urban area, while for the industrial area the figures were 6.4 and 7.0, respectively. In the rural area, the reverse was found: mean family sizes were 6.3 for women with primary education and 6.0 for illiterate women.

With regard to occupation, urban women who had clerical or professional occupations showed lower mean family sizes than did housewives. In the rural and industrial areas the number of women in these occupations was too small for valid comparisons to be made.

Table 2.B.5 shows means family sizes at marriage. The earlier she was married, the more children a women had. In the highest reported age group (35–39 years), women who were married before 15 years of age had the highest mean family sizes, the figures being 5.9, 6.4, and 7.7 for the urban, rural, and industrial areas, respectively. Women who married later usually had smaller families.

TABLE 2.B.5. MEAN FAMILY SIZE BY AGE OF ELIGIBLE WOMEN, RESIDENCE, AND AGE AT MARRIAGE*

Residence and age at marriage	Mean family size at age:					Number (all ages)
	<20	20–24	25–29	30–34	35–39	
Urban						
<15	(1.5)	2.5	3.6	4.6	5.9	397
15–19	0.5	1.5	3.1	4.1	5.6	1340
20–24	—	0.7	1.6	3.2	5.5	301
25–44	—	—	(0.6)	(1.7)	9.0	51
Unknown						8
Rural						
<15	1.0	2.3	3.2	4.6	6.4	587
15–19	0.4	1.4	2.8	3.8	5.0	1239
20–24	—	(0.8)	1.7	2.8	4.6	245
25–44	—	—	(0.8)	(6.4)	4.7	51
Unknown						23
Industrial						
<15	(1.0)	(3.0)	(4.0)	4.3	7.7	42
15–19	0.7	1.6	3.0	4.8	6.3	486
20–24	—	0.6	1.3	3.7	8.8	82
25–44	—	—	(1.7)	(0.7)	(4.0)	8
Unknown						11

* Figures in parentheses refer to fewer than 25 eligible women.

121

C. PAKISTAN

M. Saeed Qureshi

Family Structure

Of all the families included in the study 63.6% were nuclear and 36.4% were extended families. The proportion of nuclear families was higher in the semi-urban (71.3%) than in the urban area (56.2%). Nuclear families were also more frequent among the low status group than among the middle status group for both semi-urban and urban residents. These differences might be due to economic factors and also to the fact that the houses in semi-urban areas were smaller than those in urban areas.

Age at Marriage

In Pakistan, according to the Muslim Family Law promulgated in 1961, the minimum age for marriage is 18 years for men and 16 years for women. The average age at marriage for females was found in earlier studies to be 16.3 years in 1953 and 19.4 years in 1969.

The present study shows that on the average the women in the study areas were married at the age of 17.6 years. However, considerable differences were found between the semi-urban and urban populations. The women in the semi-urban population were married at the age of 16.7 years while the mean age at marriage of women in the urban population was 18.3 years. In the urban population, age at marriage did not differ much by social status. In contrast, in the semi-urban population women in the low SES group married nearly one year earlier than the women in the middle SES group. The mean age at marriage in the middle and low status groups was 17.3 and 16.2 years, respectively. In the semi-urban area, it was 18.5 and in the urban area it was 18.1 years. However, the mean age at marriage increased with an increase in the level of education in both the semi-urban and the urban population. A distinct difference of 4–5 years was observed between women who were illiterate or had no schooling and those who were educated at the college level.

Table 2.C.1 presents the distribution of age at marriage for the urban and semi-urban populations by social status. A high proportion of women in both the semi-urban and urban areas, i.e., 87.7% and 71.7%, respectively, were married before attaining the age of 20. The remaining 12.3% in the semi-urban area and 28.0% in the urban area were married between 20 and 29 years of age. Only 0.3% of the women married after the age of 30 years in the urban population.

The difference in mean age at marriage was examined according to social status in both the urban and the semi-urban areas. It was observed that women of low social status married earlier than those of middle social status. About 92% of women of low social status in both the semi-urban and the urban areas married before the age of 20 years, compared with 83.3% and 70% for middle status women in the semi-urban and urban areas, respectively. The differences

122

TABLE 2.C.1.   PERCENTAGE DISTRIBUTION OF ELIGIBLE WOMEN BY RESIDENCE, AGE AT MARRIAGE AND SOCIAL CHARACTERISTICS

Social characteristic and residence	Percentage of eligible women who married at age:					Number (all ages)
	10–14	15–19	20–24	25–29	30–34	
Social status						
Semi-urban						
Middle	23.4	59.9	14.6	2.1	—	1189
Low	35.1	56.9	7.0	1.0	—	1199
Both categories	29.3	58.4	10.8	1.5	—	2388
Urban						
Middle	15.5	54.5	25.1	4.6	0.3	2294
Low	40.8	51.4	6.7	1.1	—	179
Both categories	17.4	54.3	23.7	4.3	0.3	2473
Education of EW						
Semi-urban						
Illiterate + no schooling	34.4	56.3	8.4	0.9	—	1678
Primary	20.7	66.3	10.7	2.3	—	515
Secondary	9.8	61.2	26.2	2.8	—	142
College +	3.7	39.6	47.3	9.4		53
Urban						
Illiterate + no schooling	32.7	53.8	11.1	2.2	0.2	827
Primary	16.4	63.6	17.9	1.9	0.2	706
Secondary	6.8	59.4	28.6	4.9	0.3	514
College +	1.6	33.6	58.3	1.8	0.7	426
Occupation of EW						
Semi-urban						
Housewife	29.1	58.9	10.6	1.4	—	2276
Clerical/professional	20.5	46.1	23.1	10.3	—	40
Agricultural/janitorial/industrial	41.4	46.5	12.1	0.0	—	59
Other	16.7	58.3	16.7	8.3	—	13
Urban						
Housewife	17.7	55.1	23.6	3.3	0.3	2368
Clerical/professional	7.1	23.8	35.7	32.3	1.2	84
Agricultural/janitorial/industrial	16.8	72.2	5.5	5.5	0.9	18
Other	—	100.0	—	—	—	3

between the middle and low status groups in the percentage of women married before the age of 20 was found to be statistically significant at the 0.01 level in both the semi-urban and urban areas.[1]

The table also depicts the percentage distribution of women by educational level, and shows a positive relationship between education and the age at marriage. With an increase in the level of education, the proportion marrying in the earlier age group (i.e., before aged 20) declined. Among the semi-urban

---

[1] For many of the tables in this text a large number of statistical tests were performed. Only a few of the more important results are mentioned in the text. Where a test is statistically significant at a probability level of 0.01 or 0.05 this is indicated in parentheses following the summary of the data (e.g., $P < 0.01$).

women the respective proportions were 90.7% for those with no education, 87% for women with primary education, 71% for those with secondary level education, and 43.3% for those with college education. The corresponding proportions in the urban area were 86.5%, 80.0%, 66.1%, and 35.2%, respectively. In both areas, the differences between women with no education and those with some education in regard to the percentage who married before the age of 20 were statistically significant at the 0.01 level.

As regards occupation of women, a high proportion (96%) reported their occupation as housewife and only 4% were engaged in clerical or other professions. Consequently, no further analysis for this variable was undertaken.

Gravidity

The 4861 women included in the present study experienced 24 213 pregnancies up to the time of the interview, yielding an average of 5.0 pregnancies per woman. The women in the semi-urban area had experienced, on the average, 5.4 pregnancies, while urban women had experienced 4.6 pregnancies. This does not account for any recall lapse or underreporting due to fetal losses, miscarriages, abortions, etc. As expected, the mean number of pregnancies was higher among low status than among middle status women in both the residential areas.

Looking at the pregnancy pattern, it is obvious that the mean number of pregnancies increased with the rise in age group. In all the age groups, semi-urban women had a higher number of pregnancies than urban women. However, in the last age group, 40–44, where it is assumed that women complete their fertility, the difference between the two residential groups in regard to total number of pregnancies was not so large as for the younger age groups. The semi-urban women had experienced 8.1 pregnancies, whereas the urban women had experienced 7.6 pregnancies at the last stage of their fertile period (Table 2.C.2 and Fig. 2.C.1 and 2.C.2).

TABLE 2.C.2.   MEAN GRAVIDITY BY AGE OF ELIGIBLE WOMEN, RESIDENCE, AND SOCIAL STATUS*

Residence and social status	Mean gravidity at age:						Number (all ages)
	<20	20–24	25–29	30–34	35–39	40–44	
Semi-urban							
Middle	0.85	1.96	4.21	5.83	6.97	7.59	1189
Low	0.87	2.35	4.64	6.62	7.69	8.58	1199
Both categories	0.86	2.11	4.43	6.29	7.36	8.08	2388
Urban							
Middle	0.81	1.78	3.28	5.11	6.14	7.52	2294
Low	(1.00)	2.37	4.54	6.83	8.17	8.36	179
Both categories	0.81	1.81	3.36	5.26	6.30	7.59	2473

* Figures in parentheses refer to fewer than 25 eligible women.

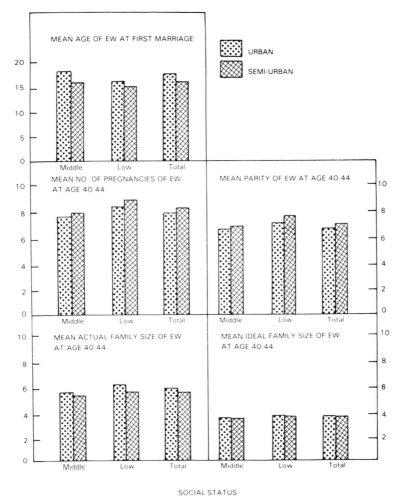

FIG. 2.C.1. FAMILY FORMATION BY SOCIAL CHARACTERISTICS

SOCIAL STATUS

Parity

Table 2.C.3 presents the parity distribution of women by residence, social status, education of eligible women and education of their husbands. The table indicates that there were more live births among semi-urban than among urban women. The semi-urban women had an average of 4.8 live births whereas urban women had an average of 4.0 live births up to the time of the survey. Furthermore, the mean number of children born to women in all age groups was higher for semi-urban than for urban residents. The difference in births increased progressively from 0.13 for women in the age group less than 20 years to 1.01 in the age group 30–34 years. However, in the last age group (40–44) the difference narrows down to 0.5 births ($P < 0.05$). The higher

125

FIG. 2.C.2. FERTILITY VARIABLES SPECIFIC FOR AGE, BY RESIDENCE AND SOCIAL STATUS

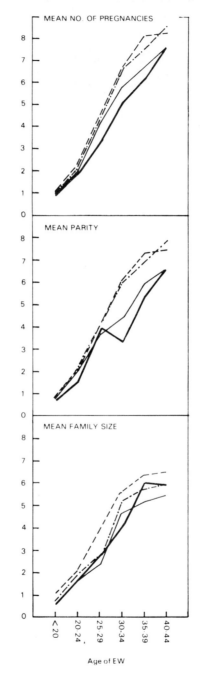

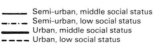

Semi-urban, middle social status
Semi-urban, low social status
Urban, middle social status
Urban, low social status

differentials for the younger age groups are probably a result of variations in age structure. The table further shows that in both residential groups at all ages low status women had more births than middle status women.

The differentials in mean number of children by education are also pronounced. The findings clearly indicate that education has a strong negative association with fertility. Educated women had lower parity than uneducated

TABLE 2.C.3. MEAN PARITY BY AGE OF ELIGIBLE WOMEN, RESIDENCE, AND SOCIAL CHARACTERISTICS*

Social characteristic and residence	Mean parity at age:						Number (all ages)
	<20	20–24	25–29	30–34	35–39	40–44	
Social status							
Semi-urban							
Middle	0.72	1.73	3.69	4.38	5.92	6.63	1189
Low	0.74	2.08	4.14	5.99	6.85	7.75	1199
Both categories	0.73	1.86	3.91	5.64	6.43	7.18	2388
Urban							
Middle	0.60	1.58	3.90	3.28	5.33	6.60	2294
Low	(1.00)	2.15	4.07	6.29	7.37	7.45	179
Both categories	0.60	1.62	2.98	4.63	5.49	6.67	2473
Education of EW							
Semi-urban							
Illiterate + no schooling	0.79	2.03	4.04	5.75	6.51	7.25	1680
Primary	0.74	1.88	3.98	5.57	6.22	7.00	513
Secondary	(0.50)	1.64	3.34	(4.21)	(5.23)	(5.00)	142
College +	(0.00)	1.06	(2.06)	(4.33)	0.00	(3.00)	53
All categories	0.73	1.86	3.92	5.64	6.43	7.18	2388
Urban							
Illiterate + no schooling	(0.55)	2.03	3.71	5.50	6.13	7.07	827
Primary	0.74	1.75	3.45	5.00	5.80	6.50	706
Secondary	0.55	1.76	2.75	4.01	4.30	5.46	514
College +	(0.56)	1.00	2.09	2.92	3.13	(4.26)	426
All categories	0.60	1.62	2.98	4.63	5.49	6.67	2473
Education of husband							
Semi-urban							
Illiterate + no schooling	0.64	2.02	4.02	5.77	6.83	7.61	847
Primary	0.65	1.88	3.80	5.78	6.50	7.14	577
Secondary	0.85	2.00	4.06	5.31	5.75	6.67	576
College +	(0.82)	1.54	3.67	5.67	6.27	6.98	388
All categori	0.73	1.86	3.91	5.64	6.43	7.18	2388
Urban							
Illiterate + no schooling	(0.67)	1.90	3.55	5.89	7.22	7.38	203
Primary	(0.70)	1.87	3.51	5.08	6.71	7.03	277
Secondary	0.59	1.67	3.40	5.05	5.45	6.92	715
College +	0.59	1.52	2.64	4.05	4.80	6.14	1278
All categories	0.60	1.62	2.98	4.63	5.49	6.67	2473

127

TABLE 2.C.3 (*continued*)

Social characteristic and residence	Mean parity at age:						Number (all ages)
	< 20	20–24	25–29	30–34	35–39	40–44	
Occupation of EW							
Semi-urban							
Housewife	0.74	1.86	3.98	5.70	6.45	7.14	2280
Clerical/professional	—	(1.54)	(2.10)	(4.42)	(4.60)	(7.05)	39
Agricultural/industrial	—	(2.00)	(3.25)	(4.50)	(7.50)	(7.83)	43
Janitorial/others	(0.5)	(4.00)	(2.33)	(4.40)	(5.22)	(9.00)	26
Urban							
Housewife	0.59	1.63	3.02	4.74	5.50	6.74	2368
Clerical/professional	(2.00)	(1.13)	2.03	(2.22)	(3.86)	(5.43)	84
Agricultural/industrial	—	—	(2.00)	(5.00)	(8.50)	(3.83)	12
Janitorial/others	—	—	—	—	—	—	9

* Figures in parentheses refer to fewer than 25 eligible women.

women. In the urban area, at the age of 40–44 years, women having no schooling had an average of 7.1 live births, while the women with college or higher education had an average of 4.3 live births. The same pattern is also observed for semi-urban residents (Table 2.C.3).

The data show that the husband's education also had an association with fertility, but it was less strong than the association with the wife's education. The women whose husbands were illiterate or had had no schooling had experienced higher parities than women whose husbands were educated. Women whose husbands were illiterate had experienced on the average 7.6 and 7.4 live births at the age of 40–44 years in the semi-urban and urban area respectively. The corresponding figures for women whose husbands had had college education were 7.0 and 6.1 live births (Table 2.C.3).

Family Size

Data on family size, i.e., mean number of living children, by age of married women, residence, and social status are presented in Table 2.C.4. It can be seen that, on the average, a woman resident in the semi-urban area had 4.1 living children while a woman resident in the urban area had 3.7 children. At all ages except 40–44 urban women had a lower number of living children than semi-urban women. As previously noted at all ages including 40–44 years parity was higher among semi-urban women than among urban women. Comparing the findings of Tables 2.C.3 and 2.C.4 it may clearly be deduced that in the semi-urban area women aged 40–44 years had, on the average, experienced 1.5 child losses up to the time of the survey, whereas in the urban area the corresponding figure was 0.8 child loss. It may therefore be concluded from these tables that infant and child mortality was higher in semi-urban than in urban areas.

TABLE 2.C.4. MEAN FAMILY SIZE BY AGE OF ELIGIBLE WOMEN, RESIDENCE, AND SOCIAL CHARACTERISTICS*

Social characteristic and residence	Mean family size at age:						Number (all ages)
	<20	20–24	25–29	30–34	35–39	40–45	
Social status							
Semi-urban							
Middle	0.68	1.57	3.36	4.66	5.21	5.45	1189
Low	0.68	1.85	3.68	5.24	5.82	5.92	1199
Both categories	0.68	1.68	3.53	4.99	5.54	5.69	2388
Urban							
Middle	0.50	1.52	2.73	4.19	6.09	5.86	2294
Low	(1.00)	2.07	3.86	5.74	6.37	6.48	179
Both categories	0.56	1.56	2.81	4.33	5.04	5.91	2473
Education of FW							
Semi-urban							
Illiterate + no schooling	0.70	1.81	0.93	5.01	5.57	5.69	1680
Primary	0.72	1.69	3.66	4.84	5.55	5.83	513
Secondary	(0.50)	1.56	3.14	(3.89)	(4.69)	(4.00)	142
College +	(0.00)	1.00	(2.00)	(4.33)	—	(3.00)	53
All categories	0.68	1.68	3.53	4.99	5.54	5.69	2388
Urban							
Illiterate + no schooling	(0.54)	1.90	3.41	4.40	5.50	6.23	827
Primary	0.67	1.71	3.21	4.74	3.36	5.66	706
Secondary	0.50	1.69	2.67	3.76	3.98	5.02	514
College +	(0.56)	0.97	1.28	2.79	3.07	(4.21)	426
All categories	0.56	1.56	2.81	4.33	5.04	5.91	2473
Occupation of EW							
Semi-urban							
Housewife	0.68	1.68	3.50	5.05	5.56	5.69	2280
Clerical/professional	—	(1.45)	(2.83)	(3.20)	(4.60)	(4.25)	39
Agricultural/industrial		(1.00)	(2.07)	(4.08)	(6.25)	(5.67)	43
Janitorial/others	(0.50)	(4.00)	(2.00)	(3.60)	(4.44)	(6.80)	26
All categories	0.68	1.68	3.53	4.99	5.54	5.69	2389
Urban							
Housewife	0.55	1.58	2.85	4.43	5.06	5.95	2368
Clerical/professional	(2.00)	(0.78)	2.00	(2.17)	(3.71)	(5.28)	84
Agricultural/industrial	—	—	(2.00)	(5.00)	(3.50)	(3.84)	12
Janitorial/others	—	—	—	—	—	—	9
All categories	0.56	1.56	2.81	4.33	5.04	5.91	2473

* Figures in parentheses refer to fewer than 25 eligible women.

The mean family size by age at marriage and residence is shown in Table 2.C.5. The table indicates that as the age at marriage increases the overall family size declines. This trend has been observed in both residential areas. In the urban area in the age group 40–44 the total family size declined from 6.3

129

for women whose age at marriage was less than 15 years to 5.2 for women whose age at marriage was 20 to 24 years, with a further reduction in family size to 1.9 years for women who married after 25 years of age. The same trend has also been noted for the semi-urban area. But one has to consider the finding with caution as the numbers involved were small for those who married at age 25 and over.

TABLE 2.C.5. MEAN FAMILY SIZE BY AGE OF ELIGIBLE WOMEN, RESIDENCE, AND AGE AT MARRIAGE*

Residence and age at marriage	Mean family size at age:						Number (all ages)
	< 20	20–24	25–29	30–34	35–39	40–45	
Semi-urban							
<15	1.07	2.64	4.34	5.31	5.77	5.76	697
15–19	0.55	1.68	3.69	5.17	5.65	5.70	1396
20–24	—	0.65	2.06	3.63	4.65	5.46	258
25 and over	—	—	(0.54)	(1.36)	(2.86)	(3.80)	37
Urban							
<15	(1.27)	2.94	4.24	5.59	6.03	6.26	429
15–19	0.47	1.77	3.38	5.13	5.39	5.93	1342
20–24	—	0.73	1.88	3.07	4.33	5.23	588
25 and over	—	—	0.52	1.51	1.97	(1.87)	114

* Figures in parentheses refer to fewer than 25 eligible women.

Ideal Family Size

When the women were asked what they considered as the ideal number of children, their replies were found to be quite consistent when they were broken down by residence, parity, education, and social status of the respondents. On the average the semi-urban residents reported an ideal family size of 3.9 children while the urban residents reported an ideal family size of 3.7 children. Among the women of parity less than two, the semi-urban residents reported an ideal family size of 3.5 compared with a figure of 3.2 for the urban residents. Among those with a parity of 5, the corresponding figures were 4.0 and 3.8, respectively. The education of the husband did not seem to have much influence on the opinion of the wife. However, the education of the wife seemed to have some influence on views about ideal family size. Semi-urban women with no education gave the ideal family size as 3.9 compared with 3.4 for those with college education, while the corresponding figures for urban residents were 4.0 and 3.3, respectively (Table 2.C.6).

The majority of women—56% in the semi-urban area and 53% in the urban area—were of the opinion that the ideal family size was about 4 children. An ideal family size of 3 or fewer children was stated by 29% of women in the semi-urban area and by 36% in the urban area (Table 2.C.7).

130

TABLE 2.C.6. MEAN IDEAL FAMILY SIZE BY POPULATION CHARACTERISTICS*

| Characteristic | Mean ideal family size by social status | | | | | |
| | Semi-urban | | | Urban | | |
	Middle	Low	Both categories	Middle	Low	Both categories
Parity						
0	3.4	3.7	3.5	3.2	(3.6)	3.2
1	3.2	3.6	3.5	3.2	(3.2)	3.2
2	3.4	3.4	3.4	3.3	(3.9)	3.3
3	4.0	3.8	3.7	3.5	(3.5)	3.5
4	3.9	3.8	2.9	3.7	(3.9)	3.7
5	4.1	3.9	4.0	2.3	(4.2)	3.8
6 and over	4.0	4.2	3.8	4.1	4.2	3.6
Parity of EW's mother						
1	(3.5)	3.9	3.8	3.7	(4.1)	3.8
2	3.6	3.8	3.7	3.6	(4.1)	3.6
3	2.6	3.9	3.9	3.6	(4.3)	3.6
4	3.6	4.1	3.8	3.6	(4.3)	3.7
5	3.7	3.7	3.7	3.6	(3.9)	3.6
6	3.7	3.9	3.8	3.5	(3.6)	3.5
7	3.8	3.8	3.8	2.6	(4.1)	3.7
8	3.8	3.9	3.8	3.6	(3.9)	3.6
9	3.9	4.0	3.9	3.6	(4.9)	3.6
10 and over	3.9	3.2	3.2	3.9	(3.7)	3.7
Education of husband						
Illiterate + no schooling	3.7	4.0	4.0	3.8	4.0	3.9
Primary	3.8	3.9	3.7	3.9	3.9	4.0
Secondary	4.0	3.8	3.8	3.7	(3.6)	3.7
College +	5.3	(3.8)	3.8	3.6	(3.8)	3.5
Education of EW						
Illiterate + no schooling	3.8	3.9	3.9	3.9	4.0	4.0
Primary	3.8	3.7	3.8	3.9	3.7	3.7
Secondary	3.5	(3.4)	3.5	3.4	(4.0)	3.4
College +	3.4	(4.0)	3.4	3.3	(—)	3.3
Occupation of EW						
Housewife	4.0	3.9	3.9	3.6	3.9	3.7
Clerical/professional	3.3	(3.5)	3.4	3.5	(4.7)	3.3
Agricultural/industrial	(4.0)	5.3	4.9	(2.7)	(3.0)	(1.9)
Janitorial/others	(3.5)	(3.4)	(3.5)	(3.5)	(4.6)	(4.1)
Age of EW						
<20	3.6	3.8	3.7	3.1	(2.3)	3.0
20–25	2.5	3.6	3.6	3.7	(3.9)	3.4
25–29	3.8	4.1	3.9	3.6	3.9	3.6
30–34	3.9	3.9	3.9	3.7	4.0	3.7
35–39	3.9	4.1	4.0	3.8	(3.9)	3.8
40–44	3.8	4.0	3.9	3.9	4.2	4.0
All ages	3.8	4.0	3.9	3.6	4.0	3.7

* Figures in parentheses refer to fewer than 25 eligible women.

TABLE 2.C.7. PERCENTAGE DISTRIBUTION OF IDEAL FAMILY SIZE BY ACTUAL FAMILY SIZE

Actual family size	Percentage of eligible women choosing ideal family size of:								Number of women[a]
	0–3	4	5	6	7	8	9	10 and over	
Semi-urban									
0	35.9	60.0	1.5	2.6	—	—	—	—	195
1	37.4	57.3	3.2	2.1	—	—	—	—	187
2	36.6	54.3	4.9	4.2	—	—	—	—	243
3	31.6	57.1	6.6	4.3	—	—	—	0.4	228
4	20.6	66.0	5.8	6.2	0.7	0.7	—	0	291
5	27.8	43.1	15.7	9.3	1.2	1.7	—	1.2	248
6 and over	22.4	54.5	7.3	9.5	2.1	2.1	0.9	1.2	524
All family sizes	28.7	55.8	6.8	6.2	0.9	0.9	0.3	0.4	1917
Urban									
0	50.8	46.3	1.2	0.8	0.4	0.4	—	—	242
1	51.4	45.8	0.8	1.2	0	0.8	—	—	253
2	47.6	46.5	2.1	2.7	0.4	0.4	—	0.3	365
3	51.0	44.5	2.9	1.2	—	0	—	0.3	339
4	16.2	78.0	1.4	3.7	—	0.7	—	—	296
5	27.8	43.7	24.5	2.4	0.4	1.2	—	—	249
6 and over	17.0	60.6	5.3	13.1	1.4	2.1	0.2	0.2	488
All family sizes	35.8	53.0	5.1	4.4	0.4	0.8	0.0	0.4	2232

[a] Exludes non-respondents.

More than one-third (36%) of the semi-urban women with no children or with 1–2 living children considered 3 or fewer children to be the ideal family size; in the urban area, the corresponding figure was about 50%. The proportion of women choosing 0–3 children as the ideal family size was lower among women who had 4 or more living children.

D. SYRIAN ARAB REPUBLIC

M. El-Jabi & A. R. Omran

Family Structure

The majority of families in the study were classified as nuclear. The proportion varied considerably by residence: 62.4% of the rural families were nuclear compared with 83.6% of families in Sweida. There was also a slight variation (5–6%) by social status in Damascus and rural Aleppo, while in Sweida this was not the case. The middle status women were found more frequently in nuclear households.

132

Age at Marriage

It was found in this study that Syrian women usually marry at a relatively young age. In all groups, the mean age at marriage for eligible women was between 15 and 19 years. In examining the percentage distribution by age at marriage (Table 2.D.1 and Fig. 2.D.1), it was found that the percentage of women marrying before age 20 was greater in rural Aleppo than in either Damascus or Sweida. These differences were statistically significant at the 0.01 level.[1] Whereas in Damascus the percentage of women marrying before age 20 was greater among those of low social status than among those of middle social status, the reverse was true for Sweida and rural Aleppo.

---

[1] For many of the following tables a large number of statistical tests were performed. Only a few of the more important results are mentioned in the text. Where a test is statistically significant at a probability level of 0.01 or 0.05 this is indicated in parentheses following the summary of the data (e.g., $P < 0.01$).

TABLE 2.D.1. PERCENTAGE DISTRIBUTION OF ELIGIBLE WOMEN BY RESIDENCE, AGE AT MARRIAGE AND SOCIAL CHARACTERISTICS*

Social characteristic and residence	Percentage of eligible women who married at age:						N^a
	10–14	15–19	20–24	25–29	30–34	35–44	
Social status							
Damascus							
Middle	12.7	57.0	23.4	5.4	1.1	0.5	1590
Low	17.4	53.8	22.1	4.7	2.1	0	385
Both categories	13.7	56.1	23.2	5.3	1.3	0.5	1975
Sweida							
Middle	7.5	57.9	27.8	5.5	0.9	0.5	1314
Low	6.8	56.7	27.5	5.8	2.5	0.8	397
Both categories	7.3	57.6	27.7	5.6	1.3	9.5	1711
Rural Aleppo							
Middle	14.7	65.7	18.3	0.9	0.4	0.0	668
Low	15.2	59.0	21.6	3.3	0.8	0.1	1267
Both categories	15.0	61.3	20.5	2.5	0.7	0.1	1935
Education of EW							
Damascus							
Illiterate + no school	15.4	57.8	21.2	4.1	1.1	0.4	1402
Primary	13.0	61.2	20.3	4.5	0.8	0.3	399
Secondary	1.4	36.4	43.4	14.7	3.5	0.7	143
College + graduate	0	(3.2)	(58.1)	(29.0)	(6.5)	(3.2)	31
Sweida							
Illiterate + no school	7.9	58.2	26.6	5.2	1.5	0.6	1388
Primary	5.7	64.5	25.7	3.3	0.4	0.4	245
Secondary	1.4	26.4	54.2	18.1	0	0	72
College + graduate	(16.7)	(50.0)	(33.3)	0	0	0	6
Rural Aleppo							
Illiterate + no school	15.0	61.4	20.4	2.5	0.7	0.1	1916
Primary	(15.8)	(64.9)	(15.8)	(3.5)	0	0	19
Secondary	—	—	—	—	—	—	—
College + graduate	—	—	—	—	—	—	—

133

TABLE 2.D.1 (continued)

Social characteristic and residence	Percentage of eligible women who married at age:						N[a]
	10–14	15–19	20–24	25–29	30–34	35–44	
Occupation of EW							
Damascus							
Housewife	14.0	58.0	22.1	4.4	1.2	0.3	1868
Clerical/professional	5.6	15.6	46.7	24.4	4.4	3.3	90
Agricult./janit./ industrial	(18.8)	(56.3)	(25.0)	0	0	0	16
Others	—	—	—	—	—	—	—
Sweida							
Housewife	7.6	59.7	26.0	4.8	1.3	0.5	1620
Clerical/professional	1.5	11.8	63.2	23.5	0	0	68
Agricult./janit./ industrial	(5.0)	(50.0)	(35.0)	(5.0)	(5.0)	0	20
Others	0	(33.3)	(66.7)	0	0	0	3
Rural Aleppo							
Housewife	15.1	62.0	19.8	2.4	0.6	0.1	1845
Clerical/professional	(21.1)	(31.6)	(36.8)	(10.5)	0	0	19
Agricult./janit./ industrial	9.5	50.8	34.9	1.6	3.2	0	63
Others	(25.0)	(50.0)	(25.0)	0	0	0	8

* Figures in parentheses refer to fewer than 25 eligible women.
[a] N = total number of eligible women in category (all ages).

However, only in rural Aleppo was the social status difference statistically significant ($P < 0.01$).

Somewhat larger variations in age at marriage were found when education was considered. Looking at the percentage distribution (Table 2.D.1), it can be seen that the age at marriage increased gradually with the educational level of women in the 3 residential categories. The majority of women still married between ages 15 and 19, but the proportion differed according to the educational status. The proportion marrying between ages 15 and 19 was the highest (61.2–64.5%) for those with primary education. It decreased for illiterate women (57.8–58.2%). The majority of women having secondary or higher education married between ages 20 and 24. In all the residential areas, a higher proportion of illiterate women than of those with some schooling married before age 20, but this difference was statistically significant only in the Damascus area ($P < 0.01$) and Sweida ($P < 0.05$). The majority of women working as housewives or in agricultural or janitorial occupations married at 15–19 years of age, while the majority of those engaged in clerical or professional occupations married later (between 20 and 24 years).

Gravidity

Table 2.D.2 and Fig. 2.D.2 show that gravidity increased steadily with age. The average age-specific mean gravidity for eligible women in rural areas was

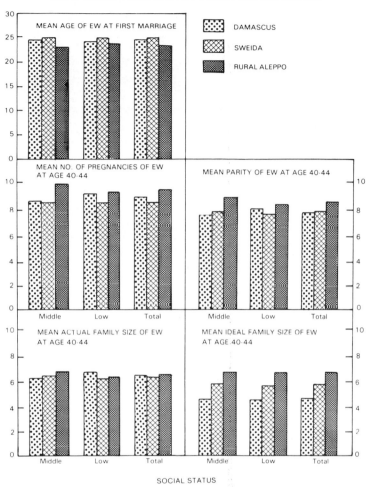

higher than for women in urban areas. At age 40–44, women in rural Aleppo had had on the average 9.6 pregnancies compared with 8.4 in Sweida and 8.7 in Damascus (Table 2.D.2 and Fig. 2.D.1 and 2.D.2). With regard to social status, the average number of pregnancies at age 40–44 revealed the expected social differential, namely that gravidity was higher among women of low social status than among those of middle status.

Parity

The pattern for parity was similar to that for gravidity (Table 2.D.3). Parity increased steadily with age and it was higher in the lower social group in urban areas and in the middle social group in the rural areas. At age 40–44 years, women in rural Aleppo had one more live birth than the women in either Damascus or Sweida ($P < 0.01$) (Table 2.D.3 and Fig. 2.D.1 and 2.D.2).

135

FIG. 2.D.2. FERTILITY VARIABLES SPECIFIC FOR AGE, BY RESIDENCE AND SOCIAL STATUS

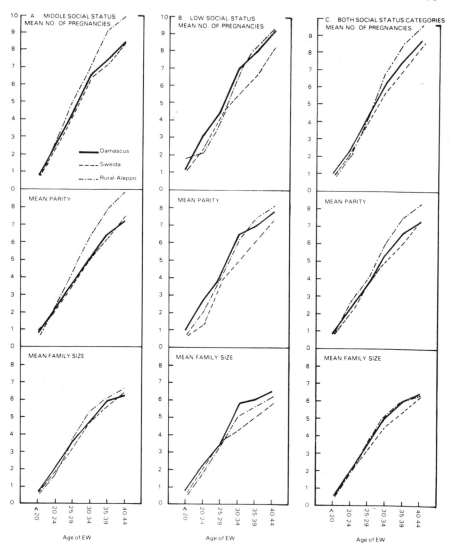

The mean parity specific for age varied inversely with the educational level of women in all areas, i.e., the more education a woman had, the fewer births she was likely to experience. There was a similar relationship between the education of the husbands and the parity of their wives. In both large and small cities, wives of college-educated husbands had the lowest mean parities, followed by those married to husbands of lower education. In rural areas, the number with secondary or college education was too small to allow meaningful comparison. In regard to occupation, women in clerical or professional jobs had the lowest mean age-specific parity. This was true in all three areas.

136

TABLE 2.D.2. MEAN GRAVIDITY BY AGE OF ELIGIBLE WOMEN, RESIDENCE, AND SOCIAL STATUS

Residence and social status	Mean gravidity at age:						N[a]
	< 20	20–24	25–29	30–34	35–39	40–44	
Damascus							
Middle	0.92	2.56	4.43	6.6	7.50	8.58	1590
Low	1.24	3.20	4.64	7.13	8.14	9.23	385
Both categories	1.00	2.66	4.34	6.25	7.66	8.74	1975
Sweida							
Middle	0.93	2.35	4.01	5.80	7.18	8.42	1314
Low	1.00[b]	2.56	4.50	5.68	6.84	8.31	397
Both categories	0.94	2.38	4.09	5.78	7.07	8.38	1711
Rural Aleppo							
Middle	0.74	2.30	5.06	7.12	9.02	10.38	668
Low	0.80	2.33	4.24	6.90	8.46	9.33	1267
Both categories	0.78	2.32	4.58	6.96	8.62	9.61	1935

[a] N = total number of eligible women in category (all ages).
[b] Refers to fewer than 25 eligible women.

TABLE 2.D.3. MEAN PARITY BY AGE OF ELIGIBLE WOMEN, RESIDENCE, AND SOCIAL CHARACTERISTICS*

Social characteristic and residence	Mean parity at age:						N[a]
	< 20	20–24	25–29	30–34	35–39	40–44	
Social status							
Damascus							
Middle	0.78	2.30	3.79	5.26	6.57	7.23	1590
Low	0.94	2.72	4.07	6.50	7.01	7.73	385
Both categories	0.82	2.36	3.83	5.48	6.68	7.36	1975
Sweida							
Middle	0.82	2.10	3.67	5.23	6.28	7.47	1314
Low	(0.07)	2.44	3.98	5.00	6.21	7.37	397
Both categories	0.80	2.14	3.72	5.18	6.26	7.44	1711
Rural Aleppo							
Middle	0.63	2.04	4.56	6.44	7.95	8.97	668
Low	0.72	2.12	3.98	6.22	7.49	8.10	1267
Both categories	0.68	2.08	4.22	6.29	7.62	8.33	1935
Education of EW							
Damascus							
Illiterate + no school	0.91	2.59	4.26	5.95	7.02	7.57	1402
Primary	0.71	2.00	3.80	5.06	6.01	6.74	399
Secondary	(0.33)	1.39	2.50	4.08	(3.80)	(5.80)	143
College + graduate	—	(1.00)	(1.09)	(2.40)	(3.57)	(1.50)	31
Sweida							
Illiterate + no school	0.76	2.24	3.95	5.40	6.35	7.44	1388
Primary	0.84	2.05	3.66	4.84	(3.67)	(8.22)	245
Secondary	(1.00)	(1.64)	1.79	(2.94)	—	(4.50)	72
College + graduate	—	(1.50)	(3.50)	(2.00)	—	(5.00)	6

TABLE 2.D.3 (continued)

Social characteristic and residence	Mean parity at age:						N[a]
	< 20	20–24	25–29	30–34	35–44	40–44	
Rural Aleppo							
Illiterate + no school	0.69	2.10	4.21	6.29	7.62	8.33	1916
Primary	(0.50)	(1.00)	(6.00)	(6.00)	—	—	19
Secondary	—	—	—	—	—	—	—
College + graduate	—	—	—	—	—	—	—
Education of husband							
Damascus							
Illiterate + no school	0.82	2.56	4.36	5.99	7.10	7.96	888
Primary	0.94	2.49	3.77	5.30	6.65	6.63	548
Secondary	0.72	2.04	3.79	5.13	5.49	5.76	335
College + graduate	(0.70)	1.98	2.76	4.50	(5.87)	(5.42)	204
Sweida							
Illiterate + no school	(0.64)	2.31	4.03	5.20	6.21	7.36	891
Primary	(0.87)	2.09	3.90	5.34	6.51	7.71	506
Secondary	(0.76)	2.05	3.13	4.79	(5.56)	(7.67)	228
College + graduate	(1.00)	(2.00)	(2.48)	(4.89)	(6.60)	(7.50)	86
Rural Aleppo							
Illiterate + no school	0.76	2.10	4.17	6.24	7.54	8.31	1617
Primary	0.47	1.92	4.45	(7.16)	(8.90)	(9.22)	191
Secondary	(0.58)	2.12	3.81	(6.13)	(9.00)	—	100
College + graduate	(0.67)	(2.38)	(6.00)	(6.50)	—	—	27
Occupation of EW							
Damascus							
Housewife	0.83	2.39	3.52	5.08	6.97	9.83	1868
Clerical/professional	—	(0.57)	1.84	3.24	(3.95)	(6.00)	90
Agricultural/industrial	(0.0)	(1.00)	(5.00)	(1.00)	(11.50)	(7.50)	12
Janitorial/others	—	(3.00)	—	—	(6.50)	(9.00)	5
Sweida							
Housewife	0.82	2.19	3.92	5.37	6.30	7.47	620
Clerical/professional	(0.0)	(1.15)	(1.52)	(2.00)	(4.00)	(3.75)	68
Agricultural/industrial	—	—	(3.33)	(4.75)	(4.00)	(7.80)	13
Janitorial/others	—	(2.66)	(2.00)	(4.00)	(3.50)	(8.50)	10
Rural Aleppo							
Housewife	0.69	2.08	4.22	6.32	7.56	8.37	1845
Clerical/professional	(1.00)	(3.00)	(2.50)	(4.50)	(8.00)	(6.86)	19
Agricultural/industrial	(0.33)	(2.33)	(5.25)	(5.62)	(8.67)	(8.88)	58
Janitorial/others	—	—	(3.67)	(6.00)	(9.50)	(6.86)	13

* Figures in parentheses refer to fewer than 25 eligible women.

[a] N = total number of eligible women in category (all ages).

Family Size

Since family size is a function of parity and child mortality, it was to be expected that the figures for family size would be smaller than those for parity. The mean family size increased with the age of the eligible woman (Table 2.D.4

TABLE 2.D.4. MEAN FAMILY SIZE BY AGE OF ELIGIBLE WOMEN, RESIDENCE, AND SOCIAL CHARACTERISTICS*

Social characteristic and residence	Mean family size at age:						N[a]
	<20	20–24	25–29	30–34	35–39	40–44	
Social status							
Damascus							
Middle	0.72	2.13	3.56	4.85	5.98	6.38	1590
Low	0.94	2.46	3.56	5.83	6.19	6.66	385
Both categories	0.77	2.18	3.56	5.03	6.03	6.45	1975
Sweida							
Middle	0.78	1.94	3.34	4.75	5.61	6.40	1314
Low	(0.67)	2.19	3.62	4.37	5.13	5.99	397
Both categories	0.77	1.97	3.39	4.66	5.46	6.24	1711
Rural Aleppo							
Middle	0.56	1.82	3.94	5.36	6.15	6.74	668
Low	0.67	1.86	3.43	5.27	6.13	6.29	1267
Both categories	0.62	1.84	3.64	5.30	6.14	6.41	1935
Education of EW							
Damascus							
Illiterate + no school	0.86	2.36	3.91	5.39	6.31	6.60	1402
Primary	0.67	1.90	3.44	4.76	5.54	5.90	399
Secondary	(0.33)	1.39	2.41	3.78	(3.67)	(5.70)	143
College + graduate	—	(1.00)	(1.09)	(2.40)	(3.29)	(1.50)	31
Sweida							
Illiterate + no school	0.71	2.02	4.68	4.82	5.53	6.23	1388
Primary	0.84	1.95	3.43	4.51	(3.44)	(7.44)	245
Secondary	(1.00)	(1.64)	1.72	(2.75)	—	(4.50)	72
College + graduate	—	(1.50)	(3.00)	(2.00)	—	(3.00)	6
Rural Aleppo							
Illiterate + no school	0.00	1.00	3.61	5.31	6.14	6.41	1016
Primary	(0.60)	(1.91)	(4.43)	(5.33)	—	—	19
Secondary	—	—	—	—	—	—	—
College + graduate	—	—	—	—	—	—	—

* Figures in parentheses refer to fewer than 25 eligible women.
[a] N = total number of eligible women in category (all ages).

and Fig. 2.D.1 and 2.D.2). Only small differences were observed by social status, with a tendency for smaller family sizes with increasing education.

There was a direct correlation between parity and age at marriage. In all age groups, women who had married at an early age (less than 20) had more children than those who had married later in life (Table 2.D.5). The difference was particularly marked for women who were aged 40–44, i.e., close to completed family size, at the time of interview.

TABLE 2.D.5. MEAN FAMILY SIZE BY AGE OF ELIGIBLE WOMEN, RESIDENCE AND AGE AT MARRIAGE*

Residence and age at marriage	Mean family size at age:						N^a
	< 20	20–24	25–29	30–34	35–39	40–44	
Damascus							
<15	1.35	3.47	5.07	6.95	6.93	7.51	270
15–19	0.58	2.21	3.90	5.49	6.77	7.45	1108
20–24	—	0.85	2.30	4.26	5.33	5.93	458
25–44	—	—	(0.82)	1.77	3.53	3.86	139
Sweida							
<15	(1.42)	3.44	5.11	(5.50)	(5.36)	7.86	125
15–19	0.63	2.07	3.95	5.38	6.40	6.40	986
20–24	—	1.08	2.09	3.75	5.12	6.00	474
25–44	—	—	(0.62)	(1.40)	2.76	3.77	126
Rural Aleppo							
<15	0.92	2.97	4.75	6.43	6.56	6.44	291
15–19	0.54	1.80	3.90	5.70	6.64	6.90	1186
20–24	—	0.85	2.26	4.06	5.54	6.16	396
25–44	—	—	(1.00)	(2.36)	(2.90)	(3.71)	62

* Figures in parentheses refer to fewer than 25 eligible women.
^{a} N = total number of eligible women in category (all ages).

Ideal Family Size

The ideal family size was more closely associated with residence, age, and parity than with social and educational factors. The average number of children considered ideal in rural areas (Aleppo) was about 6 and in small towns (Sweida) about 5, but in Damascus it was about 4 (Table 2.D.6). There was a steady increase in ideal family size with the age of the eligible woman, perhaps reflecting a generation effect. In each residential area and among all social status groups the mean ideal family size was directly correlated with the parity of the eligible woman. The parity of the woman's mother had no effect on ideal family size and there were only small differences by education, in that women who had had a secondary level education chose a somewhat smaller ideal family size than women with no formal education.

Table 2.D.7 shows a comparison between the ideal family size and the actual family size. A direct positive association was observed between the opinion that a woman had about ideal family size and the actual size of her family. Again, it should be noted that among all women in Damascus, 80% chose an ideal family size of 4 or fewer. In Sweida the corresponding proportion was 55% and in rural Aleppo only 17.5%. In Damascus, even among women with family sizes of 6 or more, 69% chose an ideal family size of 4 or fewer, the corresponding proportions in Sweida and rural Aleppo being 35% and 13.1%, respectively.

140

TABLE 2.D 6. MEAN IDEAL FAMILY SIZE BY POPULATION CHARACTERISTICS*

Characteristic	Damascus			Sweida			Rural Aleppo		
	Middle	Low	Both categories	Middle	Low	Both categories	Middle	Low	Both categories
All characteristics combined	3.88	3.89	3.88	4.52	5.03	4.63	6.36	6.51	6.45
Parity									
0	3.18	(3.44)	3.22	3.49	(4.29)	3.63	6.30	6.69	6.54
1	3.25	(3.26)	3.25	3.69	(3.86)	3.71	6.19	6.33	6.27
2	3.26	(3.18)	3.25	3.81	(3.88)	3.82	5.89	6.52	6.27
3	3.54	3.71	3.57	3.96	3.60	3.90	5.38	6.58	6.07
4	3.93	(4.10)	3.95	4.26	4.83	4.39	6.19	6.48	6.38
5	3.92	3.48	3.85	4.56	4.89	4.64	6.50	6.30	6.37
6 and over	4.42	4.32	4.40	5.35	5.65	5.44	6.78	6.53	6.62
Parity of EW's mother									
1	—	—	—	—	—	—	—	—	—
2	3.37	4.00	3.52	4.50	(4.55)	4.51	(6.00)	(5.56)	5.71
3	4.15	3.62	4.04	4.65	(4.68)	4.66	(7.28)	(6.26)	6.27
4	4.08	3.95	4.05	4.59	5.07	4.74	5.98	5.99	5.98
5	3.82	(4.36)	3.92	4.68	4.82	4.71	6.16	6.54	6.38
6	3.99	(3.13)	3.88	4.46	4.80	4.54	6.34	6.56	6.49
7	(3.76)	(4.11)	(3.80)	4.50	(5.31)	4.62	6.98	6.12	6.40
8	(3.83)	(3.45)	(3.77)	4.44	(4.95)	4.53	6.60	6.89	6.78
9	(3.71)	(4.14)	(3.77)	(4.58)	(5.68)	(4.75)	(6.14)	(7.27)	6.33
10 and over	(3.90)	(3.74)	(3.87)	(4.48)	(5.42)	(4.80)	6.15	6.64	6.41
Education of husband									
Illiterate + no school	4.04	3.93	4.00	4.92	5.01	4.96	6.52	6.51	6.51
Primary	3.93	(3.25)	3.92	4.53	(5.71)	4.57	6.25	(6.87)	6.33
Secondary	3.74	(3.80)	3.74	3.97	(4.00)	3.97	6.13	(5.83)	6.10
College + graduate	3.62	(3.00)	3.61	3.73	—	3.73	(5.88)	—	(5.88)

TABLE 2.D.6 (continued)

Mean ideal family size by social status

Characteristic	Damascus			Sweida			Rural Aleppo		
	Middle	Low	Both categories	Middle	Low	Both categories	Middle	Low	Both categories
Education of EW									
Illiterate + no school	4.04	3.96	4.03	4.72	5.07	4.81	6.36	6.50	6.45
Primary	3.71	3.50	3.69	4.06	(3.80)	4.05	(6.22)	(8.33)	(6.75)
Secondary	3.50	(2.67)	3.48	3.49	—	3.49	—	—	—
College + graduate	3.17	—	3.17	(2.67)	—	(2.67)	—	—	—
Occupation of EW									
Housewife	3.91	3.88	3.91	4.59	5.05	4.70	6.36	6.46	6.42
Clerical/professional	3.48	(4.20)	3.52	3.17	—	3.17	(6.67)	(7.8)	(7.18)
Agricultural/industrial	(3.00)	(3.00)	(3.00)	(6.00)	(4.00)	(5.09)	(6.23)	(8.78)	(7.27)
Janitorial/others	(3.00)	(5.00)	(4.67)	(3.88)	—	(3.88)	(6.00)	(7.75)	(7.00)
Age of EW									
<20	3.44	3.56	3.47	3.55	(4.80)	3.66	5.98	6.23	6.12
20–24	3.55	3.56	3.55	3.80	(4.17)	3.84	6.02	6.57	6.32
25–29	3.76	3.68	3.75	4.13	4.56	4.20	6.09	6.57	6.37
30–40	3.97	4.12	3.99	4.55	4.62	4.56	6.42	6.39	6.40
35–39	4.14	4.06	4.13	4.88	5.32	5.01	7.24	6.49	6.72
40–49	4.09	4.06	4.14	5.73	5.50	5.64	6.86	6.68	6.73

* Figures in parentheses refer to fewer than 25 eligible women.

TABLE 2.D.7. PERCENTAGE DISTRIBUTION OF IDEAL FAMILY SIZE BY ACTUAL FAMILY SIZE

Actual family size	Percentage of EW choosing ideal family size of:								Number of women
	0–3	4	5	6	7	8	9	10 and over	
Damascus									
0	56.3	37.9	1.9	2.9	1.0	0	0	0	103
1	56.7	35.8	4.1	2.0	0.7	0	0	0.7	148
2	56.1	34.1	6.7	0.6	1.2	1.2	0	0	164
3	40.5	45.5	9.0	5.0	0	0	0	0	200
4	19.5	67.8	6.8	4.4	0	1.5	0	0	205
5	33.3	32.8	27.2	4.1	0.5	0.5	0	1.5	195
6 and over	28.5	40.3	3.6	14.6	4.5	4.2	1.9	2.3	471
All family sizes	37.3	42.5	8.1	6.9	1.7	1.7	0.6	1.1	1486
Sweida									
0	49.5	29.5	11.4	5.7	1.0	2.9	0	0	105
1	49.7	31.4	11.1	3.3	2.6	0.7	0	1.3	153
2	38.0	34.5	15.2	7.0	2.3	1.8	0	1.2	171
3	31.2	39.9	14.8	10.4	3.3	0.5	0	0	183
4	12.0	50.9	19.2	14.3	1.8	0.4	0	1.3	224
5	12.2	21.8	46.8	13.3	3.2	1.1	1.1	0.5	188
6 and over	13.1	21.9	12.3	27.0	10.4	8.0	3.3	3.5	511
All family sizes	23.9	31.1	18.0	15.4	5.1	3.4	1.2	1.8	1535
Rural Aleppo									
0	4.2	14.4	7.6	40.7	11.9	7.6	1.7	11.9	118
1	9.2	13.8	7.3	39.4	6.4	9.2	3.7	11.0	109
2	3.2	19.4	16.9	29.8	8.1	4.8	7.3	10.5	124
3	7.4	17.3	18.5	27.2	13.6	6.2	1.2	8.6	81
4	1.9	17.3	12.5	33.7	11.5	6.7	4.8	11.5	104
5	1.0	10.5	22.9	28.6	14.3	11.4	1.9	9.5	105
6 and over	4.3	8.8	11.2	29.2	15.5	13.4	2.7	13.4	329
All family sizes	4.3	13.2	13.1	32.1	12.4	9.6	3.3	12.1	970

Chapter Three

FAMILY FORMATION AND PREGNANCY OUTCOME

INTRODUCTION

M. R. Bone, C. C. Standley & A. R. Omran

This chapter examines the relationships between pregnancy wastage on the one hand and family formation variables on the other. The family formation variables involved are: maternal age (age at termination of index pregnancy), pregnancy order, family size, and duration of the preceding pregnancy interval (the period between the end of the preceding pregnancy and the end of the index pregnancy).

In previous investigations, described in Part I, a J-shaped relationship has usually been found between pregnancy wastage and maternal age or pregnancy order. That is to say, wastage was lowest at intermediate ages and pregnancy orders and greatest for the latest ages and highest pregnancy orders. By contrast, the relationship between pregnancy wastage and the length of the preceding pregnancy interval has usually been shown to be a reverse J, i.e., wastage was greatest for the shortest intervals and lowest for those of intermediate length.

This chapter examines, first, whether the same relationships exist in the populations of the participating areas and, second, whether it is possible to indicate, in terms of the family formation variables, the most and least favourable conditions for conception to be followed by a successful pregnancy, i.e., one that results in a live-born child.

Information on pregnancy outcome was obtained by collecting from each eligible woman a detailed pregnancy history for the period between marriage and interview. Pregnancies resulting in either stillbirths or abortions were considered wasted. For the purposes of this study, stillbirths were defined as non-live births occurring 7 months or more after conception, and abortions as those occurring within 7 months of conception. Stillbirth rates, which are likely to be more reliable than abortion rates, are shown separately from the latter, and in relation to both total births and total pregnancies.

The difficulties that arise in the analysis and interpretation of the data are as follows:

1. *Interrelationships among the family formation variables.* Many of the variables are interrelated, e.g., age, pregnancy interval, and pregnancy order. First and second pregnancies and short interpregnancy intervals are likely to be most frequent among the youngest women, while pregnancies of the highest orders and long interpregnancy intervals are more likely to be found among the oldest women of childbearing age. To examine the pure relationship between any two of the variables alone, it is necessary that the other variables should be held constant. In practice, it is seldom useful to control more than one extraneous variable, since many of the subgroups thus formed would be too small to exhibit trends.

2. *The nature of the sample.* The findings are based on retrospective evidence from samples of women, and not on current evidence from samples of pregnancies. The effects of this are:

(*a*) Pregnancies that occurred to non-eligible women (e.g., those now dead or too old for inclusion) in the same areas and during the same time period are disregarded.

(*b*) Women who have had many pregnancies make a larger contribution to the results than women with fewer pregnancies; this may produce bias through differences in pregnancy outcome.

(*c*) The women's pregnancy histories cover varying periods up to some 30 years prior to the interview. During this time, the risks of pregnancy wastage may have changed and this could distort the relationships under study.

(*d*) It is unlikely that recall over periods of up to 30 years will be perfect, and there may be underreporting of pregnancies for other reasons in a single interview survey. In none of the three areas for which the information was available, however, could any differences be found between fetal wastage rates for last pregnancies and those for all pregnancies, whether analysed by maternal age or by pregnancy order. This suggests that there was no underreporting of earlier pregnancies due to lack of recall.

3. *Interpretation of the results.* Several points need to be kept in mind in interpreting some of the associations found between pregnancy wastage and the family formation variables. Firstly, a woman who wants a child and whose pregnancy ends in fetal death is likely to conceive again as soon as she can in the hope of producing a live child. If she is repeatedly unsuccessful, the statistics will show pregnancy loss following numerous, closely spaced pregnancies. The number and spacing of the pregnancies in such cases are the effects, not the causes, of pregnancy wastage. Secondly, induced abortion may be used intentionally as a method of birth control. An unsuccessful outcome of pregnancy then depends on deliberate choice by the woman, not on physiological factors.

A. COLOMBIA

A. Gil, G. Ochoa & A. R. Omran

Pregnancy Wastage and Social Characteristics

Of the 23 191 pregnancies reported by the 5270 women in the study, 1.2% terminated in stillbirths and 13.6% in abortions. That is, for all the eligible women, 15% of the pregnancies were lost between the time of initial conception and the time of delivery. Pregnancy wastage was about the same for women in both zones. However, in the OUZ women in the low social status group had a higher percentage of pregnancy wastage than women in the middle social status group, while in the NSZ this difference was not found (Table 3.A.1).

TABLE 3.A.1. PREGNANCY WASTAGE BY RESIDENCE AND SOCIAL STATUS

Residence and social status	No. of pregnancies	Stillbirths (%)	Abortions (%)	Pregnancy wastage
Old urban zone				
Middle	9128	0.9	14.0	14.9
Low	753	1.6	16.6	18.2
All OUZ	9881	0.9	14.2	15.1
Newly settled zone				
Middle	3768	1.5	13.3	14.8
Low	9542	1.4	13.0	14.4
All NSZ	13310	1.4	13.1	14.5

FIG. 3.A.1. PREGNANCY WASTAGE BY MATERNAL AGE, RESIDENCE, AND SOCIAL STATUS

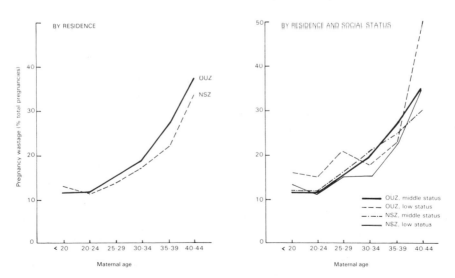

147

Pregnancy Outcome and Maternal Age

The rates of pregnancy wastage increased with maternal age after age 25, as shown in Table 3.A.2 and Fig. 3.A.1. This is true for both social status groups and both areas of residence. For women over 25 years, wastage was higher in the OUZ than in the NSZ. No consistent difference was observed between social status groups. Abortions made up the bulk of pregnancy wastage in both areas (Table 3.A.2 and Fig. 3.A.2). When the stillbirths were calculated as a percentage of the total number of births, a J-shaped relationship with maternal age was revealed, especially in the NSZ (Table 3.A.3 and Fig. 3.A.3).

FIG. 3.A.2. ABORTIONS AND STILLBIRTHS BY RESIDENCE AND MATERNAL AGE

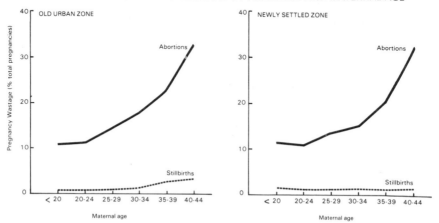

FIG. 3.A.3. STILLBIRTHS AS A PERCENTAGE OF TOTAL BIRTHS, BY RESIDENCE AND MATERNAL AGE

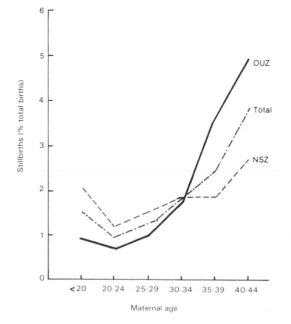

TABLE 3.A.2. PREGNANCY OUTCOME BY RESIDENCE, SOCIAL STATUS, AND MATERNAL AGE

Residence, social status and maternal age	Total no. of pregnancies	Pregnancy outcome as percentage of all pregnancies			
		Live births	Stillbirths	Abortions	Pregnancy wastage
Old urban zone					
Middle					
<20	1250	88.1	0.6	11.3	11.9
20–24	3413	88.0	0.5	11.5	12.0
25–29	2716	84.6	0.9	14.5	15.4
30–34	1298	80.4	1.3	18.3	19.6
35–39	398	73.1	3.0	23.9	26.9
40–44	53	64.2	3.8	32.1	35.9
Total	9128	85.1	0.9	14.0	14.9
Low					
<20	115	83.5	2.6	13.9	16.5
20–24	255	84.7	2.0	13.3	15.3
25–29	220	79.1	0.5	20.5	21.0
30–34	118	82.2	2.5	15.3	17.8
35–39	37	78.4	—	21.6	21.6
40–44	8	50.0	—	50.0	50.0
Total	753	81.8	1.6	16.6	18.2
All OUZ					
<20	1365	87.9	0.8	11.5	12.3
20–24	3668	87.8	0.6	11.6	12.2
25–29	2936	84.2	0.9	15.0	15.8
30–34	1416	80.6	1.4	18.0	19.4
35–39	435	73.6	2.8	23.7	26.5
40–44	61	62.3	3.3	34.4	37.7
Total	9881	84.9	0.9	14.2	15.1
Newly settled zone					
Middle					
<20	623	87.8	2.4	9.8	12.2
20–24	396	88.3	1.1	10.8	12.0
25–29	1014	84.8	1.5	13.7	15.8
30–34	510	79.6	1.4	19.0	20.4
35–39	195	75.9	1.0	23.1	24.1
40–44	30	70.0	—	30.0	30.0
Total	3768	85.2	1.5	13.3	14.8
Low					
<20	1344	85.7	1.6	12.1	14.3
20–24	2366	88.3	1.1	10.6	11.7
25–29	2719	85.7	1.3	13.0	14.3
30–34	1557	83.6	1.7	14.8	16.5
35–39	574	78.2	1.6	20.2	21.8
40–44	82	64.6	2.4	32.9	35.4
Total	9542	85.6	1.4	13.0	14.4
All NSZ					
<20	1967	86.4	1.8	11.8	13.6
20–24	4662	88.2	1.1	10.7	11.8
25–29	3733	85.5	1.3	13.2	14.5
30–34	2067	82.6	1.6	15.8	17.4
35–39	769	77.6	1.4	20.9	22.3
40–44	112	66.1	1.8	32.1	33.9
Total	13310	85.5	1.4	13.1	14.5

TABLE 3.A.3. STILLBIRTHS AS A PERCENTAGE OF TOTAL BIRTHS, BY RESIDENCE AND MATERNAL AGE

Maternal age	Old urban zone		Newly settled zone	
	Total births	Stillbirths (%)	Total births	Stillbirths (%)
<20	1208	0.9	1735	2.1
20–24	3243	0.7	4165	1.2
25–29	2496	1.0	3241	1.5
30–34	1161	1.7	1740	1.9
35–39	332	3.6	608	1.8
40–44	40	5.0	74	2.7

To examine the possibility of memory lapses, the outcome of the last pregnancy was studied separately. Fig. 3.A.4 compares the patterns of wastage for the last pregnancy and for the total number of pregnancies in relation to maternal age and pregnancy order. The trends of the two rates conform fairly closely, suggesting that underreporting was more or less uniform and that the association between pregnancy wastage and family formation is reflected fairly accurately in women's recollections of their past experiences.

Pregnancy Outcome and Pregnancy Order

The data relating unfavourable outcome of pregnancy and pregnancy order show a positive relationship for abortions (Table 3.A.4 and Fig. 3.A.5) and a J-shaped relationship for stillbirths (although there were fluctuations) in the NSZ. Only small differences were observed between the residential zones.

Wastage by Both Pregnancy Order and Maternal Age

For a given age of the mother, a positive relationship was evident between gravidity and pregnancy wastage, except for women aged 35 and over. It is also noteworthy that the risk of wastage was higher for teenage pregnancies than for pregnancies at age 20–24 for every pregnancy order.

For individual pregnancy orders, the highest risks of wastage were evident at the two extremes of reproductive age, namely under 20 and over 35. The relationship to maternal age was J-shaped for the first 3 pregnancies, and a reversed-J for the subsequent ones (Table 3.A.5 and Fig. 3.A.6).

When both age and gravidity were taken into consideration, the highest risks of wastage were found to be associated with high-order pregnancies of 4–5 and over occurring at a young age, especially under 20 (Table 3.A.5 and Fig. 3.A.6).

150

FIG. 3.A.4. PREGNANCY WASTAGE BY RESIDENCE, MATERNAL AGE, AND PREGNANCY ORDER, FOR TOTAL PREGNANCIES AND FOR LAST PREGNANCY

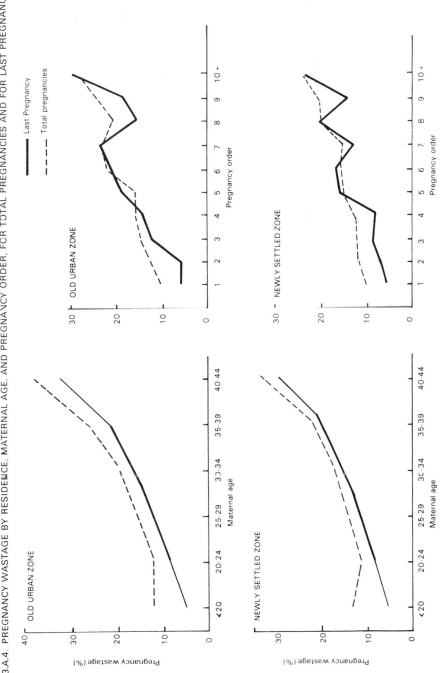

TABLE 3.A.4. PREGNANCY OUTCOME BY RESIDENCE AND PREGNANCY ORDER

Residence	Pregnancy order	Total no. of pregnancies	Pregnancy outcome as percentage of total pregnancies			
			Live births	Stillbirths	Abortions	Pregnancy wastage
Old urban zone	1	2417	89.6	0.9	9.6	10.5
	2	1984	87.5	0.7	11.8	12.5
	3	1505	85.6	0.7	13.8	14.5
	4	1135	84.2	1.0	14.8	15.8
	5	825	84.2	0.8	14.9	15.7
	6	608	78.5	0.8	20.7	21.5
	7	436	77.3	1.6	21.1	22.7
	8	336	79.8	2.4	17.9	20.3
	9	216	76.4	0.9	22.7	23.6
	10 and over	419	71.6	2.1	26.3	28.4
Newly settled zone	1	2447	89.4	1.7	8.9	10.6
	2	2157	88.2	1.2	10.6	11.8
	3	1830	87.6	1.3	11.1	12.4
	4	1524	86.9	0.9	12.1	13.0
	5	1243	84.6	1.0	14.4	15.4
	6	1013	84.2	1.2	14.6	15.8
	7	804	84.3	1.5	14.2	15.7
	8	631	79.7	2.4	17.9	20.3
	9	482	79.5	1.7	18.9	20.6
	10 and over	1179	75.8	1.6	22.6	24.2

FIG. 3.A.5. PREGNANCY WASTAGE BY RESIDENCE AND PREGNANCY ORDER

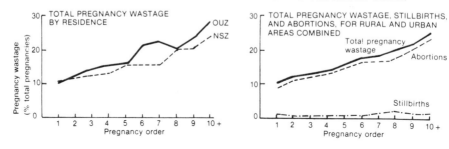

TABLE 3.A.5. PREGNANCY WASTAGE BY PREGNANCY ORDER AND MATERNAL AGE
FOR OLD URBAN AND NEWLY SETTLED ZONES COMBINED

Maternal age	Pregnancy wastage (%) for pregnancy order:					
	1	2	3	4	5	6 and over
<20	11.2	14.3	15.0	21.4	33.3	42.9
20–24	9.3	10.3	11.9	13.0	14.4	23.6
25–29	11.3	13.0	13.4	13.1	14.2	18.7
30–34	12.6	13.6	16.1	17.5	16.3	19.6
35–44	32.0	29.7	24.4	20.0	30.9	22.1

FIG. 3.A.6. PREGNANCY WASTAGE BY MATERNAL AGE AND PREGNANCY ORDER, FOR
URBAN AND RURAL AREAS COMBINED

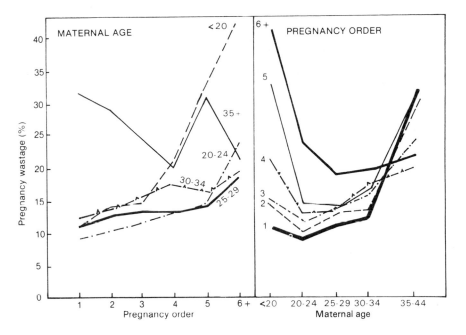

FIG. 3.A.7. PREGNANCY WASTAGE BY DURATION OF PRECEDING PREGNANCY INTERVAL
FOR BOTH RESIDENTIAL AREAS COMBINED

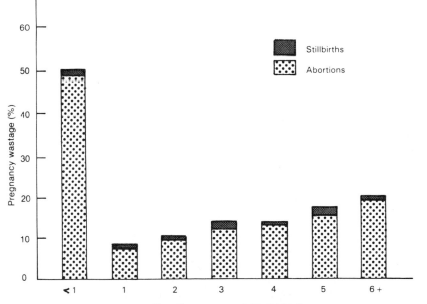

153

Wastage by Preceding Pregnancy Interval

The preceding pregnancy interval is defined as the period between the end of the preceding pregnancy and the end of the index pregnancy. According to this definition, the first pregnancy is excluded from the analysis. There was a reversed J-shaped relationship between pregnancy wastage and preceding pregnancy interval (Table 3.A.6 and Fig. 3.A.7). For an interval of less than one year, the risk of poor pregnancy outcome was very high (50.6%) and the percentage of women having an abortion was 49.5%. For longer intervals, the risks decreased dramatically, with slight rises for intervals of 5 or more years, probably because of the older maternal age.

TABLE 3.A.6. PREGNANCY WASTAGE BY DURATION OF PRECEDING PREGNANCY INTERVAL FOR NEWLY SETTLED AND OLD URBAN ZONES COMBINED

Preceding pregnancy interval (years)	Pregnancy outcome as percentage of total pregnancies			Total pregnancies other than the first
	Stillbirths	Abortions	Total pregnancy wastage	
< 1	1.1	49.5	50.6	2673
1–2	1.1	6.8	7.9	10086
2–3	1.2	8.5	9.7	3030
3–4	1.2	12.0	13.3	1130
4–5	0.7	12.6	13.3	547
5–6	2.2	15.2	17.5	269
6 and over	1.2	18.6	19.8	242

B. EGYPT

A. F. El-Sherbini, H. M. Hammam, A. Omran,
M. A. El-Torky & S. I. Fahmy

Pregnancy Outcome

Out of the 24 979 pregnancies reported by 4861 women, 434 (1.74%) were stillbirths and 2111 (8.45%) were abortions.

Pregnancy Wastage and Social Characteristics

Table 3.B.1 shows that the three areas exhibited some differences in regard to pregnancy wastage (i.e., pregnancies terminating in death of the babies). Pregnancy wastage in both the urban and the industrial areas was higher than in the rural area. The rates were 9.3%, 10.9%, and 10.7% in the rural, urban, and industrial areas, respectively. In the industrial area, pregnancy wastage among women of middle social status was more than double that among women of low social status (16.9% and 7.8%, respectively). A smaller difference existed between the two social classes in the urban area: 11.5% and 10.2% for women of middle and low social status, respectively. No differences by social status were noted in the rural area.

TABLE 3.B.1. PREGNANCY WASTAGE BY RESIDENCE AND SOCIAL STATUS

Residence and social status	No. of pregnancies	Stillbirths (%)	Abortions (%)
Rural			
Middle	3595	1.6	7.5
Low	7227	1.8	7.6
Both categories	10822	1.7	7.6
Urban			
Middle	6627	1.6	9.9
Low	4705	2.0	8.2
Both categories	11332	1.7	9.2
Industrial			
Middle	908	3.4	13.5
Low	1917	1.3	6.5
Both categories	2825	2.0	8.7

Abortion was responsible for 81.7% of total pregnancy wastage among rural women, 84.4% among urban women, and 81.3% among industrial women. Women of middle social status had more abortions than those of low social status in both the industrial area (13.5% and 6.5%, respectively) and the urban area (9.9% and 8.2%, respectively). In the rural area, both social classes had nearly the same percentage of abortions.

Pregnancy Wastage and Maternal Age

Table 3.B.2 shows that there was a J-shaped relationship between pregnancy wastage and maternal age for all areas (Fig. 3.B.1). The maternal age that was associated with the lowest pregnancy wastage was 20–29 years, while the highest wastage was at 40–44 years (17.8% for rural, 23.5% for urban, and 30.3% for industrial areas). In addition, the table shows that stillbirth rates are also independently related to maternal age in a J-shaped fashion.

For each age group, urban women had the highest pregnancy wastage, followed by rural women and then those from the industrial area. At age 40–44 years, urban women had 23.5% pregnancy loss, compared with 17.8% for rural women. The number of women in the 40–44 age group in the industrial area was too small to permit valid comparisons to be made, but pregnancy wastage at each age group in the industrial area was lower than in either the urban or the rural area. Women of middle social status in the urban area had higher pregnancy wastage than those in the low social status group at all ages (Table

155

TABLE 3.B.2. PREGNANCY OUTCOME BY RESIDENCE, SOCIAL STATUS, AND MATERNAL AGE*

Residence, social status, and maternal age	Total no. of pregnancies	Pregnancy outcome as percentage of all pregnancies			
		Live births	Stillbirths	Abortions	Pregnancy wastage
Rural					
Middle					
<20	965	92.7	2.3	5.0	7.3
20–24	882	93.1	1.8	5.1	6.9
25–29	873	91.2	0.7	7.4	8.1
30–34	490	88.2	1.4	10.4	11.8
35–39	243	85.6	1.6	11.9	13.5
40–44	53	77.4	—	22.6	22.6
Unknown	89				
Low					
<20	1778	90.3	2.4	7.0	9.4
20–24	1818	91.3	1.6	6.7	8.3
25–29	1791	91.9	1.4	6.2	7.6
30–34	1089	89.5	1.7	8.2	9.9
35–39	500	87.6	2.4	8.8	11.2
40–44	104	84.6	1.0	14.4	15.4
Unknown	147				
Both categories					
<20	2743	91.2	2.3	6.3	8.6
20–24	2700	91.9	1.7	6.2	7.9
25–29	2664	91.7	1.2	6.6	7.8
30–34	1579	89.1	1.6	8.9	10.5
35–39	743	86.9	2.2	9.8	12.0
40–44	157	82.2	0.6	17.2	17.8
Unknown	236				
Urban					
Middle					
<20	1604	90.0	2.1	7.9	10.0
20–24	1785	89.2	1.6	9.2	10.8
25–29	1682	90.5	1.1	8.2	9.3
30–34	934	86.6	1.7	11.0	12.7
35–39	421	81.9	1.9	16.2	18.1
40–44	81	70.4	3.7	25.9	29.6
Unknown	120				
Low					
<20	1055	89.8	2.1	7.6	9.7
20–24	1180	89.9	2.8	6.7	9.5
25–29	1191	91.1	2.1	6.6	8.7
30–34	719	89.1	1.0	9.2	10.2
35–39	370	85.7	0.8	12.4	13.2
40–44	76	80.3	1.3	15.8	17.1
Unknown	114				
Both categories					
<20	2659	89.9	2.1	7.8	9.9
20–24	2965	89.5	2.1	8.2	10.3
25–29	2873	90.7	1.5	7.6	9.1
30–34	1653	87.7	1.4	10.2	11.6
35–39	791	83.7	1.4	14.4	15.8
40–44	157	75.2	2.5	21.0	23.5
Unknown	234				

TABLE 3.B.2 (continued)

Residence, social status, and maternal age	Total no. of pregnancies	Pregnancy outcome as percentage of all pregnancies			
		Live births	Stillbirths	Abortions	Pregnancy wastage
Industrial					
Middle					
<20	393	92.9	1.0	6.1	7.1
20–24	579	93.8	0.5	5.7	6.2
25–29	481	92.7	1.1	6.2	7.3
30–34	303	91.4	3.3	5.3	8.6
35–39	134	91.8	—	8.2	8.2
40–44	20	(65.0)	(10.0)	(25.0)	(35.0)
Unknown	7				
Low					
<20	154	91.6	2.6	5.8	8.4
20–24	213	92.0	1.4	6.6	8.0
25–29	205	94.1	0.5	5.4	5.9
30–34	148	87.8	2.0	10.2	12.2
35–39	87	95.4	2.3	2.3	(4.6)
40–44	3	(100.0)	(—)	(—)	(—)
Unknown	98				
Both categories					
<20	547	92.5	1.5	6.0	7.5
20–24	792	93.3	0.8	5.9	6.7
25–29	686	93.1	0.9	6.0	6.9
30–34	451	90.2	2.9	6.9	9.8
35–39	221	93.2	0.9	5.9	6.8
40–44	23	(69.7)	(8.6)	(21.7)	(30.3)
Unknown	105				

* Figures in parentheses refer to fewer than 25 eligible women.

3.B.2 and Fig. 3.B.2). Rural women showed a similar pattern at all ages except those under 20 years of age. Women in the industrial area showed an inconsistent pattern.

Abortions again accounted for by far the greatest part of pregnancy wastage: 96.6% and 89.4% of total wastage among rural and urban women aged 40–44 years, respectively. Abortions showed a direct relationship with maternal age. In rural and urban areas, abortions occurred more frequently among middle than among low social status women, while in the industrial area the women showed an inconsistent pattern. The greater pregnancy wastage among women of middle social status, in both rural and urban areas could be accounted for by a larger number of induced abortions. It should also be noted that underreporting of pregnancy wastage may have been a factor, and that the extent of underreporting may have been greater in the rural area and among low social status women.

Table 3.B.2 shows that the stillbirth rate was independently related to maternal age in a U-shaped manner. When the stillbirth rate was calculated in

FIG. 3.B.1. ABORTIONS AND STILLBIRTHS BY RESIDENCE AND MATERNAL AGE

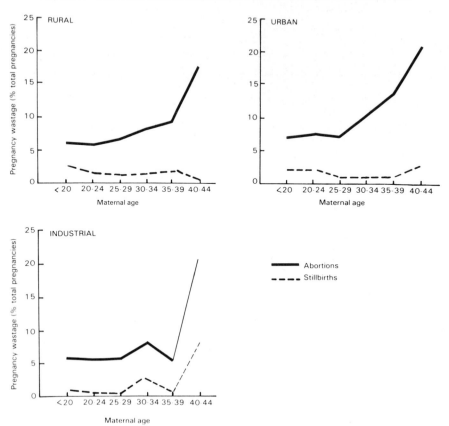

TABLE 3.B.3. STILLBIRTHS AS A PERCENTAGE OF TOTAL BIRTHS BY RESIDENCE AND
MATERNAL AGE

Maternal age	Rural		Urban		Industrial	
	Total births	Stillbirths (%)	Total births	Stillbirths (%)	Total births	Stillbirths (%)
<20	2501	2.6	2390	2.3	506	1.6
20–24	2481	1.8	2653	2.3	739	0.8
25–29	2443	1.2	2607	1.7	639	0.9
30–34	1407	1.7	1450	1.5	407	3.2
35–39	646	2.4	662	1.6	206	0.9
40–44	129	0.8	118	3.3	16	(12.5)[a]
Unknown	74		66		14	

[a] Refers to fewer than 25 eligible women.

158

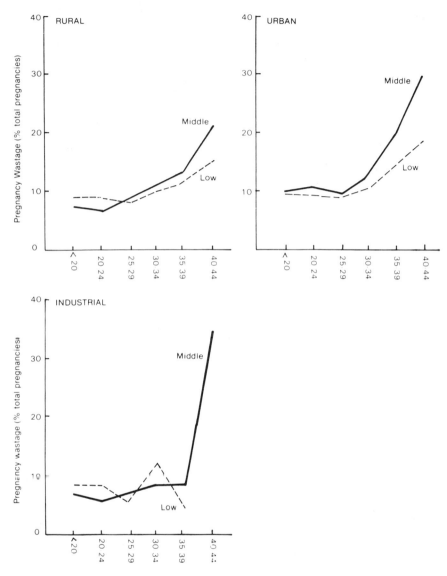

the more traditional way (by relating it to births) a similar pattern was revealed (Table 3.B.3 and Fig. 3.B.3). Stillbirths accounted for a small percentage of total wastage. The rates were highest in the youngest age group (less than 20 years) (at least in the urban and rural areas) and in the older age groups (over 35), resulting in an inverse J-shaped or U-shaped curve. There was little variation in the percentages of stillbirths by residence and social status in most of the maternal age groups.

FIG. 3.B.3. STILLBIRTHS AS A PERCENTAGE OF TOTAL BIRTHS, BY RESIDENCE AND
MATERNAL AGE

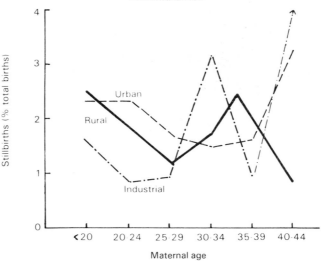

Pregnancy Wastage and Pregnancy Order

Table 3.B.4 shows that, on the whole, total pregnancy wastage increased with pregnancy order. The first 5 birth orders were associated with the least wastage; at birth orders 7, 8, and 9, pregnancy wastage was moderate; and birth orders of 9 and 10 or more were associated with the highest pregnancy wastage. The rise in wastage with increasing pregnancy order was mostly due

FIG. 3.B.4. ABORTIONS AND STILLBIRTHS BY RESIDENCE AND PREGNANCY ORDER

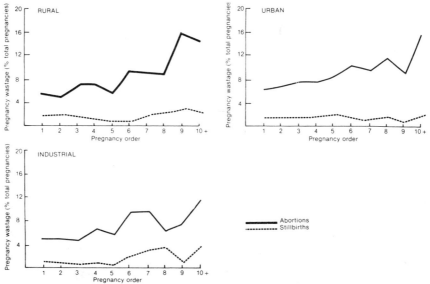

to more frequent abortion. The percentages of stillbirths were low and they fluctuated with birth order. They tended to increase at higher birth orders (7 or more) and there was a slight increase at the first two birth orders (Fig. 3.B.4).

Pregnancy Wastage by Both Pregnancy Order and Maternal Age

Table 3.B.5 shows three patterns. The first was the presence of a decrease in pregnancy wastage with increase in birth order among mothers aged less than

TABLE 3.B.4. PREGNANCY OUTCOME BY RESIDENCE AND PREGNANCY ORDER

Residence	Pregnancy order	Total no. of pregnancies	Pregnancy outcome as percentage of total pregnancies			
			Live births	Stillbirths	Abortions	Pregnancy wastage
Rural						
	1	1840	92.5	1.8	5.6	7.4
	2	2708	93.3	1.9	4.8	6.7
	3	1509	91.5	1.7	6.4	8.1
	4	1338	91.8	1.3	6.6	7.9
	5	1141	91.9	1.2	5.9	7.1
	6	927	89.1	1.1	9.4	10.5
	7	730	88.4	1.9	8.9	10.8
	8	558	87.8	2.0	8.9	10.9
	9	377	80.9	2.9	15.4	18.3
	10 and over	243	82.3	2.1	14.4	16.5
	Unknown	451				
Urban						
	1	1852	91.9	1.8	6.1	7.9
	2	1719	90.7	1.8	6.9	8.7
	3	1534	90.1	1.8	7.7	9.5
	4	1336	89.9	1.9	7.7	9.6
	5	1148	88.7	2.1	8.3	10.4
	6	945	86.3	1.6	10.9	12.5
	7	756	88.8	1.2	9.5	10.7
	8	599	85.5	1.8	11.8	13.6
	9	443	88.9	0.9	9.5	10.4
	10 and over	322	81.7	1.9	15.8	17.7
	Unknown	678				
Industrial						
	1	449	94.2	1.1	4.7	5.8
	2	418	94.3	0.9	4.8	5.7
	3	375	94.9	0.5	4.3	4.8
	4	325	92.6	0.9	6.5	7.4
	5	289	93.8	0.3	5.9	6.2
	6	237	88.6	2.1	9.3	11.4
	7	198	87.4	3.0	9.6	12.6
	8	161	90.7	3.1	6.2	9.3
	9	121	91.8	0.8	7.4	8.2
	10 and over	78	84.6	3.8	11.6	15.4
	Unknown	174				

20 years. (It should be noted, however, that very few women under 20 years of age had 4 or more children.) The second pattern was a biphasic one at age group 20–24 years: there was an increase in wastage up to the third or fourth birth order, followed by a decrease in wastage up to a birth order of 6 or more. Among women aged 30 years and over there was an increase in wastage with an increase in birth order and this increase was particularly marked between birth orders 5 and 6.

TABLE 3.B.5. PREGNANCY WASTAGE BY PREGNANCY ORDER AND MATERNAL AGE

Residence and maternal age	Pregnancy wastage (%) for pregnancy order:						Total no. of pregnancies
	1	2	3	4	5	6 and over	
Rural							
< 20	3.7	2.3	1.1	0.5	0.1	0.5	2743
20–24	0.7	1.1	2.0	1.9	1.2	1.0	2700
25–29	0.3	0.4	0.9	1.2	1.1	4.1	2664
30–34	0.1	—	0.2	0.5	0.9	9.1	1579
35–44	—	0.1	—	0.3	0.4	13.0	900
Unknown	—	—	—	—	—	—	236
Urban							
< 20	4.2	2.9	1.4	0.7	0.3	0.5	2652
20–24	0.8	1.6	2.9	2.1	1.7	1.5	2965
25–29	0.2	0.6	1.1	1.0	1.3	4.9	2873
30–34	0.1	0.1	1.3	1.8	1.8	20.5	1653
35–44	0.1	0.3	0.3	—	0.5	15.4	948
Unknown	—	—	—	—	—	—	241
Industrial							
< 20	3.4	2.7	1.1	0.2	—	—	547
20–24	0.9	1.0	1.4	2.3	0.5	0.6	792
25–29	—	0.1	0.1	0.6	1.9	4.1	686
30–34	—	—	—	0.2	0.2	9.3	451
35–44	—	—	—	—	—	9.0	244
Unknown							105

Pregnancy wastage at birth order 6 or more increased with an increase in maternal age up to the age of 35 years in the urban and industrial areas and beyond this age in the rural area.

Pregnancy Wastage by Preceding Pregnancy Interval

Preceding pregnancy interval is defined as the period between the end of the preceding pregnancy and the end of the index pregnancy. Thus, the first pregnancy is excluded from the analysis.

There was an inverted J-shaped relationship between pregnancy wastage and pregnancy interval. Table 3.B.6 shows that the highest pregnancy wastage occurred when the interval was less than two years (29.8%), then the pregnancy wastage decreased to 14.3%, 7.6%, 5.2% and 4.2% for intervals 2,

162

3, 4, and 5 years, respectively, subsequently increasing to 7.0% for an interval of 6 or more years (Fig. 3.B.5).

Since abortions accounted for most pregnancy wastage, the percentage of abortions by preceding pregnancy interval exhibited a trend almost identical with that for total pregnancy wastage.

A high percentage of pregnancies terminated in abortions when the interval was less than 2 years. A preceding pregnancy interval is, by definition, shorter when the index pregnancy ends in abortion than when it goes to full term. For intervals of 3–5 years, a low percentage of abortions was shown, whereas at

TABLE 3.B.6. PREGNANCY WASTAGE BY DURATION OF PRECEDING PREGNANCY
INTERVAL FOR RURAL AND URBAN AREAS COMBINED

Preceding pregnancy interval (years)	Pregnancy outcome as percentage of total pregnancies			Total pregnancies other than the first
	Stillbirths	Abortions	Total pregnancy wastage	
<2	3.2	26.6	29.8	1054
2–3	2.4	11.9	14.3	6210
3–4	1.4	6.2	7.6	7176
4–5	1.3	3.9	5.2	2742
5–6	0.8	3.4	4.2	952
6 and over	0.7	6.3	7.0	396

FIG. 3.B.5. PREGNANCY WASTAGE BY DURATION OF PRECEDING PREGNANCY INTERVAL,
FOR ALL RESIDENTIAL AREAS COMBINED

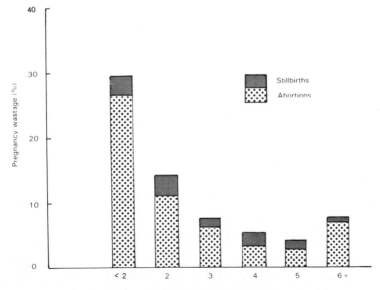

163

intervals of 6 or more years the percentage moved upwards. The increase in wastage with a longer pregnancy interval might have been due in part to increased age of the mother.

Stillbirths do not appreciably shorten the preceding pregnancy interval since, by definition, they occur mostly near the end of a full-term pregnancy. Stillbirth rates show an inverse relationship with pregnancy interval.

From this analysis, the highest risks obtain for intervals of less than 2 years. There is also a high risk for intervals of 2–3 years, and again an increasing risk when the interval is greater than 6 years.

C. PAKISTAN

M. Saeed Qureshi & A. R. Omran

Pregnancy Outcome

Most of the studies in developing countries have shown that data on pregnancy wastage are usually deficient in quality and coverage. In traditional societies with high illiteracy, especially among women, one should expect slightly more underreporting of pregnancy wastage. Such was the case in this study.

Out of the 24 213 pregnancies reported by 4856 women included in this study, 511 (2.1%) terminated in stillbirths and 2327 (9.6%) in abortions. This yielded a pregnancy wastage rate of 11.7% (Table 3.C.1).

TABLE 3.C.1. PREGNANCY WASTAGE BY RESIDENCE AND SOCIAL STATUS

Residence and social status	No. of pregnancies	Stillbirth (%)	Abortions (%)
Semi-urban			
Middle	5786	2.4	10.4
Low	7135	2.2	8.1
Both categories	12921	2.3	9.1
Urban			
Middle	10217	1.9	10.5
Low	1075	2.1	7.5
Both categories	11292	1.9	10.2

Pregnancy Wastage and Social Characteristics

Pregnancy wastage among semi-urban women was found to be less than among urban women. The proportions were 11.4% and 12.1%. respectively. Within each residential group, women of middle social status had experienced more pregnancy wastage than had women in the low status group. The pregnancy wastage rates for middle status women were 12.8% and 12.4% for semi-urban and urban areas, respectively, while the corresponding rates for the low status group were 10.3% and 9.7%, respectively.

The differences in wastage rates by residence were due to the higher proportion of abortions among urban women (10.3%) than among semi-urban women (9.1%). There were also more abortions among middle status women than among low status women. On the other hand, the stillbirths were higher (2.3%) among semi-urban women than among urban women (1.9%). The data might be deficient in quality, as has been noticed in other such studies in developing countries (Table 3.C.2 and Fig. 3.C.1). Some of the reported abortions might have been induced, a fact that could not be ascertained in the survey.

FIG. 3.C.1. PREGNANCY WASTAGE BY MATERNAL AGE, SOCIAL STATUS, AND RESIDENCE

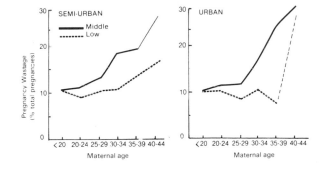

Pregnancy Wastage and Maternal Age

The pregnancy wastage pattern has been found to increase consistently with maternal age. The average wastage rate increased steadily at early ages and then rose sharply after 30 years of age. The wastage rate among urban women increased from 10.2% for the age group less than 20 to 37.1% for the age group 40–44. In semi-urban women the wastage rate first declined slightly from 10.9% for the age group less than 20 to 10.1% for the age group 20–24, and then increased to 19.6% for women aged 40–44. A similar pattern, with some variations, was observed by social status.

At all maternal ages, low status women reported lower wastage rates than higher status women in both residential areas. For semi-urban women stillbirths increased steadily with increasing maternal age, but no definite trend was evident in the data for urban women. However, the abortion rate increased directly with increasing maternal age in both the residential areas (Table 3.C.2 and Fig. 3.C.2).

165

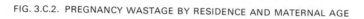

FIG. 3.C.2. PREGNANCY WASTAGE BY RESIDENCE AND MATERNAL AGE

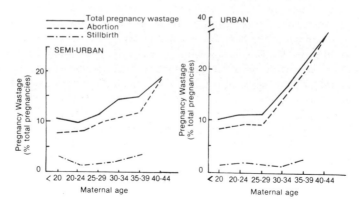

TABLE 3.C.2. PREGNANCY OUTCOME BY RESIDENCE, SOCIAL STATUS, AND MATERNAL AGE*

Residence, social status, and maternal age	Total no. of pregnancies	Pregnancy outcome as percentage of all pregnancies			
		Live births	Stillbirths	Abortions	Pregnancy wastage
Semi-urban					
Middle status					
<20	1414	89.0	2.5	8.5	10.9
20–24	2027	88.9	2.1	9.0	11.1
25–29	1414	86.9	2.3	10.8	13.1
30–34	712	81.3	2.8	15.9	18.7
35–39	204	80.4	3.9	15.7	19.6
40–44	15	(73.3)	—	(26.7)	(26.7)
All ages	5786	87.2	2.4	10.4	12.8
Low status					
<20	1845	89.2	3.2	7.5	10.8
20–24	2319	90.6	1.6	7.5	9.1
25–29	1727	89.5	1.8	8.7	10.5
30–34	886	89.3	2.2	8.5	10.7
35–39	327	86.5	3.1	10.4	13.5
40–44	31	83.8	—	16.2	16.2
All ages	7135	89.7	2.2	8.1	10.3
Both social groups					
<20	3259	89.1	2.9	7.9	10.9
20–24	4346	89.9	1.8	8.2	10.1
25–29	3141	88.4	2.0	9.6	11.6
30–34	1598	85.7	2.5	11.8	14.3
35–39	531	84.2	3.4	12.4	15.8
40–44	46	80.4	—	19.6	19.6
All ages	12921	88.6	2.3	9.1	11.4

TABLE 3.C.2. PREGNANCY OUTCOME BY RESIDENCE, SOCIAL STATUS, AND MATERNAL AGE*

Residence, social status, and maternal age	Total no. of pregnancies	Pregnancy outcome as percentage of all pregnancies			
		Live births	Stillbirths	Abortions	Pregnancy wastage
Urban					
Middle status					
<20	2159	89.7	1.6	8.7	10.3
20–24	3789	88.5	2.2	9.3	11.4
25–29	2625	88.4	1.7	9.8	11.6
30–34	1256	83.5	1.6	14.9	16.5
35–39	363	75.7	3.1	21.2	24.3
40–44	25	60.0	—	40.0	40.2
All ages	10217	87.6	1.9	10.5	12.4
Low status					
<20	288	90.0	2.0	8.0	10.1
20–24	356	89.9	1.4	8.7	10.1
25–29	238	91.6	2.9	5.5	8.4
30–34	138	89.9	2.2	8.0	10.2
35–39	51	92.2	3.9	3.9	7.8
40–44	4	(75.0)	—	(25.0)	(25.0)
All ages	1075	90.3	2.1	7.5	9.7
Both social groups					
<20	2447	89.7	1.6	8.6	10.2
20–24	4145	88.6	2.1	9.3	11.4
25–29	2863	88.7	1.8	9.5	11.3
30–34	1394	84.1	1.6	14.2	15.9
35–39	414	77.8	3.1	19.1	22.2
40–44	29	62.1	—	37.9	37.9
All ages	11292	87.8	1.9	10.3	12.1

* Numbers in parentheses refer to fewer than 25 eligible women.

The ratio of stillbirths to the total number of live births was 2.3%. In the urban and semi-urban areas the corresponding proportions were 2.1% and 2.5%, respectively. The pattern of stillbirths by maternal age was found to be J-shaped in the semi-urban area whereas an increase with age was noted for the urban area (Table 3.C.3 and Fig. 3.C.3).

To examine the possibility of memory lapses, the outcome of the last pregnancy was studied separately. Fig. 3.C.4 compares the patterns of wastage for the last pregnancy and for the total number of pregnancies in relation to maternal age and pregnancy order. The trends conform fairly closely, suggesting that underreporting was more or less uniform, and the association between pregnancy wastage and family formation is a reasonable reflection of the state of affairs when women recall their past experiences. On the figures for maternal age, the rates for the last pregnancy are lower than those for total experience, which may be a reflection of improved health conditions for the most recent pregnancy.

167

TABLE 3.C.3. STILLBIRTHS AS A PERCENTAGE OF TOTAL BIRTHS, BY RESIDENCE AND MATERNAL AGE

Maternal age	Semi-urban		Urban		Both areas	
	Total births	Stillbirths (%)	Total births	Stillbirths (%)	Total births	Stillbirths (%)
< 20	3001	3.2	2236	1.8	5237	2.6
20–24	3989	2.0	3761	2.3	7750	2.1
25–29	2838	2.2	2592	2.0	5430	2.1
30–34	1410	2.8	1196	1.9	2606	2.4
35–39	465	3.9	335	3.9	800	3.9
40–44	37	0.0	18	0.0	55	0.0

FIG. 3.C.3. STILLBIRTHS AS A PERCENTAGE OF TOTAL BIRTHS, BY RESIDENCE AND MATERNAL AGE

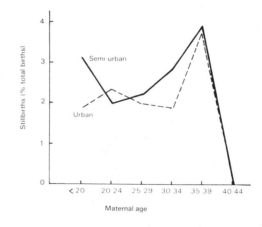

Pregnancy Outcome and Pregnancy Order

Table 3.C.4 depicts pregnancy outcome by residence and pregnancy order. The findings indicate that on the whole, pregnancy wastage increased with increase in pregnancy order.

The rise in pregnancy wastage was due mainly to the increase in abortions. The table indicates that the proportion of abortions increased with increase in pregnancy order whereas the proportion of stillbirths showed no such trend. On passing from pregnancy order 1 to pregnancy order 10 or more, the proportion of abortions increased from 6.3% to 18.6% in the semi-urban area and from 7.8% to 25.1% in the urban area, respectively (Table 3.C.4 and Fig. 3.C.4).

In the semi-urban area, stillbirth rates demonstrated a U-shaped relationship with pregnancy order (i.e., high stillbirth rates were associated with pregnancy orders 1 and 4 and over). In the urban area, there was a progressive increase in stillbirth rates with pregnancy order.

168

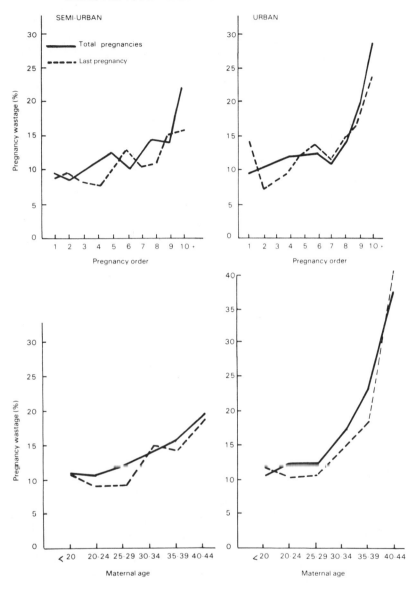

FIG. 3.C.4. PREGNANCY WASTAGE BY RESIDENCE, MATERNAL AGE, AND PREGNANCY ORDER, FOR TOTAL PREGNANCIES AND FOR LAST PREGNANCY

Pregnancy Wastage by Pregnancy Order and Maternal Age

Table 3.C.5 shows the pregnancy wastage by pregnancy order and maternal age. Controlling for the age of the mothers, the pregnancy wastage increased with increased pregnancy order. However, some deviations and a see-saw pattern have been observed in the higher age groups which may be due to the very small numbers involved.

169

TABLE 3.C.4. PREGNANCY OUTCOME BY RESIDENCE AND PREGNANCY ORDER

Residence	Pregnancy order	Total no. of pregnancies	Pregnancy outcome as percentage of total pregnancies			
			Live births	Stillbirths	Abortions	Pregnancy wastage
Semi-urban						
	1	2215	90.6	3.1	6.3	9.4
	2	2038	91.6	1.9	6.5	8.4
	3	1836	90.3	1.7	7.9	9.6
	4	1634	88.6	2.3	9.1	11.4
	5	1400	87.6	2.2	10.2	12.3
	6	1140	87.3	1.7	10.8	12.6
	7	881	87.7	2.0	10.2	12.2
	8	648	85.1	2.3	12.5	14.8
	9	451	85.8	2.7	11.5	14.2
	10 or more	678	77.9	3.5	18.6	22.1
	Total	12921	88.6	2.3	9.1	11.4
Urban						
	1	2260	90.5	1.6	7.8	9.5
	2	2013	89.7	1.9	8.4	10.3
	3	1692	88.6	1.9	9.5	11.4
	4	1382	88.4	1.3	10.3	11.6
	5	1102	87.5	1.9	10.6	12.5
	6	874	87.4	1.8	10.7	12.6
	7	665	89.0	0.9	10.1	11.0
	8	486	85.6	3.7	10.7	14.4
	9	323	81.1	3.4	15.4	18.9
	10 or more	495	71.3	3.6	25.1	28.7
	Total	11292	87.9	1.9	10.2	12.1

TABLE 3.C.5. PREGNANCY WASTAGE BY PREGNANCY ORDER AND MATERNAL AGE

Residence and maternal age	Pregnancy wastage (%) for pregnancy order:					
	1	2	3	4	5	6 and over
Semi-urban						
<20	9.6	10.7	11.9	19.0	20.9	14.3
20–24	8.8	5.6	9.4	11.3	13.0	16.6
25–29	2.9	7.4	15.4	9.1	14.0	13.4
30–34	—	10.6	9.4	9.8	9.8	15.3
35–44	—	—	—	15.4	5.2	16.2
Urban						
<20	8.2	11.9	13.3	16.5	20.0	—
20–24	10.8	8.7	11.6	12.2	14.1	15.5
25–29	11.9	11.2	9.8	8.8	10.6	13.3
30–34	19.0	15.8	4.0	14.8	13.2	16.8
35–44	—	40.0	42.9	20.0	17.6	22.2

At almost all pregnancy orders, the wastage rate was high for mothers of age less than 20, and then decreased for mothers of ages 20–24 and 25–29 years. In both urban and semi-urban areas, these two age groups consistently showed the lowest wastage rates (Table 3.C.5 and Fig. 3.C.5).

Pregnancy Wastage by Preceding Pregnancy Interval

The data presented in Table 3.C.6 show that the risk of pregnancy wastage was highest when the interval between the two pregnancies was short. Total

TABLE 3.C.6. PREGNANCY OUTCOME BY DURATION OF PRECEDING PREGNANCY INTERVAL FOR BOTH RESIDENTIAL AREAS COMBINED

Preceding pregnancy interval (years)	Pregnancy outcome as percentage of total pregnancies			Total pregnancies other than the first
	Stillbirths	Abortions	Total pregnancy wastage	
<1	1.3	61.9	63.2	543
1–2	3.0	14.7	7.7	6939
2–3	1.7	5.6	7.3	7443
3–4	1.0	4.8	5.8	2653
4–5	1.0	4.1	5.1	1153
5–6	1.9	4.9	6.8	485
6 and over	2.2	8.4	10.6	462

FIG. 3.C.5. PREGNANCY WASTAGE BY RESIDENCE, MATERNAL AGE, AND PREGNANCY ORDER

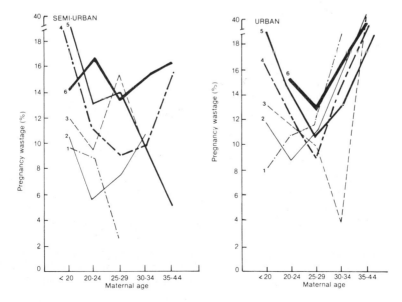

171

pregnancy wastage was very high (63.2%) when the preceding pregnancy interval was less than one year; the rate then dropped steeply to 7.7% for an interval between 1 and 2 years, and fell further to a minimum of 5.1% for an interval between 4 and 5 years. For longer intervals it increased again. Particularly at higher birth orders, this increase may be attributed to higher age. Thus there appears to be a reverse-J relation between length of preceding pregnancy interval and pregnancy wastage.

FIG. 3.C.6. PREGNANCY WASTAGE BY DURATION OF PRECEDING PREGNANCY INTERVAL FOR BOTH RESIDENTIAL AREAS COMBINED

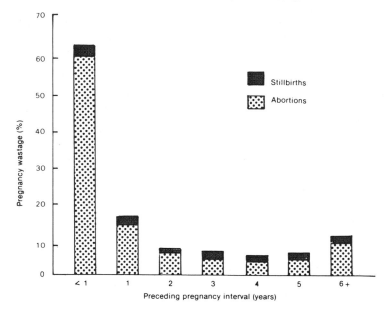

D. SYRIAN ARAB REPUBLIC

G. Ghebe, N. Hallak & A. R. Omran

Pregnancy Outcome

Of the 31 567 pregnancies reported by the 5621 women in the study, 656 (2.1%) terminated in stillbirths and 3029 (9.6%) in abortions. That is, for the eligible women as a whole, 11.7 out of every 100 pregnancies were wasted.

Pregnancy Wastage by Residence and Social Characteristics

Wastage was somewhat lower for Sweida women (10.6%) than for women in other areas. Although the differences were relatively small, women of middle social status within each residential group (except in Sweida) tended to report

172

higher pregnancy wastage rates than those of low social status. The reverse
was observed for Sweida women and their wastage rates for each social status
group were also lower than those of the corresponding social status groups in
other areas (Table 3.D.1).

TABLE 3.D.1. PREGNANCY WASTAGE BY RESIDENCE AND SOCIAL STATUS

Residence and social status	No. of pregnancies	Stillbirths (%)	Abortions (%)
Damascus			
Middle	8466	1.7	11.5
Low	2455	1.6	11.9
Both categories	10921	1.6	11.6
Sweida			
Middle	6856	2.3	8.3
Low	2527	3.8	6.9
Both categories	9383	2.7	7.9
Rural Aleppo			
Middle	3714	2.2	9.3
Low	7549	1.9	9.0
Both categories	11263	2.0	9.1

Stillbirth rates were lower in Damascus than in the other areas. The reverse
was true for abortion rates. The stillbirth rate was higher among the low than
among the high social status groups in Sweida, while the differences between
the other two residential areas were small. On the other hand, abortion was
higher in the middle status than in the low status groups in the small towns,
while the differences between the social status groups in the other areas were
small.

Pregnancy Wastage and Maternal Age

The results showed a characteristic relationship between pregnancy wastage
and maternal age. In all residential areas, starting at a relatively high rate for
women under 20 years, pregnancy wastage rates first declined with age and
then rose to a level higher than the initial rate to give a J-shaped curve (Table
3.D.2 and Fig. 3.D.1). This was also generally true for both components of
wastage, namely stillbirths and abortions. At all maternal ages, Damascus
reported higher wastage rates than the other two residential areas, which had
more or less similar rates. The maternal age group associated with the lowest
risks of wastage was 20–24 for women of all residential areas. No definite
trends in pregnancy wastage were evident among different social status groups
(Table 3.D.2 and Fig. 3.D.2).

The greater part of pregnancy wastage was accounted for by abortions.
Abortion rates showed a J-shaped relationship to maternal age in all three
residential areas, with the large city rates being higher than the rates for the
other areas. For all maternal ages, the middle status women in Sweida tended

173

TABLE 3.D.2. PREGNANCY OUTCOME BY RESIDENCE, SOCIAL STATUS, AND MATERNAL AGE

Residence, social status, and maternal age	Total no. of pregnancies	Pregnancy outcome as percentage of all pregnancies			
		Live births	Stillbirths	Abortions	Pregnancy wastage
Damascus					
Middle					
<20	1615	88.6	2.1	9.2	11.3
20–24	2773	89.1	1.5	9.4	10.9
25–29	2194	86.3	1.5	12.2	13.7
30–34	1256	86.1	1.6	12.3	13.9
35–39	530	77.4	1.3	21.3	22.6
40–44	98	68.4	4.1	27.5	31.6
All ages	8466	86.9	1.6	11.5	13.1
Low					
<20	434	87.1	0.9	12.0	12.9
20–24	716	86.9	1.4	11.7	13.1
25–29	592	89.7	2.5	7.8	10.3
30–34	441	88.2	1.1	10.7	11.8
35–39	214	87.5	1.4	20.1	21.5
40–44	58	62.1	3.4	34.5	37.9
All ages	2455	86.5	1.6	11.9	13.5
Both categories					
<20	2049	88.3	1.9	9.8	11.7
20–24	3489	88.7	1.5	9.9	11.4
25–24	2786	87.0	1.8	11.2	13.0
30–34	1697	86.6	1.5	11.9	13.4
35–39	744	77.7	1.3	21.0	22.3
40–44	156	66.0	3.8	30.1	33.9
All ages	10921	86.8	1.6	11.6	13.2
Sweida					
Middle					
<20	1194	89.5	2.3	8.2	10.5
20–24	2249	92.0	2.0	6.0	8.0
25–29	1791	90.5	2.0	7.5	9.5
30–34	1083	86.7	3.0	10.3	13.3
35–39	444	82.9	3.2	14.0	17.2
40–44	95	67.4	3.2	29.5	32.7
All ages	6856	89.4	2.3	8.3	10.6
Low					
<20	345	89.6	3.8	6.7	10.5
20–24	729	91.5	3.3	5.2	8.5
25–29	648	89.8	4.3	5.9	10.2
30–34	487	88.7	4.5	6.8	11.3
35–39	256	84.4	3.1	12.5	15.6
40–44	62	79.0	3.2	17.7	20.9
All ages	2527	89.2	3.8	6.9	10.7
Both categories					
<20	1539	89.5	2.6	7.9	10.5
20–24	2978	91.9	2.3	5.8	8.1
25–29	2439	90.3	2.6	7.1	9.7
30–34	1570	87.3	3.4	9.2	12.6
35–39	700	83.4	3.1	13.4	16.5
40–44	157	72.0	3.2	24.8	28
All ages	9383	89.4	2.7	7.9	10.6

TABLE 3.D.2 (continued)

Residence, social status, and maternal age	Total no. of pregnancies	Pregnancy outcome as percentage of all pregnancies			
		Live births	Stillbirths	Abortions	Pregnancy wastage
Rural Aleppo					
Middle					
<20	746	88.5	2.7	8.8	11.6
20–24	1206	91.9	2.2	6.0	8.2
25–29	863	88.6	1.7	9.6	11.3
30–34	549	87.1	1.8	11.1	12.9
35–39	281	84.0	2.1	13.9	16.0
40–44	69	59.4	4.3	36.2	40.5
All ages	3714	88.5	2.2	9.3	11.5
Low					
<20	1274	90.5	2.5	7.0	9.5
20–24	2254	91.1	1.6	7.4	9.0
25–29	1884	90.6	1.7	7.7	9.4
30–34	1327	86.9	2.0	11.2	13.2
35–39	645	82.3	2.2	15.5	17.7
40–44	165	80.0	3.0	17.0	20.0
All ages	7549	89.1	1.9	9.0	10.9
Both categories					
<20	2020	89.8	2.6	7.7	10.3
20–24	3460	91.4	1.8	6.9	8.7
25–29	2747	90.0	1.7	8.3	10.0
30–34	1876	86.9	1.9	11.1	13.0
35–39	926	82.8	2.2	15.0	17.2
40–44	234	73.9	3.4	22.6	26.0
All ages	11263	88.9	2.0	9.1	11.1

to have higher abortion rates than low status women. In the other residential areas, no well-defined trend was evident.

The pattern of stillbirths was also noteworthy. Women in the small towns had somewhat higher stillbirth rates than did the others. In all residential areas, the highest stillbirth rates occurred among women who were less than 20 or over 40 years of age.

When stillbirths were calculated as a percentage of total births, a notable increase occurred in the age-group 40–44 (Table 3.D.3 and Fig. 3.D.3).

To examine the possibility that the findings may have been biased by selective underreporting or memory lapses, the outcome of the last (and most easily remembered) pregnancy was analysed separately. As shown in Fig. 3.D.4, the patterns for pregnancy wastage by maternal age were similar for the last pregnancy to those for total pregnancies. This suggests that underreporting was more or less uniform and that the pattern of association of pregnancy wastage with family formation may not have been unduly distorted.

175

FIG. 3.D.1. PREGNANCY WASTAGE BY RESIDENCE AND MATERNAL AGE

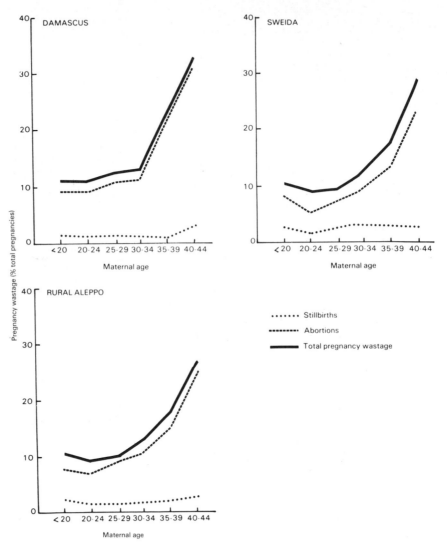

.... Stillbirths
--------- Abortions
━━━━━━━ Total pregnancy wastage

FIG. 3.D.2. PREGNANCY WASTAGE BY RESIDENCE, MATERNAL AGE, AND SOCIAL STATUS

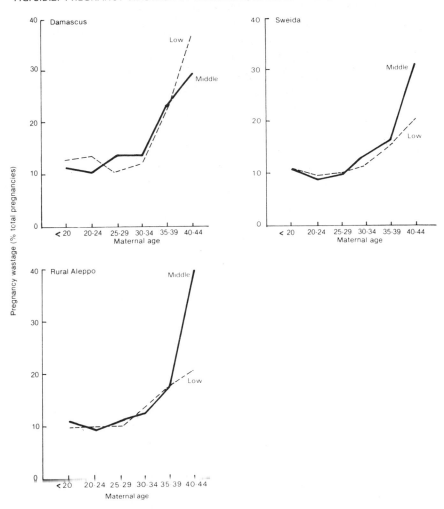

TABLE 3.D.3. STILLBIRTHS AS A PERCENTAGE OF TOTAL BIRTHS BY RESIDENCE AND
MATERNAL AGE

Maternal age	Damascus		Sweida		Rural Aleppo	
	Total births	Stillbirths (%)	Total births	Stillbirths (%)	Total births	Stillbirths (%)
<20	1848	2.1	1418	2.8	1865	2.8
20–24	3145	1.6	2805	2.4	3222	1.9
25–29	2473	2.0	2267	2.8	2519	1.9
30–34	1495	1.7	1425	3.8	1667	2.2
35–39	588	1.7	606	3.6	787	2.5
40–44	109	5.5	118	4.2	181	4.4

177

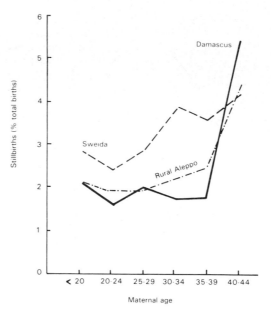

It is noteworthy that pregnancy wastage was high among mothers of younger age (under twenty), dropped among those aged 20–24, then increased gradually with increasing age of the mother, as shown in Tables 3.D.2 and 3.D.3. The same trend is shown also in Tables 3.D.4 and 3.D.5, which relate pregnancy wastage to pregnancy order, which in turn is parallel to the functional as well as to the chronological age of the mother. This phenomenon might be explained by the viability of the zygote, genotype changes with age, and maturity or degeneration of the endometrium. The histological biochemical, and functional changes of the endometrium vary; it might show prematurity among teenagers or degeneration at advanced ages. Such features of the maternal endometrium might be detrimental to the viability of the implanted zygote or might act as a mutagenic factor producing lethal genotyping of the zygote. Either phenomenon would terminate pregnancy early and result in pregnancy wastage.

Pregnancy Wastage and Pregnancy Order

Despite the fluctuations observed, the curve relating pregnancy wastage to pregnancy order exhibited a flattened J-shape in all residential groups, but the rates were higher for Damascus women than for women of the other residential

178

FIG. 3.D.4. PREGNANCY WASTAGE BY RESIDENCE, MATERNAL AGE, AND PREGNANCY
ORDER FOR TOTAL PREGNANCIES AND FOR LAST PREGNANCY

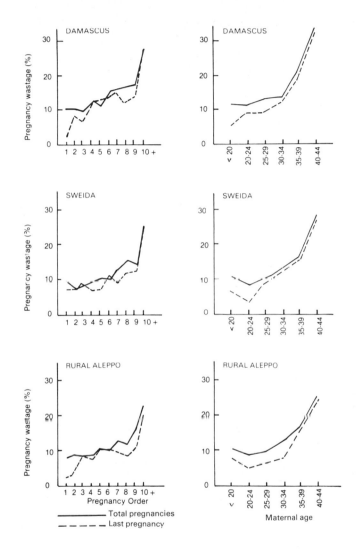

179

TABLE 3.D.4. PREGNANCY OUTCOME BY RESIDENCE AND PREGNANCY ORDER

Residence	Pregnancy order	Total no. of pregnancies	Pregnancy outcome as percentage of total pregnancies			
			Live births	Stillbirths	Abortions	Pregnancy wastage
Damascus						
	1	1837	89.6	2.2	8.2	10.4
	2	1690	89.9	1.7	8.4	10.1
	3	1534	90.5	1.4	8.0	9.4
	4	1327	88.3	1.4	10.3	11.7
	5	1120	87.0	1.0	12.1	13.1
	6	926	85.0	2.1	13.0	15.1
	7	740	84.1	1.1	14.9	16.0
	8	564	83.3	1.8	14.9	16.7
	9	414	83.1	1.2	15.7	16.9
	10 and over	769	72.3	2.1	25.6	27.7
Sweida						
	1	1604	90.5	3.3	6.2	9.5
	2	1490	92.8	1.5	5.6	7.1
	3	1340	91.9	2.4	5.7	8.1
	4	1180	91.1	2.2	6.7	8.9
	5	978	90.0	2.2	7.8	10.0
	6	815	89.0	2.7	8.3	10.0
	7	618	87.1	3.6	9.4	13.0
	8	485	84.5	4.3	11.1	15.4
	9	352	84.4	4.0	11.6	14.6
	10 and over	521	75.6	3.5	20.9	24.4
Rural Aleppo						
	1	1752	91.7	2.6	5.8	8.4
	2	1610	91.1	2.2	6.6	8.8
	3	1436	91.6	1.9	6.5	8.4
	4	1281	91.2	2.0	6.8	8.8
	5	1152	89.1	1.6	9.2	10.8
	6	1016	90.1	1.2	8.8	10.0
	7	834	87.2	1.0	11.9	12.9
	8	676	88.3	1.2	10.5	11.7
	9	516	84.3	1.9	13.8	15.7
	10 and over	990	76.8	3.2	20.0	23.2

groups (Table 3.D.4 and Fig. 3.D.5). Although this pattern was again due to the abortion figures, which formed the main component of pregnancy wastage rates, the stillbirth rates followed the same pattern.

Again, the last pregnancy was analysed separately and, as with maternal age, the pattern of the relationship between birth order and outcome of the last pregnancy was similar to that between birth order and outcome of total pregnancies (Fig. 3.D.4).

180

TABLE 3.D.5 PREGNANCY WASTAGE BY PREGNANCY ORDER AND MATERNAL AGE

Residence and maternal age	Pregnancy wastage (%) for pregnancy order:					
	1	2	3	4	5	6 and over
Damascus						
<20	11.0	11.5	13.2	13.6	23.5	0
20–24	8.5	8.8	8.8	12.4	14.5	23.6
25–29	13.5	9.9	7.5	10.4	11.0	17.8
30–34	10.0	13.2	10.7	7.5	12.4	14.0
35–44	7.7	15.4	10.5	25.0	22.2	25.2
Sweida						
<20	10.4	8.1	11.5	19.6	33.3	50.0
20–24	7.1	6.6	6.9	7.9	9.3	19.9
25–29	11.2	7.1	8.0	8.8	8.0	12.5
30–34	7.4	7.5	10.9	8.7	10.6	14.0
35–44	40.0	8.3	20.0	10.7	18.2	18.7
Rural Aleppo						
<20	8.9	11.4	11.1	18.4	20.0	0
20–24	6.9	6.9	7.8	8.8	12.6	15.0
25–29	9.1	8.2	7.5	7.5	10.4	11.9
30–34	5.9	12.5	13.7	12.2	7.3	13.9
35–44	25.0	0	7.7	7.7	14.7	19.4

Wastage by both Pregnancy Order and Maternal Age

When pregnancy order was held constant, a J- or U-shaped relationship was found between pregnancy wastage and maternal age in all three residential areas. This means that teenage pregnancies and pregnancies at age 35 and over had poorer outcomes than pregnancies at intermediate ages. When maternal age was kept constant, there was an increase in the risk of wastage with increasing pregnancy order. Occasionally, there was also an increased risk for first pregnancies.

Pregnancy wastage by both pregnancy and maternal age is shown in Table 3.D.5.

Pregnancy Wastage by Preceding Pregnancy Interval

Preceding pregnancy interval is defined as the period between the end of the preceding pregnancy and the end of the index pregnancy. Hence, the first pregnancy must be excluded from the analysis. As shown in Table 3.D.6, the risk of poor pregnancy outcome was highest when the interval was less than 1 year (22.8%), and dropped steeply for intervals between 1 and 2 years (7.6%) and between 2 and 3 years (4.6%). Thereafter, the risk increased gradually, giving a U-shaped relationship between pregnancy wastage and preceding pregnancy interval (Fig. 3.D.6).

181

FIG. 3.D.5. PREGNANCY WASTAGE BY RESIDENCE AND PREGNANCY ORDER

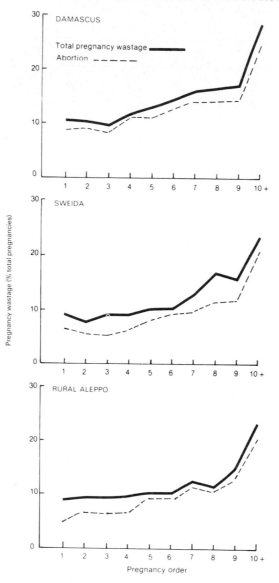

A higher proportion of pregnancies terminated in abortions when the preceding pregnancy interval was less than 1 year. It should be noted, however, that a preceding interval was, by definition, shorter after an abortion than it otherwise would have been if the index pregnancy had been carried to term. Although the U-shaped relationship was mostly accounted for by abortions, stillbirths were highest when the interval was less than 1 year (2.6%) and between 4 and 5 years (2.3%).

TABLE 3.D.6. PREGNANCY WASTAGE BY DURATION OF PRECEDING PREGNANCY INTERVAL
FOR ALL RESIDENTIAL AREAS COMBINED

Preceding pregnancy interval (years)	Pregnancy outcome as percentage of total pregnancies			Total pregnancies other than the first
	Stillbirths	Abortions	Total pregnancy wastage	
<1	2.6	20.2	22.8	8510
1–2	1.8	5.8	7.6	12517
2–3	1.0	3.6	4.6	3814
3–4	1.6	5.2	6.8	866
4–5	2.3	6.0	8.3	298
5–6	2.2	8.1	10.3	136
6 and over	0.6	11.5	12.1	157

FIG. 3.D.6. PREGNANCY WASTAGE BY DURATION OF PRECEDING PREGNANCY INTERVAL
FOR ALL RESIDENTIAL AREAS COMBINED

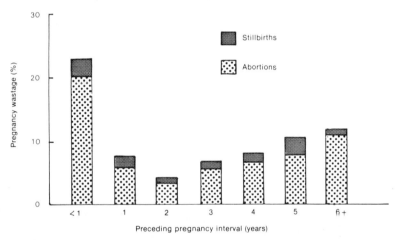

Short birth intervals usually mean poor restoration of body resources. When this is accompanied by breastfeeding, further depletion of maternal resources occurs, especially in poor women whose nutrition is inadequate with regard to animal protein supplies. Under such circumstances pregnancy wastage may increase.

Chapter Four

FAMILY FORMATION
AND CHILDHOOD MORTALITY

INTRODUCTION

M. R. Bone, C. C. Standley & A. R. Omran

In the present chapter the relationship between family formation variables and child mortality is examined for 5 periods of risk: the first month; the second to the eleventh month; the first year; the first to the fifth year; and the first 5 years of life, the object being to find out whether the relationships discovered elsewhere also held for the participating areas.

The family formation variables are those already referred to: maternal age, birth order, and preceding pregnancy interval. The data concerned were collected from each eligible woman at interview as an extension of the detailed pregnancy history mentioned in the Introduction to chapter 3. For each live birth, the informant was asked whether the child was still living, and, if not, how long after birth it had died.

The problems of analysis and interpretation are for the most part similar to those described for pregnancy outcome.

The difficulties created by the interrelationships among family formation variables need not be discussed again here. It has to be remembered, however, that, as in all retrospective pregnancy history studies, the child mortality rates derived differ from those obtained in conventional demographic studies. In particular, infant mortality rates are usually based on the total live births occurring in a defined population during one calendar year. Those in the present enquiry are based, instead, on the number of children ever born to the eligible women. The study mortality rates differ from conventional rates in the following ways:

1. Live births to the eligible women exclude some births occurring in the area population during a given time period but include others: births to non-eligible women (e.g., those now dead or too old) that took place during the same period and in the same area are excluded; conversely, births to eligible women who were living outside the area at the time are included.

2. During the period of some 30 years over which the births occurred, the risks may have changed. This not only complicates comparisons between the study rates and conventional mortality rates, but may also distort the relationships between mortality and the family formation variables. An attempt has been made to overcome this problem by considering only births that occurred in the last 10 years.

3. All births for each eligible woman are included, which means that the more fertile the women, the larger their contribution to the results. If the risks of a chiid's dying are related to the mother's fertility, then death rates based on all births that have ever occurred in a population of women will differ from those that would have been derived from births occurring in a specific year (even if the risks did not change over time).

4. Another problem common to most child mortality studies is that mortality rates are shown for risk periods of 1 month, 1 year, and 5 years following birth. Whilst the great majority of births will have occurred more than one year before the interview and almost all more than one month previously, a considerable proportion will have taken place within the preceding 5 years. Children born less than 5 years before the interview will not have been exposed to the hazard of death for 5 full years; if they are only 4 years old, for example, they may yet die before their 5th birthday. It is especially for the 1–4-year period that the rates may be artificially low.

5. The retrospective nature of the enquiry means that some underreporting of births—particularly those of children who died shortly after birth—is probable. However, this is likely to be less than in the case of pregnancies, and a comparison between mortality for recent births and that for all births did not suggest selective underreporting of earlier deaths. In most cases, as will be shown, there appeared to have been a decline in child mortality over the generations. Such a decline would not be detectable had there been gross underreporting of earlier deaths. Moreover, a prospective study being undertaken in Gandhigram supports the evidence of the present study.

The investigators were well aware from the outset of the above considerations and of the fact they not only render comparisons with conventional mortality rates difficult but also complicate the relationships to be examined and qualify the comparisons made between subgroups. In the analyses in chapter 4 an attempt is made, wherever possible, to disentangle the relationships of interest by holding the confounding factors constant.

The difficulties are best illustrated in the case of preceding pregnancy interval. Generally, mortality rates decline as the preceding pregnancy interval lengthens. The question of interest is whether a short preceding interval depresses a child's chances of survival. For instance, the duration of interpregnancy intervals is related to maternal age, which is related, in turn, to child mortality; it is the youngest mothers who are most likely to experience the shortest intervals, as was confirmed in the samples investigated. It is therefore necessary to hold maternal age constant if one wishes to discover the relationship between interval length and mortality. But interval length is also likely to be related to parity. Women who have many births are likely to have shorter interpregnancy intervals than those who have few. Hence, parity, or birth order, must also be controlled.

A third problem, which is particularly troublesome when carrying out retrospective studies, arises from the relationship of interval length to the age of the preceding child at death. If it died soon after birth, the next pregnancy is likely to occur earlier than it would have done if the preceding child had survived longer. This may in part be voluntary, as an attempt to replace the dead child, and in part physiological, since if breastfeeding (but not contraception) is commonly practised in the area, its curtailment in the case of a child who dies young will also curtail the period of postpartum sterility. This is relevant to the present problem if a child's chances of survival are related to the survival of preceding children born to the same woman. That is to say, some women may experience short intervals because their children die young and not vice versa, a question discussed in more detail in chapter 8. As shown in chapter 7, interpregnancy intervals following the birth of children who died within a month were indeed considerably more likely to be short (under 1 year or between 1 and 2 years) than those succeeding the birth of a child who survived until the date of interview. The problem in a retrospective study is complicated by the possibility that short intervals for women who frequently lose children unduly weight the total of short intervals: it may be the repeated experience of poor reproducers and not the short intervals that determines the pattern. In order to examine this possibility it would also be necessary to control the outcome of the preceding pregnancy.

A further difficulty arises from the retrospective nature of the enquiry. Since, on average, the shortest interpregnancy intervals occur to the youngest mothers and many of the women were no longer young when interviewed, the information often related to pregnancies that had occurred years before. Because there is evidence in some areas that child mortality rates have declined over the years, a disproportionate number of these pregnancies, compared with those to older women having longer interpregnancy intervals, will have been subject to the higher risks of death prevailing at an earlier period. Consequently, the relationship found between child mortality and preceding pregnancy interval cannot be taken by itself as evidence that short preceding intervals hamper children's chances of survival.

One factor that may confound these relationships is possible changes in child mortality risks during the women's lifetime. In an attempt to mitigate the effects of such changes, analyses have also been made of data relating only to pregnancies occurring within the 10 years preceding interview. Since neither the date of birth nor the date of the interview was recorded, this 10-year period was situated approximately from the women's age at interview and the ages at which they had experienced their pregnancies. Thus, for a woman aged 30–34 at interview, pregnancies during the preceding 10 years were taken as those occurring while she was in the age groups 25–29 and 30–34.

Although this procedure reduced the distortion resulting from changes in mortality over time, it does increase that due to truncated risk periods. That is, the proportion of children born less than 1 month, 1 year, or 5 years before interview is greater amongst the births of the previous 10 years than amongst all births. The effect is to reduce death rates below what they will eventually be to a greater extent among children born in the last 10 years than in the case of all births. The artefactual reduction in mortality will be greatest for deaths under 5 years and least for those under 1 month.

At the beginning of each area report, the proportions of the women's children who had died within the specified risk periods are given for the area samples. These are of immediate interest, and where there are differences between groups the question arises whether these are due to differences in family formation patterns or are of cultural origin. The cultural differences may themselves be related to socioeconomic circumstances, as expressed by social status, for which mortality rates are also given.

If the differences between groups are entirely due to family formation variables, then, when these are controlled, there should be no difference between cultural groups. Other things being equal, mortality for each maternal age group, as well as the pattern of their relationship, should be identical. In fact, other things are not equal and, as already discussed, it is not possible to hold constant all the other variables concerned: if birth order, preceding birth interval, and time were all to be controlled, subgroups would dwindle to negligible numbers. We can therefore only begin to examine the question by finding out, for example, whether the differences between subgroups are maintained when child mortality rates are made specific for maternal age.

This consideration also applies to comparisons between the participating areas, and, of course, to any made between them and data from other investigations.

A. COLOMBIA

A. Gil, G. Ochoa & A. R. Omran

Child Mortality by Residence and Social Status

The 5270 eligible women in the study reported a total of 19 768 live births over their years of marriage. Of these live births, 2% died within the first month of life, 3.8% during the first year, and 4.9% during the first 5 years.

Child mortality for all social status groups and for all periods of risk was higher in the NSZ than in the OUZ; the rates for mortality under 5 years were 5.7% and 3.7%, respectively (Table 4.A.1 and Fig. 4.A.1). In other words, there was a difference of two child deaths per 100 reported live births. The differences between the OUZ and the NSZ and between social status groups were very small for mortality under 1 month (neonatal) and became much more marked for older ages. The differences by social class were not as large as expected.

188

TABLE 4.A.1. CHILD MORTALITY BY RESIDENCE AND SOCIAL STATUS

Residence and social status	Deaths per 100 reported live births at:					Total reported live births
	<1 month	1–11 months	<1 year	1–4 years	<5 years	
Old urban zone						
Middle	1.9	1.1	3.0	0.6	3.6	7771
Low	1.8	1.6	3.4	1.5	4.9	616
All OUZ	1.9	1.2	3.1	0.6	3.7	8387
Newly settled zone						
Middle	2.3	2.1	4.4	1.3	5.7	3211
Low	1.9	2.3	4.2	1.3	5.5	8170
All NSZ	2.0	2.3	4.3	1.4	5.7	11381

FIG. 4.A.1. CHILD MORTALITY BY RESIDENCE AND SOCIAL STATUS

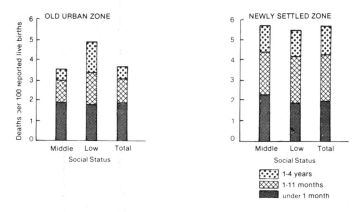

Child Mortality and Maternal Age

For both regions, the risk of child mortality was high for women less than 20 years old and did not change significantly for older women.

For most maternal ages, mortality among the children of women in the NSZ was higher than among those of women in the OUZ. This is readily evident when the figures for mortality under 5 are compared (Table 4.A.2).

One of the factors that may affect the association between childhood mortality and maternal age is the change in mortality risk over time. Births in the study population occurred over a period of 30 years preceding the interview. Some of the births delivered by women when they were under 20 years of age occurred up to 30 years before the interview, whereas births delivered by women at maternal age of 40 and over had taken place within the preceding 5 years. It is therefore informative to analyse the data according to both maternal age (or age of woman at the birth of the child) and current age or age of the woman at the time of the interview.

189

TABLE 4.A.2. CHILD MORTALITY BY RESIDENCE AND MATERNAL AGE (TOTAL EXPERIENCE)

Residence and maternal age	Reported live births	Deaths per 100 reported live births at:				
		<1 month	1–11 months	<1 year	1–4 years	<5 years
Old urban zone						
<20	1196	2.2	1.3	3.5	0.7	4.1
20–24	3216	1.8	1.1	2.9	0.8	3.7
25–29	2469	1.5	1.0	2.5	0.5	3.0
30–34	1140	2.5	1.4	3.9	0.6	4.5
35–39	320	2.2	0.9	3.1	0.6	3.7
40–44	38	5.3	0.0	5.3	2.6	7.9
All OUZ	8379	1.9	1.2	3.1	0.6	3.7
Newly settled zone						
<20	1699	2.5	2.2	4.7	2.1	6.8
20–24	4112	2.0	2.4	4.4	1.6	6.0
25–29	3191	1.7	2.1	3.8	0.9	4.7
30–34	1707	2.3	2.1	4.4	1.2	5.6
35–39	595	1.8	2.5	4.3	1.2	5.5
40–44	74	2.7	0.0	2.7	0.0	2.7
All NSZ	11378	2.0	2.3	4.3	1.4	5.7

Table 4.A.3 shows the rates of child mortality according to maternal age and the age of the mother at interview for 3 age groups as follows: (1) less than 25, (2) those from 25–34 years, and (3) those aged 35 and over. In this way, an approximate control is introduced for changes in risk factors over time.

It is evident from the table that the child mortality rates have declined over the last 10 years, especially in the NSZ. For example, women in the NSZ over 35 years of age at interview had lost, within one month of birth, 2.5% of the children born to them when they were under 25, while those women under 25 years of age at interview had lost only 1.5% of their children within the first month of life. The pattern in the OUZ was similar, although not consistent.

The direction of the association between child mortality and maternal age can be seen from the figures above the diagonal lines representing mortality among recent births to women of each age group (within the 10 years preceding the interview). The effect of pooling the experience of different generations is shown in the rows for total mortality rates (all age groups pooled).

Using this method of analysis, the mortality experience for children born during the 10 years preceding the interview is shown in Table 4.A.4 and Fig. 4.A.2. The patterns were similar to those for the total child mortality experience, which suggests that the reporting of child mortality in our study population was reasonably reliable. For most age-risk periods in the OUZ, child mortality rates described the characteristic J-shaped relationship with maternal age.

TABLE 4.A.3. CHILD MORTALITY BY MATERNAL AGE, RESIDENCE, AND AGE AT INTERVIEW

Residence and age of child at death	Age of mother at interview	Deaths as percentages of live births at maternal age:		
		<25	25–34	35–44
Old urban zone				
under 1 month	<25	1.5	—	—
	25–34	1.2	0.8	—
	35–44	2.6	2.2	2.5
	Total	1.9	1.8	2.5
1–11 months	<25	0.9	—	—
	25–34	0.9	0.8	—
	35–44	1.5	1.3	0.8
	Total	1.2	1.1	0.8
under 1 year	<25	2.4	—	—
	25–34	2.1	1.6	—
	35–44	4.1	3.5	3.3
	Total	3.1	2.9	3.3
1–4 years	<25	0.0	—	—
	25–34	0.6	0.0	—
	35–44	1.1	0.8	0.8
	Total	0.7	0.6	0.8
under 5 years	<25	2.4	—	—
	25–34	2.7	1.6	—
	35–44	5.2	4.3	4.1
	Total	3.8	3.5	4.1
Newly settled zone				
under 1 month	<25	1.5	—	—
	25–34	2.0	2.1	—
	35–44	2.5	1.8	1.9
	Total	2.1	1.9	1.9
1–11 months	<25	1.3	—	—
	25–34	1.9	0.6	—
	35–44	3.4	2.6	0.2
	Total	2.3	2.1	2.2
under 1 year	<25	2.8	—	—
	25–34	3.9	2.7	—
	35–44	5.9	4.4	4.1
	Total	4.4	4.0	4.1
1–4 years	<25	0.9	—	—
	25–34	1.3	0.4	—
	35–44	2.6	1.2	1.0
	Total	2.7	1.0	1.0
under 5 years	<25	3.7	—	—
	25–34	5.2	3.1	—
	35–44	8.6	5.6	5.1
	Total	6.1	5.0	5.1

TABLE 4.A.4. CHILD MORTALITY DURING THE 10 YEARS PRECEDING THE INTERVIEW, BY RESIDENCE AND MATERNAL AGE

Residence and maternal age	Reported live births	Deaths per 100 reported live births at:				
		<1 month	1–11 months	<1 year	1–4 years	5 years
Old urban zone						
<20	187	2.1	0.5	2.7	0.0	2.7
20–24	987	1.1	0.6	1.7	0.2	1.9
25–29	956	0.6	0.9	1.6	0.0	1.6
30–34	617	2.3	1.1	3.6	0.2	3.7
35–39	320	2.2	0.9	3.1	0.6	3.8
40–44	38	5.3	0.0	5.3	2.6	7.9
All OUZ	3105	1.4	0.8	2.3	0.2	2.5
Newly settled zone						
<20	404	1.7	1.7	3.5	1.2	4.7
20–24	1363	1.2	1.5	2.6	0.9	3.5
25–29	1327	2.2	1.3	3.5	0.1	4.1
30–34	954	1.7	1.3	2.9	0.6	3.6
35–39	595	1.8	2.5	4.4	1.2	5.5
40–44	74	2.7	0.0	2.7	0.0	2.7
All NSZ	4717	1.7	1.5	3.2	0.8	4.0

FIG. 4.A.2. CHILD MORTALITY BY RESIDENCE AND MATERNAL AGE: TOTAL AND DURING PRECEDING 10 YEARS

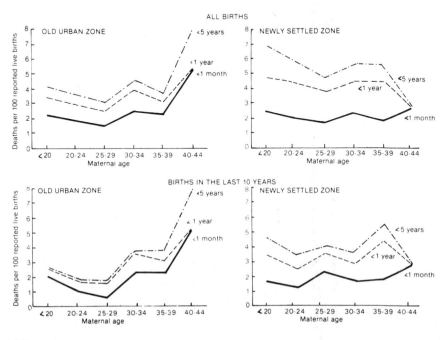

192

Child Mortality and Birth Order

The total pregnancy history experience of the woman and her experience during the 10 years preceding the interview are given in Table 4.A.5 and Fig. 4.A.3. In general, there was increased risk of child mortality for the birth orders higher than the fourth. In some cases, the second child born was at a slightly higher risk of death than either the first- or third-born children. This was particularly evident for neonatal and infant (<1 year) deaths.

TABLE 4.A.5. CHILD MORTALITY BY RESIDENCE AND BIRTH ORDER (TOTAL EXPERIENCE AND BIRTHS WITHIN 10 YEARS PRECEDING INTERVIEW)

Residence and birth order	Reported live births	Deaths per 100 reported live births at:				
		<1 month	1–11 months	<1 year	1–4 years	<5 years
Old urban zone						
Total experience						
1	2379	1.4	0.9	2.3	0.4	2.7
2	1889	1.9	1.1	3.0	0.5	3.5
3	1324	1.5	1.0	2.5	1.1	3.6
4	943	1.5	1.2	2.7	0.9	3.6
5	653	2.1	1.5	3.6	0.6	4.2
6 and over	1191	3.4	1.6	5.0	0.8	5.8
All birth orders	8379	1.9	1.1	3.0	0.7	3.1
Within 10 years preceding interview						
1	948	0.7	0.8	1.6	0.1	1.7
2	704	2.0	0.4	2.4	0.3	2.7
3	437	1.1	0.5	1.6	0.0	1.6
4	302	0.7	1.3	2.0	0.0	2.0
5	223	0.9	0.9	1.8	0.0	1.8
6 and over	491	2.9	1.4	4.3	0.6	4.9
All birth orders	3105	1.4	0.8	2.3	0.2	2.4
Newly settled zone						
Total experience						
1	2420	1.8	1.7	3.5	1.2	4.7
2	2095	2.2	2.0	4.2	1.4	5.6
3	1696	1.6	2.1	3.7	1.7	5.4
4	1365	1.7	2.9	4.6	1.6	6.2
5	1065	2.3	2.3	4.6	1.8	6.4
6 and over	2737	2.4	2.7	5.1	1.1	6.1
All birth orders	11378	2.0	2.3	4.3	1.4	5.7
Within 10 years preceding interview						
1	850	1.5	0.7	2.2	1.1	3.3
2	792	1.5	1.1	2.7	0.8	3.4
3	626	1.3	1.8	3.0	0.5	3.5
4	519	1.9	0.6	2.5	0.6	3.1
5	413	1.9	1.9	3.9	1.7	5.6
6 and over	1517	2.0	2.2	4.2	0.7	5.0
All birth orders	4717	1.7	1.5	3.2	0.8	4.0

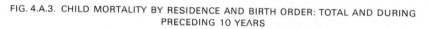

FIG. 4.A.3. CHILD MORTALITY BY RESIDENCE AND BIRTH ORDER: TOTAL AND DURING PRECEDING 10 YEARS

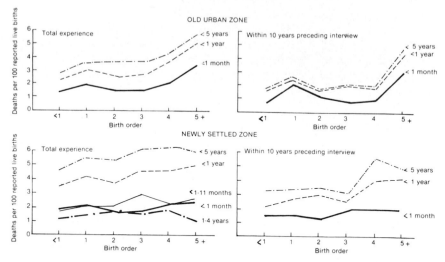

Child Mortality, Birth Order, and Maternal Age

The percentages of death within one year of birth did not show any clear relationship to birth order in either of the two residential zones (Table 4.A.6). The values were too small for any valid conclusions to be drawn.

TABLE 4.A.6. INFANT MORTALITY (DEATHS UNDER 1 YEAR) DURING 10 YEARS PRECEDING THE INTERVIEW, BY RESIDENCE, BIRTH ORDER, AND MATERNAL AGE

Residence and maternal age	Deaths per 100 reported live births at birth order:						Total live births in past 10 years
	1	2	3	4	5	6 and over	
Old urban zone							
<20	1.6	1.1	0.0	—	—	—	187
20–24	0.5	0.9	0.4	0.0	0.0	0.1	987
25–29	0.6	0.4	0.0	0.3	0.1	0.1	956
30–34	0.2	0.4	0.3	0.5	0.5	1.6	617
35–39	0.0	0.0	0.5	0.0	0.0	4.3	320
40–44	2.6	14.2	0.0	0.0	0.0	2.6	38
Newly settled zone							
<20	2.5	1.7	0.5	0.0	—	—	404
20–24	1.2	1.0	0.7	0.3	0.3	0.2	1363
25–29	0.4	0.5	0.6	0.1	0.7	1.6	1327
30–34	0.0	0.0	0.1	0.2	0.6	2.5	954
35–39	0.2	0.0	0.0	0.2	0.7	4.5	595
40–44	0.0	0.0	50.0	—	0.0	1.4	74

194

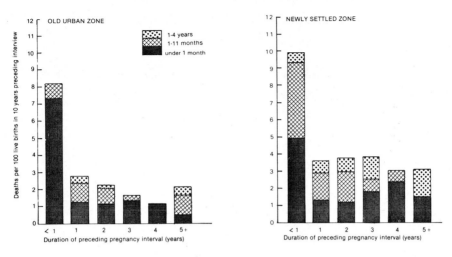

Child Mortality and Duration of Preceding Pregnancy Intervals

In both the NSZ and the OUZ, the risk was highest when the preceding pregnancy intervals were short, i.e., under 2 years (Table 4.A.7).

TABLE 4.A.7. CHILD MORTALITY DURING 10 YEARS PRECEDING INTERVIEW, BY RESIDENCE AND DURATION OF PREGNANCY INTERVAL

Residence and duration of preceding pregnancy interval (years)	Deaths per 100 live births in 10 years preceding interview, at:					Total live births in past 10 years
	<1 month	1–11 months	<1 year	1–4 years	<5 years	
Old urban zone						
<1	7.3	0.9	8.3	0.0	8.3	109
1–2	1.3	1.1	2.4	0.3	2.8	908
2–3	1.2	1.0	2.1	0.2	2.3	520
3–4	1.4	0.3	1.7	0.0	1.7	292
4–5	1.2	0.0	1.2	0.0	1.2	164
5 and over	0.6	1.1	1.7	0.6	2.2	181
Newly settled zone						
<1	5.0	4.3	9.4	0.7	10.0	299
1–2	1.4	1.6	3.0	0.7	3.7	2221
2–3	1.3	1.8	3.0	0.8	3.8	800
3–4	1.9	0.6	2.6	1.3	3.9	311
4–5	2.5	0.6	3.1	0.0	3.1	160
5 and over	1.6	0.0	1.6	1.6	3.2	125

195

B. EGYPT

A. H. A. Zaraour, S. I. Fahmy, A. F. Moustafa & A. R. Omran

Child Mortality by Residence and Social Status

Table 4.B.1 shows that out of 22 154 live-born children, 6.7% died during the first month of life, 14.5% during the first year, 10.8% at 1–4 years of age, and 25.3% before they attained their fifth birthday. These high percentages are similar to those that are found in many developing countries.

Rural children had the highest infant and child mortalities: 8.4% for infants under 1 month, 15.7% from birth to less than 1 year, 12.8% at 1–4 years, and 28.5% under 5 years. Children in the industrial area had the lowest mortalities: 2.8%, 10.6%, 5.3%, and 15.9%, respectively. Mortality among urban children was slightly lower than among rural children (Fig. 4.B.1). The breakdown of infant mortality among rural children of low social class showed higher neonatal than post-neonatal mortality. This could be attributed to the mother's faulty memory. Mothers in the rural area might not have been able to recall accurately whether their infants died at 3 or 5 weeks of life, and the ratio between neonatal and post-neonatal mortality might have been affected as a result. Of course, other factors, such as poor midwifery techniques, might also have resulted in increased neonatal mortality.

Mortality in all 5 age-risk periods was higher in the low than in the middle social status group in all 3 areas; however, in the rural area infant mortality was almost the same among both social classes (Table 4.B.1).

TABLE 4.B.1. CHILD MORTALITY BY RESIDENCE AND SOCIAL STATUS

Residence and social status	Deaths per 100 reported live births at:					Total reported live births
	<1 month	1–11 months	<1 year	1–4 years	<5 years	
Rural						
Middle	7.3	8.3	15.6	10.9	26.5	3226
Low	8.7	7.0	15.7	13.8	29.5	6455
Both categories	8.4	7.3	15.7	12.8	28.5	9681
Urban						
Middle	5.6	7.8	13.4	9.3	22.7	5813
Low	6.8	8.9	15.7	11.6	27.3	4133
Both categories	6.1	8.3	14.4	10.2	24.6	9946
Industrial						
Middle	2.0	7.5	9.5	4.6	14.1	759
Low	3.1	7.9	11.0	5.7	16.7	1768
Both categories	2.8	7.8	10.6	5.3	15.9	2527

FIG. 4.B.1. CHILD MORTALITY BY RESIDENCE AND SOCIAL STATUS

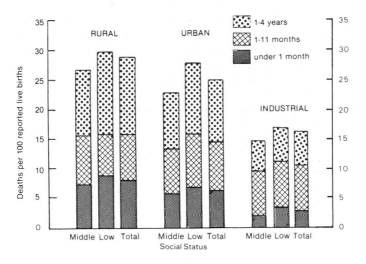

TABLE 4.B.2. CHILD MORTALITY BY RESIDENCE AND MATERNAL AGE (TOTAL EXPERIENCE)

Residence and maternal age	Reported live births	Deaths per 100 reported live births at:				
		<1 month	1–11 months	<1 year	1–4 years	<5 years
Rural						
<20	2508	10.4	9.6	20.0	15.8	35.8
20–24	2488	9.9	9.7	19.6	17.7	37.3
25–29	2451	7.2	6.2	13.4	10.6	24.0
30–34	1409	6.2	4.1	10.3	8.4	18.7
35–39	647	5.6	4.8	10.4	6.2	16.5
40–44	120	3.1	1.6	4.7	2.0	8.6
Unknown	50					
Urban						
<20	2400	7.6	11.0	18.7	13.5	32.1
20–24	2660	7.7	10.6	18.3	13.4	31.8
25–29	2619	4.8	5.7	10.6	8.9	19.5
30–34	1455	4.0	5.8	9.8	6.0	15.8
35–39	663	3.6	5.3	8.9	2.4	11.3
40–44	119	3.4	5.0	8.4	1.7	10.1
Unknown	30					
Industrial						
<20	504	4.0	12.3	16.3	6.7	23.0
20–24	737	2.2	8.3	10.5	5.6	16.1
25–29	638	1.9	5.6	7.5	4.4	11.9
30–34	405	4.2	6.2	10.4	1.7	12.1
35–39	204	2.4	6.4	8.8	2.9	11.7
40–44	16	—	6.2	6.2	—	6.2
Unknown	22					

197

Child Mortality and Maternal Age

Table 4.B.2 shows that in each of the 3 areas, the highest mortality in each of the 5 risk periods was among mothers in the two youngest age groups (less than 20 years and 20–24 years). After the age of 25, mortality decreased with increase in maternal age, except that a small rise occurred for infants and children under 5 years of age at 30–34 years in the industrial area (Fig. 4.B.2). The decline in infant and child mortality for women giving birth at 40 years and over in rural areas was based on a small sample size.[1]

In most of the maternal age groups, the mortality of children at the 5 risk periods in the rural group was higher than the corresponding figures for the urban and industrial areas. Rates for the urban group were intermediate, and the industrial group had the lowest figures.

---

[1] The data needed for conducting cohort analysis, as was done at the other centres, were not available. It was thus not possible to distinguish between the effect of young age of mother and that of the higher mortality prevalent several decades ago.

FIG. 4.B.2. CHILD MORTALITY BY RESIDENCE AND MATERNAL AGE (TOTAL EXPERIENCE)

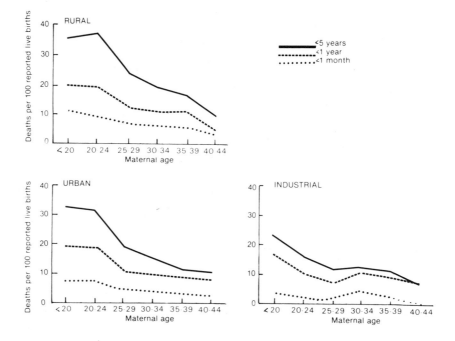

C. PAKISTAN

M. Saeed Qureshi & A. R. Omran

Child Mortality by Residence and Social Status

The 2389 semi-urban and 2473 urban women included in the present study experienced 11 443 and 9923 live births, respectively, up to the time of the interview. Of those live-born children, 1456 in the semi-urban and 616 in the urban area died before they reached their 5th birthday. Three-quarters of these deaths occurred during infancy. The data indicate that semi-urban women experienced more infant and child deaths (12.8%) than urban women (7.2%). Expressed as a percentage of total live births during the reproductive span of the woman (up to the time of the interview), the figures for infant deaths were 8.9% for the semi urban area and 5.3% for the urban area. In both areas, children of all ages experienced a higher mortality risk in the low social status group than in the middle status group (Table 4.C.1 and Fig. 4.C.1).

TABLE 4.C.1. CHILD MORTALITY BY RESIDENCE AND SOCIAL STATUS

Residence and social status	Deaths per 100 reported live births at:					Total reported live births
	<1 month	1–11 months	<1 year	1–4 years	<5 years	
Semi-urban						
Middle	3.5	4.5	8.0	3.1	11.1	5044
Low	4.3	5.3	9.6	4.6	14.2	6399
Both categories	4.0	4.9	8.9	3.9	12.8	11443
Urban						
Middle	2.5	2.7	5.3	1.8	7.0	8952
Low	2.5	3.0	5.5	3.0	8.4	971
Both categories	2.5	2.8	5.3	1.9	7.2	9923

FIG. 4.C.1. CHILD MORTALITY BY RESIDENCE AND SOCIAL STATUS

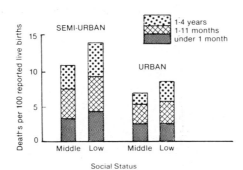

199

Child Mortality and Maternal Age

The findings indicate that child mortality at different periods of risk, i.e., neonatal, post-neonatal, and 1–4 years, was high when the mother was under 20 years of age. With increased maternal age, child mortality steadily declined, but above 30–34 years it increased again. In other words, mothers of less than 20 years of age and mothers of 40–44 years experienced the highest child mortality while mothers aged between 25 and 34 years lost the minimum proportion of children. This is evident from the U-shaped curves depicted in Fig. 4.C.2, more distinctly so in the semi-urban than in the urban group. The

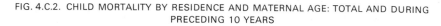

FIG. 4.C.2. CHILD MORTALITY BY RESIDENCE AND MATERNAL AGE: TOTAL AND DURING PRECEDING 10 YEARS

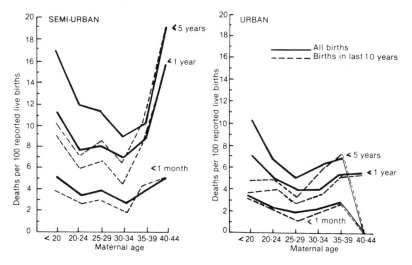

percentages of child deaths at all maternal ages and at different risk periods were higher among children of semi-urban residents than among those of urban residents and were also higher for the low status group than for the middle status group (Table 4.C.2).

The differentials observed by age of mother could have been the result of changes in mortality over time because child mortality has fallen in the region during recent years. To study the changes in mortality and its relation to the age of the mother, mortality rates have been computed for 3 broad maternal age groups according to the corresponding maternal ages at child death, as shown in Table 4.C.3. The figures clearly indicate a decline in mortality over a period of time. For example, in the semi-urban area the women who were aged 35–44, 25–34 and <25 years at the time of the interview had lost, respectively, 20%, 10.8%, and 8.9% of their total live-born children when their maternal age was less than 25 years. A similar mortality trend has been observed for the urban area. The decline in mortality was, however, greater in urban than in semi-urban areas.

200

TABLE 4.C.2. CHILD MORTALITY BY RESIDENCE AND MATERNAL AGE (TOTAL EXPERIENCE)

Residence and maternal age	Reported live births	Deaths per 100 reported live births at:				
		<1 month	1–11 months	<1 year	1–4 years	<5 years
Semi-urban						
<20	2901	5.3	6.3	11.6	5.4	17.0
20–24	3910	3.4	4.4	7.8	4.1	11.9
25–29	2771	3.8	4.5	8.3	3.2	11.5
30–34	1377	2.7	4.1	6.8	2.3	9.1
35–39	447	4.0	4.7	8.7	1.7	10.4
40–44	37	5.4	10.8	16.2	2.7	18.9
All ages	11443	4.0	4.9	8.9	3.8	12.7
Urban						
<20	2190	3.6	3.7	7.3	3.1	10.4
20–24	3675	2.3	2.8	5.1	1.7	6.8
25–29	2536	2.0	2.0	4.0	1.3	5.3
30–34	1172	2.2	2.0	4.2	2.0	6.2
35–39	322	2.8	2.8	5.6	1.5	7.1
40–44	18	—	5.6	5.6	—	5.6
All ages	9923	2.5	2.8	5.3	1.9	7.2

In Table 4.C.3, the figures above the diagonal lines show mortality rates for children born recently to women in each cohort. It can be seen that the patterns of the relationship between maternal age and child mortality thus revealed differ somewhat from those obtained when births from all periods are included.

Changes in child mortality experienced by cohorts of women over a period of 20 years were studied by questioning the women in a given age group about their history of child losses. For example, in semi-urban areas those women who were aged 35–44 years at the time of interview had experienced a child mortality of 20% before reaching the age of 25. When the same cohort was in the 25–34 years age group, they had experienced a child mortality of only 12.1%, a reduction of 40%. Ten years later, when the cohort had reached 35–44 years, a further but much smaller reduction (7.4%) in child mortality had occurred, to a figure of 11.2%. A similar trend was observed in the urban area.

When data on infant and child mortality were restricted to the 10 years preceding the interview, lower rates were obtained than those for the entire period of the woman's reproductive age (Table 4.C.4 and Fig. 4.C.2). In the semi-urban area, the proportion of infant deaths (<1 year) declined from 9.0% for mothers under 20 years of age to 4.6% for mothers aged 30–34 and then increased to 16.2% for mothers aged 40–44. However, child mortality (1–4 years) increased with increasing maternal age. In the urban area, infant mortality declined from 3.8% for women under 20 years of age to 2.8% for mothers aged 25–29 and then increased to 5.6% for mothers aged 35–39. Again, there was an increase in child mortality as maternal age increased.

201

TABLE 4.C.3. CHILD MORTALITY BY MATERNAL AGE, RESIDENCE AND AGE AT INTERVIEW

Residence and age of child at death	Age of mother at interview	Deaths as percentages of live births at maternal age:		
		<25	25–34	35–44
Semi-urban				
under 1 month	<25	3.6	—	—
	25–34	3.5	2.9	—
	35–44	5.3	3.7	4.2
	Total	4.2	3.4	4.1
1–11 months	<25	4.3	—	—
	25–34	4.0	3.6	—
	35–44	7.1	4.8	5.2
	Total	5.2	4.3	5.2
under 1 year	<25	7.9	—	—
	25–34	7.5	6.5	—
	35–44	12.4	8.5	9.4
	Total	9.4	7.7	9.3
1–4 years	<25	1.0	—	—
	25–34	3.3	1.7	—
	35–44	7.6	3.6	1.8
	Total	4.7	2.8	1.8
under 5 years	<25	8.9	—	—
	25–34	10.8	8.2	—
	35–44	20.0	12.1	11.2
	Total	14.1	10.5	11.2
Urban				
under 1 month	<25	2.2	—	—
	25–34	2.7	1.0	—
	35–44	3.1	2.7	2.7
	Total	2.8	2.1	2.6
1–11 months	<25	0.9	—	—
	25–34	3.0	1.6	—
	35–44	4.0	2.3	3.0
	Total	3.1	2.0	3.0
under 1 year	<25	3.1	—	—
	25–34	5.7	2.6	—
	35–44	7.1	5.0	5.7
	Total	5.9	4.1	5.6
1–4 years	<25	0.5	—	—
	25–34	1.2	0.6	—
	35–44	3.9	2.1	1.5
	Total	2.2	1.6	1.5
under 5 years	<25	3.6	—	—
	25–34	6.9	3.2	—
	35–44	11.0	7.1	7.2
	Total	8.1	5.7	7.1

TABLE 4.C.4.   CHILD MORTALITY DURING THE 10 YEARS PRECEDING THE INTERVIEW, BY RESIDENCE AND MATERNAL AGE*

Residence and maternal age	Reported live births	Deaths per 100 reported live births at:				
		<1 month	1–11 months	<1 year	1–4 years	<5 years
Semi-urban						
<20	508	3.9	5.1	9.0	1.2	10.2
20–24	1311	2.9	3.2	6.1	1.2	7.3
25–29	1322	3.0	3.8	6.8	2.0	8.8
30–34	782	2.0	2.6	4.6	2.0	6.6
35–39	442	4.1	4.8	8.9	1.8	10.7
40–44	37	5.4	10.8	16.2	.2.7	18.9
All ages	4402	3.0	3.7	6.7	1.7	8.4
Urban						
<20	365	3.0	0.8	3.8	1.1	4.9
20–24	1413	2.1	1.9	4.0	0.6	4.6
25–29	1151	1.0	1.8	2.8	0.5	3.3
30–34	627	1.9	1.6	3.5	2.2	5.7
35–39	319	2.8	2.8	5.6	1.7	7.3
40–44	18	—	(5.6)	(5.6)	—	(5.6)
All ages	3893	1.9	1.8	3.7	1.0	4.7

* Figures in parentheses refer to fewer than 25 live births.

Child Mortality and Birth Order

In both residental areas, mortality rates for children under 5 years of age were highest at birth order 1: 13.9% and 8.8%, for the semi-urban and urban groups, respectively. The rates then decreased to 11.2% and 5.4%, respectively, for birth order 3, subsequently increasing as birth order increased. They thus exhibited a U-shaped relationship to birth order. Mortality rates under 1 month, at 1–11 months, and under 1 year followed the same pattern. However, some variations were observed for children aged 1–4 years. In the semi-urban group, mortality for this age group was highest (5%) for birth order 2 but showed no consistent relationship with birth order. On the other hand, in the urban group, child deaths were highest (2.1%) for birth order 1, decreased slightly to 1.7% for birth order 4, and then increased to a maximum of 2.1% for birth order 6 and over (Table 4.C.5 and Fig. 4.C.3).

The table also compares infant and child mortality over the 10 years preceding the interview with that for the whole span of the mother's reproductive age. It can be seen that child mortality (1–4 years) was lower in the 10 years preceding the interview than over the longer period. The reduction was 33% in the semi-urban area and 27% in the urban area. This decline was particularly marked for the lower birth orders in the semi-urban area: the mortality fell from 3.4% to 0.4% for birth order 1, from 5% to 1.5% for birth order 2, and from 3.7% to 0.5% for birth order 3.

TABLE 4.C.5.   CHILD MORTALITY BY RESIDENCE AND BIRTH ORDER (TOTAL EXPERIENCE AND BIRTHS WITHIN 10 YEARS PRECEDING INTERVIEW)

Residence and birth order	Reported live births	Deaths per 100 reported live births at:				
		<1 month	1–11 months	<1 year	1–4 years	<5 years
Semi-urban						
Total experience						
1	2206	5.4	5.1	10.5	3.4	13.9
2	1996	3.5	4.6	8.1	5.0	13.1
3	1767	2.9	4.6	7.5	3.7	11.2
4	1515	3.2	4.8	8.0	3.8	11.8
5	1242	3.6	4.7	8.3	4.0	12.3
6 and over	2767	4.3	5.3	9.6	3.6	13.2
All birth orders	11443	4.0	4.9	8.9	3.8	12.7
Within 10 years preceding interview						
1	562	4.3	4.8	9.1	0.4	9.4
2	551	2.7	3.6	6.4	1.5	7.8
3	558	1.4	2.7	4.1	0.5	4.7
4	568	2.6	3.5	6.2	1.2	7.4
5	568	2.5	3.2	5.7	2.1	7.8
6 and over	1595	3.6	5.9	7.6	2.6	10.1
All birth orders	4402	3.0	3.7	6.7	1.7	8.4
Urban						
Total experience						
1	2215	3.7	3.0	6.7	2.1	8.8
2	1941	2.1	2.9	5.0	1.9	6.9
3	1586	1.5	2.9	3.5	1.9	5.4
4	1269	2.3	2.9	5.1	1.7	6.8
5	939	2.1	2.8	4.9	1.8	6.7
6 and over	1973	2.7	2.7	5.4	2.1	7.5
All birth orders	9923	2.5	2.8	5.3	1.9	7.2
Within 10 years preceding interview						
1	911	2.9	1.8	4.7	0.9	5.6
2	727	2.2	2.1	4.3	0.9	5.3
3	574	1.2	1.2	2.5	1.2	3.7
4	457	1.3	1.9	3.3	0.2	3.5
5	356	0.6	1.4	2.0	0.3	2.3
6 and over	868	2.4	3.5	5.9	1.8	7.6
All birth orders	3893	1.9	1.8	3.7	1.0	4.7

Infant Mortality, Birth Order, and Maternal Age

When infant mortality during the 10 years preceding the interview was classified by birth order and maternal age, the rates were found to be higher for women under 20 years of age of birth order 1 and, more especially, for women aged 30 years and over of birth order 6 and above (Table 4.C.6). However, no conclusive findings can be drawn from the table as the numbers involved in each case were very small.

FIG. 4.C.3. CHILD MORTALITY BY RESIDENCE AND BIRTH ORDER (TOTAL AND DURING PRECEDING 10 YEARS)

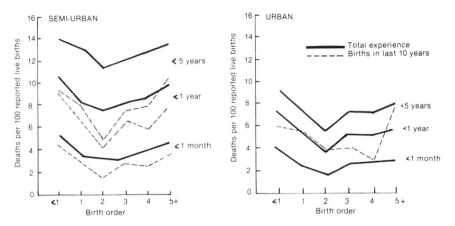

TABLE 4.C.6. INFANT MORTALITY (DEATHS UNDER 1 YEAR) DURING THE 10 YEARS PRECEDING THE INTERVIEW, BY RESIDENCE, BIRTH ORDER, AND MATERNAL AGE

Residence and maternal age	Deaths per 100 reported live births at birth order:						Total live births in past 10 years
	1	2	3	4	5	6 and over	
Semi-urban							
<20	6.7	1.8	0.2	0.2	0.2	—	508
20–24	1.1	1.6	0.8	1.2	0.9	0.4	1311
25–29	0.2	0.4	0.6	1.0	1.2	3.3	1322
30–34	—	—	0.4	0.3	0.3	3.7	782
35–39	—	—	—	0.7	—	7.0	442
40–44	—	—	—	—	2.7	13.5	37
Urban							
<20	2.5	1.1	—	—	—	—	365
20–24	1.3	1.3	0.4	0.5	0.3	0.1	1413
25–29	0.2	0.3	0.3	0.5	0.3	1.2	1151
30–34	0.3	0.2	—	0.3	—	2.7	627
35–39	—	—	0.3	—	—	5.3	319
40–44	—	—	—	—	—	5.6	18

Child Mortality and Duration of Preceding Pregnancy Interval

It has been shown in various studies that the preceding pregnancy interval is closely related to the risk of infant and child mortality. Infant and child mortality rates are inversely related to the duration of the pregnancy interval. The findings in this study indicate that the infant and child mortality rates during the 10 years preceding the interview were, in general, highest for intervals of less than two years, with mortality risks declining as pregnancy intervals increased. The same trends were observed in both urban and

205

semi-urban areas, with the exception of the pregnancy intervals of 5 years and over in the semi-urban areas, where the risks again increased (Table 4.C.7 and Fig. 4.C.4).

TABLE 4.C.7. CHILD MORTALITY DURING 10 YEARS PRECEDING INTERVIEW, BY RESIDENCE AND DURATION OF PRECEDING PREGNANCY INTERVAL

Residence and duration of of preceding pregnancy interval (years)	Deaths per 100 live births in 10 years preceding interview, at:					Total live births in past 10 years
	<1 month	1–11 months	<1 year	1–4 years	<5 years	
Semi-urban						
<1	1.4	1.4	2.9	0.0	2.9	69
1–2	4.3	5.4	9.7	2.7	12.4	1238
2–3	3.1	3.2	6.3	1.6	8.0	1519
3–4	0.8	1.9	2.6	1.6	4.2	644
4–5	1.5	1.5	3.0	0.0	3.0	264
5 and over	2.6	2.6	5.3	2.1	7.4	189
Urban						
<1	0.0	8.0	8.0	0.0	8.0	25
1–2	2.0	2.4	4.4	1.1	5.6	1045
2–3	1.4	2.4	3.7	1.1	4.8	1106
3–4	2.5	1.6	4.1	1.4	5.5	487
4–5	0.9	0.4	1.3	0.9	2.2	225
5 and over	1.3	0.4	1.7	0.0	1.7	230

FIG. 4.C.4. CHILD MORTALITY DURING THE 10 YEARS PRECEDING INTERVIEW, BY RESIDENCE AND DURATION OF PRECEDING PREGNANCY INTERVAL

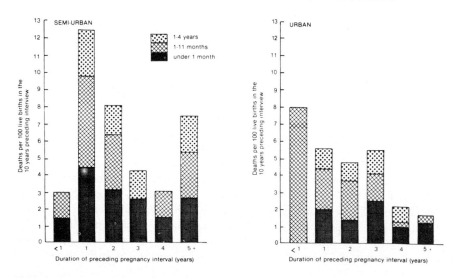

D. SYRIAN ARAB REPUBLIC

N. Ghabra, N. Hallak & A. R. Omran

Child Mortality by Residence and Social Status

Of the 27 882 live-born children reported by the eligible women in the three areas, 2.6% had died within a month of birth, 8.3% within a year and 12.4% within 5 years.

For almost all risk periods, the highest loss occurred among rural Aleppo and the lowest among Damascus children. In both Damascus and Sweida, children from low status families had a higher rate of mortality than those from middle status families. Among children from rural areas, the social differential disappeared or was even reversed. Mortality rates for children born to middle status families in these areas were slightly higher than those for children from poorer families. For both social status groups, the mortality rates were high (Table 4.D.1 and Fig. 4.D.1).

TABLE 4.D.1. CHILD MORTALITY BY RESIDENCE AND SOCIAL STATUS

Residence and social status	Deaths per 100 reported live births at:					Total reported live births
	<1 month	1–11 months	<1 year	1–4 years	<5 years	
Damascus						
Middle	2.3	3.5	5.8	2.3	8.1	7355
Low	2.5	4.3	6.8	4.3	11.1	2124
Both categories	2.4	3.7	6.1	2.7	8.8	9479
Sweida						
Middle	2.2	5.3	7.5	2.5	10.0	6131
Low	2.6	7.6	10.2	5.0	15.2	2255
Both categories	2.3	5.9	8.2	3.2	11.4	8386
Rural Aleppo						
Middle	3.7	7.5	11.2	6.7	17.9	3288
Low	3.0	7.3	10.3	6.2	16.5	7629
Both categories	3.2	7.4	10.6	6.4	17.0	10017

Child mortality is usually high for maternal ages of under 20 years and over 35 years. In this study, the initially high mortality for teenage mothers was very apparent in all areas. The expected later increase at ages of 35 and over was absent in all areas (Table 4.D.2 and Fig. 4.D.2).

It is possible for the relationship between child mortality and maternal age to be distorted by changes in risk factors over time resulting from better health services, increased amount of child care, and better social conditions. Under such circumstances, children born at an earlier period suffer higher mortality than those more recently born. In order to introduce an approximate control for such changes, the women were divided into 3 age cohorts: those aged under

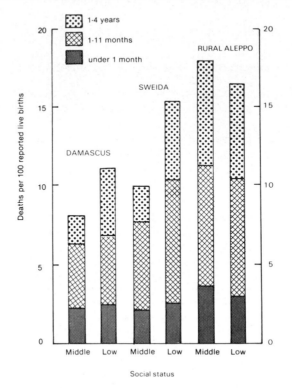

FIG. 4.D.1. CHILD MORTALITY BY RESIDENCE AND SOCIAL STATUS

25 years at interview, those aged between 25 and 34, and those aged 35 years and over.

Table 4.D.3 compared child mortality for those three groups according to their corresponding age groups at childbirth. It is evident that the reported percentage of deaths of children born to women aged under 25 years at the time of giving birth has declined over the last 10 years. For example, rural women over 35 at interview had lost, within one month of birth, 4.0% of the children born to them when they were under 25, while those women aged under 25 at interview had lost 2.8% of their children within the first month. Although the decline, particularly for deaths under 5 years, may be exaggerated by the shortening of the period of exposure to risk, the fact that an intermediate rate was found for women aged 25–34 at interview does indicate a downward trend.

In Table 4.D.3, the rows giving total mortality rates show the relationship between maternal age and child mortality for each residential group and correspond to the curves shown in Fig. 4.D.2. The figures above the diagonal lines show mortality rates for children born recently to women in each cohort, and it can be seen that the patterns of the relationship between maternal age and child mortality differ from those obtained when births from all periods were included.

208

TABLE 4.D.2. CHILD MORTALITY BY RESIDENCE AND MATERNAL AGE (TOTAL EXPERIENCE)

Residence and maternal age	Reported live births	Deaths per 100 reported live births at:				
		<1 month	1–11 months	<1 year	1–4 years	<5 years
Damascus						
<20	1810	3.5	4.9	8.4	3.8	13.3
20–24	3094	2.3	4.3	6.6	3.1	9.7
25–29	2424	2.1	3.3	5.4	2.5	7.9
30–34	1469	1.9	2.5	4.4	2.0	6.4
35–39	578	2.1	1.7	3.8	1.2	5.0
40–44	103	1.9	1.0	2.9	0	2.9
All ages	9478	2.4	3.7	6.1	2.8	8.9
Sweida						
<20	1378	2.8	7.8	10.6	3.7	14.3
20–24	2736	2.2	6.2	8.4	3.1	11.5
25–29	2201	2.3	5.1	7.4	3.7	11.1
30–34	1370	2.3	5.5	7.8	2.6	10.4
35–44	584	1.9	4.5	6.4	2.2	8.6
40–44	113	4.4	1.8	6.2	3.6	9.8
All ages	8382	2.4	5.9	8.3	3.2	11.5
Rural Aleppo						
<20	1813	4.4	10.3	14.7	7.9	22.6
20–24	3159	2.9	7.7	10.6	7.9	18.5
25–29	2472	2.8	6.6	9.4	5.7	15.1
30–34	1631	3.1	5.8	8.9	5.1	14.0
35–39	767	3.4	6.6	10.0	2.9	12.9
40–44	173	2.3	4.0	6.3	3.5	9.8
All ages	10015	3.2	7.4	10.6	6.4	17.0

FIG. 4.D.2. CHILD MORTALITY BY RESIDENCE AND MATERNAL AGE: TOTAL AND DURING PRECEDING 10 YEARS

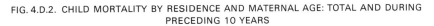
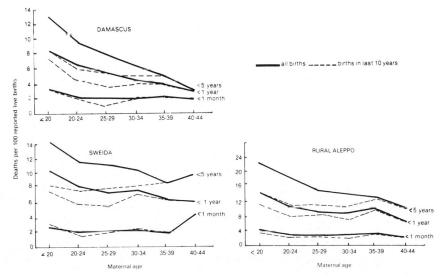

TABLE 4.D.3. CHILD MORTALITY BY MATERNAL AGE, RESIDENCE, AND AGE AT INTERVIEW

Residence and age of child at death	Age of mother at interview	Deaths as percentages of live births at maternal age:		
		<25	25–34	35–44
Damascus				
under 1 month	<25	3.1	—	—
	25–34	2.1	1.5	—
	35–44	3.5	2.3	2.1
	All ages	2.8	2.0	2.1
1–11 months	<25	3.4	—	—
	25–34	4.3	2.5	—
	35–44	5.5	3.4	1.6
	All ages	4.6	3.0	1.6
under 1 yeer	<25	6.5	—	—
	25–34	6.4	4.0	—
	35–44	9.0	5.7	3.7
	All ages	7.4	5.0	3.7
1–4 years	<25	0.9	—	—
	25–34	2.4	1.4	—
	35–44	6.0	2.9	0.9
	All ages	3.4	2.3	0.9
under 5 years	<25	7.4	—	—
	25–34	8.8	5.4	—
	35–44	15.0	8.6	4.6
	All ages	10.8	7.3	4.6
Sweida				
under 1 month	<25	2.6	—	—
	25–34	2.5	2.1	—
	35–44	2.2	2.4	2.3
	All ages	2.4	2.3	2.3
1–11 months	<25	4.3	—	—
	25–34	5.3	3.4	—
	35–44	9.9	6.3	4.1
	All ages	6.8	5.2	4.1
under 1 year	<25	6.9	—	—
	25–34	7.8	5.5	—
	35–44	12.1	8.7	6.4
	All ages	9.2	7.5	6.4
1–4 years	<25	0.9	—	—
	25–34	2.3	2.0	—
	35–44	5.5	3.9	2.4
	All ages	3.2	3.3	2.4
under 5 years	<25	7.8	—	—
	25–34	10.1	7.5	—
	35–44	17.6	12.6	8.8
	All ages	12.4	10.8	8.8

TABLE 4.D.3 (continued)

Residence and age of child at death	Age of mother at interview	Deaths as percentages of live births at maternal age:		
		<25	25–34	35–44
Rural Aleppo				
under 1 month	<25	2.8	—	—
	25–34	3.3	2.3	—
	35–44	4.0	3.3	3.2
	All ages	3.5	2.9	3.2
1–11 months	<25	5.9	—	—
	25–34	7.7	5.4	—
	35–44	11.0	6.8	6.1
	All ages	8.6	6.3	6.1
under 1 year	<25	8.7	—	—
	25–34	11.0	7.7	—
	35–44	15.0	10.1	9.3
	All ages	12.1	9.2	9.3
1–4 years	<25	2.2	—	—
	25–34	6.1	2.5	—
	35–44	13.0	7.1	3.0
	All ages	7.9	5.4	3.0
under 5 years	<25	—	—	—
	25–34	17.1	10.2	—
	35–44	28.0	17.2	12.3
	All ages	20.0	14.6	12.3

Child mortality experience in the 10 years preceding the interview is shown in Table 4.D.4. Some changes in trends are evident for this period when the mortality rates are compared with those for the total time period preceding the interview. Mortality rates under 1 month among children born to mothers in the 10 years preceding the interview exhibited a reverse J-shaped relationship with age in almost all areas. This indicated a high risk associated with teenage pregnancy and a somewhat increased risk at the other end of the reproductive span. For mortality rates at other child ages (under 1 month and under 5 years), the most consistent relationship was a high mortality rate associated with young maternal age.

Child mortality rates by residence showed a negative relationship with maternal age in large cities for ages 1–11 months and under 5 years (see Fig. 4.D.2). In small towns, there was no consistent pattern for mortality for the period 1–11 months, but for deaths under 5 years, the relationship was described by a J-shape. In rural areas, no consistent trend was observed.

Child Mortality and Birth Order

As with maternal age, the relationship between child mortality rates and birth order was found to be distorted by the effects of changes in mortality over

211

TABLE 4.D.4. CHILD MORTALITY DURING THE 10 YEARS PRECEDING THE INTERVIEW, BY RESIDENCE AND MATERNAL AGE

Residence and maternal age	Reported live births	Deaths per 100 reported live births at:				
		<1 month	1–11 months	<1 year	1–4 years	<5 years
Damascus						
<20	521	3.6	4.0	7.6	1.0	8.6
20–24	1115	2.1	2.6	4.7	1.5	6.2
25–29	1155	1.2	2.5	3.7	1.7	5.4
30–34	904	1.9	2.2	4.1	0.9	5.0
35–39	578	2.1	1.7	3.8	1.2	5.0
40–44	103	1.9	1.0	0	0	0
All ages	4376	2.0	2.5	4.5	1.3	5.8
Sweida						
<20	304	3.3	4.6	7.9	0.6	8.5
20–24	1014	1.7	4.3	6.0	1.7	7.7
25–29	1005	2.0	3.7	5.7	2.3	8.0
30–34	738	2.3	4.9	7.2	1.2	8.4
35–39	581	1.9	4.5	6.4	2.2	8.6
40–44	113	4.4	1.8	6.2	3.6	9.8
All ages	3755	2.1	4.0	6.1	1.8	7.9
Rural Aleppo						
<20	516	3.5	7.6	11.1	2.3	13.4
20–24	1157	2.3	5.8	8.1	2.9	11.0
25–29	1127	2.4	5.9	8.3	2.8	11.1
30–34	1000	2.1	5.1	7.2	3.4	10.6
35–39	764	3.4	6.5	9.9	2.9	12.8
40–44	173	2.3	4.0	6.3	3.5	9.8
All ages	4737	2.6	5.9	8.5	2.9	11.4

TABLE 4.D.5. CHILD MORTALITY BY RESIDENCE AND BIRTH ORDER (TOTAL EXPERIENCE AND BIRTHS WITHIN 10 YEARS PRECEDING INTERVIEW)

Residence and birth order	Reported live births	Deaths per 100 reported live births at:				
		<1 month	1–11 months	<1 year	1–4 years	<5 years
Damascus						
Total experience						
1	1830	3.9	3.6	7.5	2.8	10.3
2	1647	1.9	4.4	6.3	3.4	9.7
3	1467	1.6	3.2	4.8	3.2	8.0
4	1241	2.1	5.4	7.5	2.6	10.1
5	1007	2.1	2.7	4.8	3.0	7.8
6 and over	2286	2.3	3.3	5.6	2.0	7.6
All birth orders	9478	2.4	3.7	6.1	2.8	8.9

TABLE 4.D.5 (continued)

Residence and birth order	Reported live births	Deaths per 100 reported live births at:				
		<1 month	1–11 months	<1 year	1–4 years	<5 years
10-year cohort						
1	609	3.4	1.5	4.9	0.8	5.7
2	599	2.0	4.2	6.2	1.7	7.9
3	602	1.3	1.5	2.8	1.0	3.8
4	554	1.6	3.2	4.8	1.8	6.6
5	505	2.0	2.4	4.4	1.0	5.4
6 and over	1501	1.6	2.3	3.9	1.3	5.2
All birth orders	4370	1.9	2.5	4.4	1.3	5.7
Sweida						
Total experience						
1	1592	3.3	5.6	8.9	2.9	11.8
2	1464	2.0	6.8	8.8	3.7	12.5
3	1285	2.2	6.5	8.7	2.9	11.6
4	1119	2.1	6.6	8.7	3.3	12.0
5	890	2.2	5.4	7.6	4.0	11.6
6 and over	2032	2.2	4.9	7.1	3.1	10.2
All birth orders	8382	2.4	5.9	8.3	3.2	11.5
10-year cohort						
1	459	2.8	3.3	6.1	1.5	7.6
2	514	1.4	5.0	6.4	1.6	8.0
3	504	1.8	4.4	6.2	1.6	7.7
4	528	2.3	4.5	6.8	1.7	8.5
5	436	3.0	3.9	6.9	1.4	8.3
6 and over	1314	1.8	2.4	4.2	1.4	5.6
All birth orders	3755	2.1	3.6	5.7	1.5	7.2
Rural Aleppo						
Total experience						
1	1745	4.2	9.2	13.4	7.5	20.9
2	1581	3.2	8.2	11.4	7.4	18.8
3	1380	2.5	7.0	9.5	7.5	17.0
4	1210	3.3	6.9	10.2	8.2	18.4
5	1075	3.3	6.2	9.5	5.8	15.3
6 and over	3024	2.9	6.8	9.7	4.3	14.0
All birth orders	10015	3.2	7.4	10.6	6.4	17.0
10-year cohort						
1	487	3.5	7.8	11.3	2.7	14.0
2	551	2.5	5.3	7.8	2.0	9.8
3	514	2.3	4.9	7.2	2.5	9.7
4	507	3.4	4.9	8.3	4.9	13.2
5	540	2.6	5.5	8.1	3.9	12.0
6 and over	2388	2.7	6.6	9.3	2.7	12.0
All birth orders	4987	2.8	6.1	8.9	3.0	11.9

213

FIG. 4.D.3. CHILD MORTALITY BY RESIDENCE AND BIRTH ORDER: TOTAL AND DURING
PRECEDING 10 YEARS

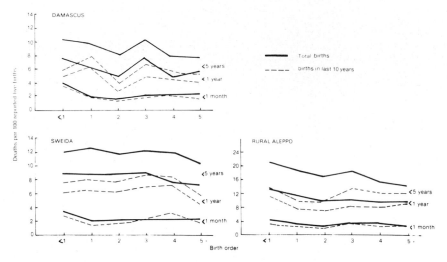

TABLE 4.D.6. INFANT MORTALITY (DEATHS UNDER 1 YEAR) DURING 10 YEARS PRECEDING
INTERVIEW, BY RESIDENCE, BIRTH ORDER, AND MATERNAL AGE

Residence and maternal age	Deaths per 100 reported live births at birth order:						Total live births in past 10 years
	1	2	3	4	5	6 and over	
Damascus							
<20	3.5	3.5	0.4	0.4	—	—	521
20–24	0.8	1.5	0.6	1.0	0.4	0.3	1115
25–29	0.1	0.2	0.3	0.9	1.0	1.1	1155
30–34	0.1	0.2	0.2	0.3	0.4	2.8	904
35–39	0.2	0	0.5	0	0.2	2.9	578
40–44	0	0	0	0	0	3.0	103
Sweida							
<20	5.3	2.0	0.3	0.3	0	0	304
20–24	1.1	2.0	1.5	1.0	0.4	0.1	1014
25–29	0.1	0.3	0.9	1.4	1.5	1.6	1005
30–34	0	0.5	0.9	0.9	1.1	3.7	738
35–39	0	0	0	0.7	0.5	5.0	581
40–44	0	0.9	0	0	0	5.3	113
Rural Aleppo							
<20	7.4	3.1	0.4	0.2	0	0	516
20–24	1.2	1.6	1.7	1.9	0.7	0.8	1157
25–29	0.3	0.4	0.8	1.4	1.5	3.7	1127
30–34	0.1	0.1	0.2	0	0.8	1.6	1000
35–39	0	0	0.5	0.3	0.8	8.4	764
40–44	0	0	0	0	0	6.4	173

time. Table 4.D.5 and Fig. 4.D.3 show, according to birth order, both the mortality rate for the total period of observation, and deaths among children born during the 10 years preceding the interview. The latter figures indicate that the lowest risks were experienced, in general, by children of the third order, fluctuations notwithstanding.

Child Mortality, Birth Order, and Maternal Age

When child mortality rates were analysed by birth order and maternal age simultaneously, the figures for deaths under 1 month and for 1–11 months become too small for valid conclusions to be drawn. For this reason, only the rates for deaths occurring under 1 year of age have been given in Table 4.D.6.

FIG. 4.D.4. CHILD MORTALITY DURING 10 YEARS PRECEDING INTERVIEW, BY DURATION OF PRECEDING PREGNANCY INTERNAL

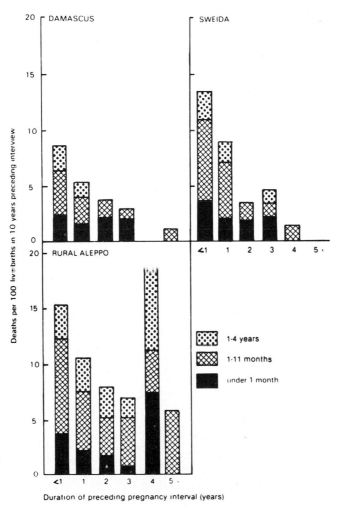

215

Two important findings are: (a) Teenage mothers sustained high infant mortality, especially among first-born children. It is striking that the risk to first-born children dropped significantly for maternal ages 20–24 and 25–29. (b) At the other extreme of birth order, i.e., among children of 6th or higher birth order, the risk of dying during the first year was also high.

Child Mortality and Duration of Preceding Pregnancy Interval

The relationship between child mortality and the preceding pregnancy interval was a negative one for all the components of child mortality. As shown in Table 4.D.7 and Fig. 4.D.4, the highest risks of mortality were observed for pregnancy intervals of less than 1 year or 1–2 years. This trend was observed in all three residential areas. In rural Aleppo, the mortality risk also increased for pregnancy intervals of 4–5 years, but this should be interpreted cautiously as sample sizes were small for the longer intervals.

TABLE 4.D.7. CHILD MORTALITY DURING 10 YEARS PRECEDING INTERVIEW, BY RESIDENCE AND DURATION OF PRECEDING PREGNANCY INTERVAL*

Residence and duration of preceding pregnancy interval (years)	Deaths per 100 live births in 10 years preceding interview, at:					Total live births in past 10 years
	<1 month	1–11 months	<1 year	1–4 years	<5 years	
Damascus						
<1	2.4	4.0	6.3	2.4	8.7	1231
1–2	1.7	2.3	4.0	1.4	5.4	1619
2–3	1.2	2.1	3.3	0.3	3.6	581
3–4	2.0	1.0	2.9	0.0	2.9	204
4–5	0.0	0.0	0.0	0.0	0.0	91
5 and over	0.0	1.0	1.0	0.0	1.0	97
Sweida						
<1	3.6	7.2	10.8	2.6	13.4	760
1–2	2.0	5.0	7.0	1.9	8.9	1567
2–3	0.7	1.1	1.8	1.6	3.4	703
3–4	2.2	1.1	3.3	1.1	4.4	183
4–5	0.0	1.4	1.4	0.0	1.4	70
5 and over	0.0	0.0	0.0	0.0	0.0	53
Rural Aleppo						
<1	3.9	8.4	12.3	3.0	15.3	998
1–2	2.2	5.4	7.6	3.1	10.7	2403
2–3	1.8	3.4	5.2	2.8	8.0	652
3–4	0.9	4.3	5.2	1.7	7.0	115
4–5	7.4	3.7	11.1	7.4	18.5	27
5 and over	(0.0)	(5.9)	(5.9)	(0.0)	(5.9)	17

* Figures in parentheses refer to fewer than 25 live births.

Chapter Five

FAMILY FORMATION AND CHILD DEVELOPMENT

I. CHILD GROWTH AND HEALTH

INTRODUCTION

M. R. Bone

The child mortality considered in the previous chapter may be taken as indicative of a much greater morbidity. In developing areas of the world, the combined effects of malnutrition and infections are held to be responsible for the greater part of both morbidity and mortality, besides retarding children's physical development. To the extent that malnutrition and infections are dependent on social and economic circumstances, their prevalence is likely to increase as family growth reduces the resources that can be devoted to each child. Child mortality may also be related independently to birth order, if this in turn affects children's susceptibility to the hazards of their environment.

Other studies, reviewed in Part I, have found that young children's health and growth are related to family size: the more siblings a child has, the more slowly he is likely to grow and the more prone he will be to malnutrition and infection. The variation in health and development with birth order, though less frequently investigated, shows a similar relationship: later-born children are at a disadvantage, especially in comparison with the first born.

The specific aspects of growth and health examined in the first part of this chapter are: height and weight, haemoglobin level, infections, and, for one centre in Egypt, intestinal parasites.

Most of the data were derived from clinical examination of the eligible women's children under 5 years of age, and from laboratory investigations of blood and stool specimens obtained from them. In addition, the eligible women were asked whether each of their children under 10 years had experienced fever, diarrhoea, or cough lasting for more than one day during the month preceding interview. These 3 symptoms were used as indications of infection.

Despite efforts to do so, clinical and laboratory methods were not standardized across participating areas. Because of such differences, it is not permissible to make comparisons of prevalence rates between areas.

Prevalence rates are shown as percentages of examined, or reported, children affected, and mean values are given for height, weight, and haemoglobin level.

For children aged between 6 months and 6 years, and living at sea level, anaemia is considered to exist if the haemoglobin level is below 11 grams per 100 millilitres of venous blood. At greater altitudes, higher limiting values apply.[1]

The reports from the different centres show that the expected relationships between family size and birth order, on the one hand, and morbidity and growth on the other, were found only in some cases. This may be because, for most of the areas and cultures covered, such relationships did not exist, or may have been obscured by other more dominant factors. There are, however, technical reasons why real relationships may be hidden.

(a) *The samples of children*

The intention in every area was to investigate all, or a representative sample, of eligible women's children under 5 years of age. In practice, there were considerable difficulties in persuading women to bring their children for examination and even more so in obtaining blood and stool specimens. Even though the children investigated may have been representative of all the eligible women's children under 5 in terms of age and family size, they may have differed in health. It is possible, for instance, that mothers tended to bring for examination only those children who were sick.

(b) *The numbers studied*

In most areas, the age and family size subgroups often contained fewer than 25 children and sometimes fewer than 10. With such small numbers, the presence in the group of one or two unusual children, or recording or other errors, would have produced relatively large fluctuations that may have obscured trends.

In the case of weight and height, the comparatively small numbers also meant that children had to be grouped according to years of age. At this stage of life, when growth is rapid, the resulting average value for the year will depend on the way the children's ages were distributed within the year. This, too, may produce fluctuations that conceal trends.

---

[1] WHO Scientific Group on Nutritional Anemias (1968) Report, Geneva, World Health Organization (WHO Technical Report Series No. 405).

218

A. COLOMBIA

G. Ochoa & A. Gil

Sample for Physical and Laboratory Examination

It was decided to examine all children under 5 years of age who were sons or daughters of the women selected for gynaecological examination, using a systematic sampling technique of dwelling units.

Of the 2492 children selected for examination, 2177 (87.3%) could be examined. These children represent about 47.3% of the total number of children under 5 years of age in the study population (Table 5.A.1). It should be noted that the coverage in the NSZ was greater than in the OUZ, the figures being 91.3% and 82.6%, respectively.

TABLE 5.A.1. CHILDREN UNDER 5 YEARS OF AGE COVERED BY EACH INVESTIGATION, BY RESIDENCE

Residence	Total children under 5 years	Children under 5 years in sample selected	Children submitted to physical examination (height and weight)			Children submitted to haemoglobin determination		
			No.	% of sample	% of total	No.	% of sample	% of total
Old urban zone	1903	1141	943	82.6	50.0	934	81.9	49.1
Newly settled zone	2697	1351	1234	91.3	45.8	1225	90.7	45.4
Both zones	4600	2492	2177	87.3	47.3	2159	86.6	46.9

Personnel and General Procedure

Two physicians (general practitioners), previously trained and supervised by a paediatrician, carried out the examination of the children and obtained the information on physical health using a standard format devised for recording results. All the diagnoses were reviewed and codified by the paediatrician. An auxiliary nurse took the height and weight of the children, and another nurse ran the haemoglobin test, using a micromethod.

The number of children selected for examination was marked on the list of dwelling units. During the interview of the eligible woman in the sampled household the inverviewer gave her an appointment for her own examination as well as for that of her children under 5 years of age. When an appointment was not kept, an outreach worker arranged a second appointment. Three unfulfilled appointments were considered to constitute a final refusal.

Height and Weight

(a) Height

For most age intervals, the children of low social status were shorter in stature than those of middle social status. This relationship was maintained in both zones. Boys tended to be slightly taller than girls of the same age in both social status groups (Table 5.A.2).

TABLE 5.A.2. MEAN HEIGHTS OF CHILDREN UNDER 5, BY RESIDENCE, SOCIAL STATUS, AGE, AND SEX*

Residence and social status	Mean heights (cm) of male (M), female (F), and all (T) children at specified ages (years):														
	<1			1–2			2–3			3–4			4–5		
	M	F	T	M	F	T	M	F	T	M	F	T	M	F	T
Old urban zone															
Middle	66.2	65.4	65.8	80.1	79.0	79.5	88.3	88.2	88.3	95.5	95.5	95.5	102.5	101.8	102.2
Low	(69.2)	(67.0)	(67.9)	(79.7)	(79.5)	(79.6)	(87.9)	(86.1)	(86.9)	(93.0)	(93.6)	(93.3)	(99.8)	(100.7)	(100.3)
Both categories	66.4	65.6	65.9	80.0	79.0	79.5	88.3	88.0	88.2	95.3	95.3	95.3	102.2	101.7	102.0
Newly settled zone															
Middle	66.5	66.8	66.7	79.5	(76.5)	78.1	86.4	86.8	86.7	93.5	93.6	93.6	100.5	100.3	100.4
Low	65.0	63.2	64.1	77.5	76.2	76.8	86.6	84.4	85.4	92.4	91.9	92.1	97.8	98.0	97.9
Both categories	65.5	64.4	65.0	78.0	76.3	77.1	86.5	85.1	85.7	92.7	92.3	92.5	98.5	98.6	98.6

* Figures in parentheses refer to fewer than 25 children.

The results indicate that children under 5 years of age in the NSZ were slightly shorter than those in the OUZ. The age-specific mean weights showed no linear change with family size or birth order. Nevertheless, children in decidely small families (those with one or two children) were on the average taller than those with 6 or more children. This was true for both zones and for most of the age groups. A similar pattern existed for birth order, where the first- and second-born were taller than those of the 6th or higher birth order (Table 5.A.3).

TABLE 5.A.3. MEAN HEIGHTS OF CHILDREN UNDER 5, BY RESIDENCE AND AGE, AND BY FAMILY SIZE OR BIRTH ORDER*

(a) By family size

| Residence | Age (years) | Mean heights (cm) in families of size: | | | | | | | Total no. measured in age group |
		1	2	3	4	5	6 and over	All family sizes	
Old urban zone	<1	66.9	65.6	(64.8)	(64.6)	(66.9)	(64.5)	65.9	179
	1–2	79.5	79.6	79.5	(79.9)	(80.0)	(79.0)	79.5	180
	2–3	88.6	88.3	87.4	(89.7)	(87.6)	(87.1)	88.2	183
	3–4	(94.1)	95.8	95.1	(96.1)	(95.7)	94.5	95.3	193
	4–5	(102.3)	102.7	101.7	100.9	102.3	101.7	102.0	208
Newly settled zone	<1	66.1	64.9	64.2	(62.9)	(67.2)	64.8	65.0	201
	1–2	77.6	78.4	77.4	(76.9)	(75.6)	76.1	77.1	219
	2–3	(87.0)	86.8	84.7	84.7	86.0	85.6	85.7	251
	3–4	(93.9)	94.6	92.9	92.2	92.2	91.3	92.5	265
	4–5	(102.6)	100.3	100.2	98.3	97.6	97.3	98.6	298

(b) By birth order

| Residence | Age (years) | Mean heights (cm) of children of birth order: | | | | | | | Total no. measured in age group |
		1	2	3	4	5	6 and over	All birth orders	
Old urban zone	<1	66.7	66.1	(64.2)	(64.8)	(66.6)	(64.7)	65.9	179
	1–2	79.5	79.5	79.6	(78.8)	(80.9)	(79.4)	79.5	180
	2–3	89.0	87.8	87.7	(88.8)	(87.8)	(86.9)	88.2	183
	3–4	95.5	95.1	(95.0)	(95.9)	(97.4)	93.9	95.3	193
	4–5	103.0	102.2	100.8	101.2	(102.5)	101.8	102.0	208
Newly settled zone	<1	66.3	64.7	64.1	(63.8)	(67.5)	64.6	65.0	201
	1–2	78.5	77.3	77.4	(77.9)	(75.7)	76.0	77.1	219
	2–3	87.0	86.1	84.2	85.1	(85.8)	85.6	85.7	251
	3–4	95.1	92.9	92.8	92.0	(90.8)	91.4	92.5	265
	4–5	100.7	100.2	98.5	98.8	96.4	97.4	98.6	298

* Figures in parentheses refer to fewer than 25 children.

(b) Weight

Children under 5 years of age were found to be lighter in weight in the NSZ than in the OUZ. Children of low social status were lighter than those of middle social status in both zones, and in most age groups. Two exceptions were the < 1 year age group in the OUZ and the 1–2 year age group in the NSZ.

221

TABLE 5.A.4. MEAN WEIGHTS OF CHILDREN UNDER 5, BY RESIDENCE, SOCIAL STATUS, AGE, AND SEX*

Residence and social status	Mean weights (kg) of male (M), female (F), and all (T) children at specified ages (years):														
	<1			1–2			2–3			3–4			4–5		
	M	F	T	M	F	T	M	F	T	M	F	T	M	F	T
Old urban zone															
Middle	7.4	7.1	7.3	11.5	11.0	11.2	13.3	13.2	13.3	15.2	14.9	15.0	17.4	16.5	17.0
Low	(8.0)	(6.8)	(7.3)	(10.8)	(10.5)	(10.7)	(13.0)	(12.5)	(12.7)	(14.1)	(14.0)	(14.0)	16.0	16.2	16.1
Both categories	7.5	7.1	7.3	11.4	11.0	11.2	13.3	13.2	13.2	15.1	14.8	15.0	17.3	16.5	16.9
Newly settled zone															
Middle	7.4	7.3	7.3	10.8	(9.9)	10.4	12.9	12.4	12.6	14.9	14.1	14.5	16.1	16.0	16.1
Low	7.0	6.4	6.7	10.3	9.9	10.0	12.3	11.6	11.9	13.9	13.5	13.7	15.4	15.1	15.3
Both categories	7.1	6.7	6.9	10.4	9.9	10.1	12.5	11.8	12.1	14.2	13.7	14.0	15.6	15.4	15.5

* Figures in parentheses refer to fewer than 25 children.

Boys tended to weigh more than girls of the same age in both social status groups (Table 5.A.4). Again children in families of one or two were, on the average, heavier than those in large-sized families of 6 or more. Likewise, first- and second-born children were heavier than 6th or later born in most cases (Table 5.A.5).

TABLE 5.A.5. MEAN WEIGHTS OF CHILDREN UNDER 5, BY RESIDENCE AND AGE, AND BY FAMILY SIZE OR BIRTH ORDER*

(a) By family size

| Residence | Age (years) | Mean heights (cm) in families of size: | | | | | | | Total no. weighed in age group |
		1	2	3	4	5	6 and over	All family sizes	
Old urban zone	<1	7.61	6.82	(6.56)	(5.88)	(7.71)	(6.82)	6.90	201
	1–2	10.48	10.53	10.39	(10.05)	(10.02)	(9.53)	10.15	219
	2–3	12.42	12.60	11.87	(11.71)	(12.39)	(11.89)	12.10	251
	3–4	(14.94)	14.53	14.27	(13.50)	(14.06)	13.50	13.95	265
	4–5	(17.18)	16.18	16.09	15.36	15.08	14.94	15.47	193
Newly settled zone	<1	7.51	7.11	7.03	(7.14)	(7.76)	6.79	7.28	179
	1–2	11.32	11.15	10.89	(11.09)	(10.99)	11.49	11.18	180
	2–3	(13.35)	13.42	12.83	13.57	12.66	13.12	13.24	182
	3–4	(14.44)	15.11	14.82	15.46	15.01	14.62	14.94	193
	4–5	(17.11)	17.60	16.18	16.72	17.27	16.54	16.93	209

(b) By birth order

| Residence | Age (years) | Mean weights (kg) of children of birth order: | | | | | | | Total no. weighed in age group |
		1	2	3	4	5	6 and over	All birth orders	
Old urban zone	<1	7.48	7.20	(6.86)	(7.23)	(7.64)	(6.87)	7.28	179
	1–2	11.36	11.05	10.91	(10.83)	(11.40)	(11.57)	11.18	180
	2–3	13.59	13.17	12.90	(13.21)	(12.59)	(13.22)	13.24	182
	3–4	15.17	14.58	(14.59)	(15.66)	(15.38)	14.44	14.94	193
	4–5	17.55	16.92	16.30	17.11	(17.00)	16.48	16.93	209
Newly settled zone	<1	7.64	6.76	6.56	(6.02)	(7.85)	6.76	6.90	201
	1–2	10.72	10.21	10.32	(10.26)	(10.43)	9.44	10.15	219
	2–3	12.38	12.43	11.82	11.88	(12.23)	11.90	12.10	251
	3–4	14.75	14.00	14.34	13.85	(13.32)	13.53	13.95	265
	4–5	16.29	16.01	15.67	15.52	14.93	14.89	15.47	298

* Figures in parentheses refer to fewer than 25 children.

Haemoglobin Level

Blood samples were taken from the fingertip of the middle finger. The blood samples were taken by an auxiliary nurse, previously trained to record a reading immediately on an electrical haemoglobinometer with an optical system. The mean level of haemoglobin in grams per hundred millilitres of venous blood is given in Tables 5.A.6 and 5.A.7.

223

TABLE 5.A.6. MEAN HAEMOGLOBIN LEVELS OF CHILDREN UNDER 5, BY RESIDENCE, SOCIAL STATUS, AGE, AND SEX*

Mean haemoglobin levels (g/100 ml) of male (M), female (F), and all (T) children at specified ages (years):

Residence and social status	<1			1–2			2–3			3–4			4–5		
	M	F	T	M	F	T	M	F	T	M	F	T	M	F	T
Old urban zone															
Middle	13.15	(10.63)	11.06	11.20	11.37	11.28	11.56	11.58	11.57	11.78	11.62	11.70	12.09	11.79	11.96
Low	(10.23)	(10.43)	(10.40)	(10.43)	(11.48)	(10.99)	(10.51)	(11.46)	(11.04)	(11.35)	(11.05)	(11.20)	12.43	11.87	12.23
Both categories	11.31	10.99	11.14	11.14	11.38	11.26	11.48	11.57	11.52	11.74	11.57	11.67	12.22	11.80	11.98
Newly settled zone															
Middle	11.25	11.04	11.15	10.78	10.98	10.87	11.30	11.50	11.43	11.95	11.88	11.92	12.01	12.07	12.04
Low	10.73	10.73	10.73	10.16	10.60	10.68	11.51	11.19	11.33	11.60	11.32	11.46	11.83	11.76	11.80
Both categories	10.90	10.83	10.87	10.77	10.77	10.72	11.46	11.28	11.36	11.70	11.47	11.59	11.88	11.84	11.86

* Figures in parentheses refer to fewer than 25 children.

TABLE 5.A.7.   MEAN HAEMOGLOBIN LEVELS OF CHILDREN UNDER 5, BY RESIDENCE AND AGE, AND BY FAMILY SIZE OR BIRTH ORDER*

(a) By family size

Residence	Age (years)	Mean haemoglobin levels (g/100 ml) in families of size:							Total no. examined in age group
		1	2	3	4	5	6 and over	All family sizes	
Old urban zone	<1	11.13	10.98	(11.86)	(11.99)	(11.19)	(10.46)	11.14	177
	1–2	11.46	11.10	11.02	(11.40)	(11.26)	(11.35)	11.26	177
	2–3	11.53	11.54	11.52	(11.49)	(12.06)	(11.17)	11.52	181
	3–4	(11.88)	11.70	11.57	(11.86)	(11.66)	11.40	11.67	192
	4–5	(12.20)	12.14	11.72	11.89	12.09	11.84	11.97	207
Newly settled zone	<1	10.85	10.66	11.29	(10.86)	(10.85)	10.76	10.87	198
	1–2	11.32	10.57	10.53	(11.09)	(10.33)	10.66	10.72	217
	2–3	(11.34)	11.48	11.11	11.31	11.25	11.48	11.36	250
	3–4	(11.78)	11.60	11.75	11.79	11.40	11.47	11.59	264
	4–5	(12.10)	12.02	11.69	11.89	11.89	11.83	11.86	296

(b) By birth order

Residence	Age (years)	Mean haemoglobin levels (g/100 ml) of children of birth order:							Total no. examined in age group
		1	2	3	4	5	6 and over	All birth orders	
Old urban zone	<1	11.13	11.06	(11.46)	(11.96)	(11.51)	(10.39)	11.14	177
	1–2	11.42	11.07	11.01	(11.40)	(11.63)	(11.25)	11.26	177
	2–3	11.56	11.58	(11.48)	(11.26)	(11.85)	(11.23)	11.52	181
	3–4	11.89	11.38	(11.56)	(11.95)	(11.58)	11.46	11.67	192
	4–5	12.17	11.80	12.01	12.10	(11.84)	11.82	11.92	207
Newly settled zone	<1	10.81	10.61	11.36	(10.94)	(10.78)	10.74	10.87	198
	1–2	11.36	10.41	10.52	(11.10)	(10.62)	10.57	10.72	217
	2–3	11.37	11.35	11.22	11.25	(11.78)	11.33	11.36	250
	3–4	11.69	11.64	11.95	11.45	(11.52)	11.44	11.59	264
	4–5	12.01	11.77	11.70	(12.10)	11.78	11.84	11.86	296

* Figures in parentheses refer to fewer than 25 children.

Surprisingly, a direct association was found between the haemoglobin level and the child's age (Table 5.A.7).   In both residential areas, the level of haemoglobin was lower in the lower social status group than in the middle social status group (Table 5.A.6). No consistent relation was found between the level of haemoglobin and family size and birth order (Table 5.A.7). However, children in one-child families had a higher mean haemoglobin level than those in families of 6 or more for most age groups. A similar pattern was found for birth order, with first-born having higher mean haemoglobin levels than the 6th and higher birth order children.

Prevalence of Child Morbidity

Medical examination of children under 5 revealed high general morbidity (ICD 001–998)[1] in both regions. The morbidity rates for various age groups were higher in the NSZ than in the OUZ. In relation to family size, the age-specific morbidity rates tended, in a number of age groups and with some fluctuations, to increase with family size. In some age groups the pattern was not clear (Table 5.A.8).

TABLE 5.A.8. PREVALENCE OF MORBIDITY IN CHILDREN UNDER 5, BY RESIDENCE, AGE, AND FAMILY SIZE

Residence and age (years)	Percentage of children with disease in families of size:							Total no. examined in age group
	1	2	3	4	5	6 and over	All family sizes	
Old urban zone								
<1	26.6	20.7	21.7	31.4	17.1	24.7	23.9	180
1	20.7	28.5	29.2	32.2	34.0	31.1	27.2	180
2	25.6	24.8	30.0	47.5	31.7	30.0	28.8	182
3	26.0	26.8	32.0	32.5	39.0	35.0	30.7	193
4	17.6	26.4	27.8	31.1	24.0	35.6	28.2	202
Newly settled zone								
<1	25.1	25.9	26.7	24.2	30.7	37.6	29.1	201
1	28.4	35.5	34.7	35.8	34.2	35.5	34.2	219
2	30.0	34.8	45.4	38.1	39.3	35.8	37.7	250
3	32.7	40.0	38.0	37.6	50.0	43.5	41.5	265
4	24.4	37.4	46.3	46.2	55.0	46.8	45.4	298

Likewise, the morbidity of infectious and respiratory diseases was higher in the NSZ than in the OUZ. Again, there was a tendency in some age groups for the age-specific morbidity rates (of infections and respiratory diseases) to increase with family size. In other age groups, no consistent pattern was discernible (Table 5.A.9).

Reported Occurrence of Fever and Diarrhoea Among Children Under 10

All mothers in the study were queried about the occurrence of fever and diarrhoea among their children under 10 during the month preceding the interview. The results are given in Table 5.A.10. In both zones, the reported occurrence of fever and diarrhoea was higher in very large families of (6 and over) than in smaller families. The lowest rates were reported for families with only one child. For a family of 2–5 children, no clear pattern can be seen.

A different pattern emerges for birth order. In both zones, a consistent decline in the reported occurrence of fever and diarrhoea was noted with increasing birth order, excluding birth orders of 6 and over.

---

[1] This code refers to the *Manual of the International Statistical Classification of Diseases, Injuries, and Causes of Death*, 8th revision, Geneva, World Health Organization, 1965.

TABLE 5.A.9. PREVALENCE OF INFECTIONS AND RESPIRATORY DISEASE IN CHILDREN UNDER 5, BY RESIDENCE, AGE, AND FAMILY SIZE

Residence and age (years)	Percentage of children with infection and respiratory disease in families of size:							Total no. investigated in age group
	1	2	3	4	5	6 and over	All family sizes	
Old urban zone								
<1	18.0	12.5	16.5	14.5	—	12.0	14.0	180
1	20.5	13.0	35.0	33.5	40.0	33.5	24.0	180
2	23.0	17.5	28.5	31.0	58.0	15.0	24.0	182
3	5.0	12.5	11.0	18.5	24.0	10.5	13.0	193
4	6.0	8.5	8.5	7.5	8.0	11.0	9.0	209
Newly settled zone								
<1	28.0	24.5	19.5	26.5	33.5	33.0	27.5	201
1	35.5	49.0	38.5	54.5	29.5	32.0	39.5	219
2	5.0	33.0	35.0	48.5	38.0	34.5	34.0	250
3	36.0	35.5	22.5	26.5	30.0	21.0	26.5	265
4	11.0	26.0	23.5	31.0	34.5	20.0	24.5	290

TABLE 5.A.10. REPORTED OCCURRENCE OF FEVER AND DIARRHOEA AMONG CHILDREN UNDER 10 DURING THE MONTH PRECEDING MOTHER'S INTERVIEW, BY RESIDENCE AND FAMILY SIZE OR BIRTH ORDER

(a) By residence and family size

Residence and condition	Percentage of infections reported by EW with families of size:						Total no. of children in age group
	1	2	3	4	5	6 and over	
Old urban zone							
Fever	11.4	24.6	19.0	13.0	11.2	20.7	4127
Diarrhoea	11.5	24.6	19.0	13.0	11.2	20.7	4122
Newly settled zone							
Fever	5.3	12.9	13.8	14.2	11.6	42.2	6101
Diarrhoea	5.3	12.9	13.8	14.2	11.6	42.3	6090

(b) By residence and birth order

Residence and condition	Percentage of infections reported by EW for birth order:						Total no. of children in age group
	1	2	3	4	5	6 and over	
Old urban zone							
Fever	29.5	22.0	14.5	10.4	7.7	15.9	4127
Diarrhoea	29.5	22.1	14.5	10.4	7.7	15.9	4122
Newly settled zone							
Fever	18.6	16.5	13.5	11.3	9.6	30.6	6101
Diarrhoea	18.6	16.4	13.5	11.3	9.6	30.6	6090

The reported occurrence of fever and diarrhoea showed no clear relationship to family size in the OUZ. Among families with 3 or fewer children, these symptoms occur almost twice as frequently in the OUZ as in the NSZ. In the NSZ, an increase in the prevalence of fever and diarrhoea was observed with an increase in the size of the family and with a decrease in the birth order; the prevalence of these symptoms was also inversely related to birth order in the OUZ (Table 5.A.10).

B. EGYPT

E. E. D. Eid, F. S. Hassanein, A. Z. Zaghloul, A. H. I. Guinena & A. F. Moustafa

Samples for Physical and Laboratory Examination

It was originally intended to give physical and laboratory examinations to all eligible women's children under 5 years of age.

Table 5.B.1 shows that of the total of 4382 children in rural and urban areas, 3309 (75.5%) were physically examined, 3273 (74.7%) were examined for height and weight, and 2612 (59.6%) were given blood and stool specimen examinations. No data for the industrial area are shown in the table.

TABLE 5.B.1. CHILDREN UNDER 5 YEARS INVESTIGATED, BY RESIDENCE

Residence	All EW's children under 5	Physical examination		Height and weight measurement		Haemoglobin determination	
		No.	%	No.	%	No.	%
Rural	2187	1678	76.7	1678	76.7	1199	54.8
Urban	2195	1631	74.3	1595	72.7	1413	64.4

Personnel and General Procedure

Two paediatricians and 3 physicians conducted the physical examinations and measured weights and heights in the local health centres. Two laboratory technicians took the blood samples and examined the blood and stool specimens in the laboratory of the health centre. All the results were recorded on a standard form.

Height and Weight

(a) Height

Table 5.B.2 shows that for both rural and urban areas, boys were taller than girls in the age groups under 1 year of age and 4–5 years. In the remaining age groups (1–2, 2–3, and 3–4) no consistent pattern was observed.

228

TABLE 5.B.2. MEAN HEIGHTS OF CHILDREN UNDER 5, BY RESIDENCE, SOCIAL STATUS, AGE, AND SEX

Mean heights (cm) of male (M), female (F), and all (T) children at specified ages (years):

Residence and social status	<1			1–2			2–3			3–4			4–5		
	M	F	T	M	F	T	M	F	T	M	F	T	M	F	T
Rural															
Middle	71.1	67.5	69.2	73.9	73.1	73.5	80.6	79.7	80.1	87.3	88.1	87.7	95.2	94.9	95.0
Low	68.3	64.5	66.5	69.9	71.2	70.6	75.9	76.9	76.4	84.9	82.4	83.8	93.3	92.7	93.0
Both categories	69.3	65.7	67.5	71.1	71.8	71.5	77.5	77.9	77.6	85.6	84.2	84.9	93.9	93.5	93.7
Urban															
Middle	69.8	69.7	69.7	83.4	78.9	81.4	85.1	87.2	86.1	91.7	92.4	92.0	99.3	98.3	98.8
Low	68.8	66.5	67.6	78.9	76.5	77.8	84.7	85.3	84.9	92.0	92.7	92.4	97.3	94.8	96.3
Both categories	69.4	68.5	69.4	81.5	77.8	79.8	84.9	86.5	85.6	91.8	92.5	92.1	98.4	97.0	97.8

For both rural and urban areas, boys and girls of middle social status were taller than those of low social status, except in the fourth year where children of middle social status in the urban area were slightly shorter.

Urban children were taller than rural children; moreover, the difference was more conspicuous after the first year of life. The better education of urban mothers and their exposure to mass media promoting health consciousness were reflected in their better understanding of the supplementation of breast feeding and of the essential food groups that determine the growth of children after weaning.

No consistent relationships were found between mean height and family size or birth order in either rural or urban areas (Table 5.B.3(a) and 5.B.3(b)).

TABLE 5.B.3. MEAN HEIGHTS OF CHILDREN UNDER 5, BY RESIDENCE AND AGE, AND BY FAMILY SIZE OR BIRTH ORDER*

(a) By family size

Residence	Age (years)	Mean heights (cm) in families of size:							Total no. measured in age group
		1	2	3	4	5	6 and over	All family sizes	
Rural	<1	65.4	70.2	67.6	67.5	65.4	68.2	67.5	315
	1–2	72.2	72.6	71.3	71.3	70.9	70.6	71.5	238
	2–3	78.5	77.1	78.4	79.2	76.7	76.3	77.6	363
	3–4	84.5	84.6	85.6	83.9	85.4	85.4	84.9	355
	4–5	(88.0)	92.2	91.8	96.1	95.3	93.7	93.7	405
	Unknown								2
Urban	<1	70.5	70.8	67.6	69.2	65.8	68.6	68.4	307
	1–2	79.9	81.6	76.1	82.8	80.5	78.5	79.8	258
	2–3	86.4	88.5	83.5	83.5	86.3	85.9	85.6	334
	3–4	(89.6)	93.8	91.3	91.9	92.2	92.4	92.1	361
	4–5	(89.8)	98.9	98.9	95.1	97.7	98.4	97.8	335

(b) By birth order

Residence	Age (years)	Mean heights (cm) of children of birth order:							Total no. measured in age group
		1	2	3	4	5	6 and over	All birth orders	
Rural	<1	68.6	67.4	69.8	67.7	65.5	66.7	67.5	314
	1–2	74.3	70.9	73.5	71.1	69.9	71.2	71.5	239
	2–3	80.5	75.5	77.7	80.5	75.6	76.9	77.6	363
	3–4	86.2	86.1	83.1	83.8	85.4	84.9	84.9	356
	4–5	89.9	94.5	93.5	94.6	94.6	93.7	93.2	403
	Unknown								3
Urban	<1	72.1	69.9	64.4	71.0	71.9	67.3	68.4	307
	1–2	81.0	78.9	82.1	78.8	77.7	79.5	79.8	256
	2–3	90.5	85.3	81.4	84.4	86.2	85.8	85.6	333
	3–4	94.5	89.9	92.5	91.1	92.4	92.4	92.1	360
	4–5	99.1	99.8	97.8	95.0	94.9	98.8	97.8	334
	Unknown								5

* Figures in parentheses refer to fewer than 25 children.

TABLE 5.B.4. MEAN WEIGHTS OF CHILDREN UNDER 5, BY RESIDENCE, SOCIAL STATUS, AGE, AND SEX

Mean weights (kg) of male (M), female (F), and all (T) children at specified ages (years):

Residence and social status	<1			1–2			2–3			3–4			4–5		
	M	F	T	M	F	T	M	F	T	M	F	T	M	F	T
Rural															
Middle	7.8	6.8	7.2	7.9	7.5	7.7	9.6	9.1	9.3	11.7	11.6	11.6	13.7	12.9	13.2
Low	6.6	6.7	6.6	7.4	6.9	7.1	8.8	8.5	8.6	11.1	10.2	10.7	12.8	12.4	12.6
Both categories	6.9	6.7	6.8	7.5	7.1	7.3	9.1	8.7	8.8	11.3	10.6	10.7	13.1	12.6	12.8
Urban															
Middle	7.1	6.9	6.9	9.3	8.8	9.1	9.9	10.3	10.1	11.9	12.0	11.9	13.9	13.4	13.7
Low	7.2	6.6	6.9	9.0	7.9	8.5	9.5	9.9	9.7	11.7	12.0	11.9	13.4	12.6	13.1
Both categories	7.1	6.8	6.9	9.2	8.4	8.7	9.8	10.1	9.9	11.8	12.0	11.9	13.7	13.1	13.4

231

Growth achievement as expressed by height was better in urban than in rural areas for all family sizes. The difference was small for infants but became very conspicuous in the later years of early childhood. One reason for this is evident from an examination of Table 5.B.10, which shows that the reported prevalence of diarrhoea was significantly higher in rural areas than in urban areas for all social groups of all family sizes. Children who seldom suffer from diarrhoea have substantially larger increments of height and weight than children who have diarrhoea more frequently. These findings highlight the fact that diarrhoea is a major public health problem in Egypt. Malnutrition and inferior medical care aggravate the harm done by diarrhoea.

(b) Weight

All children were weighed in their underwear only and in bare feet using a beam balance.

Table 5.B.4 shows that boys were heavier than girls at all ages, with the exception of urban girls who were slightly heavier than boys at 2 and 3 years of age.

Children of middle social status were heavier than children of low social status. However, in the first and fourth years of life, the weights of children in the two social status groups were nearly equal in the urban area.

Urban children were heavier than rural children at all ages. The difference was small during the first year but became much larger from the second year on. The reasons given above for differences in height also account for this finding.

No consistent relationship between weight and family size or birth order was found (Tables 5.B.5(a) and 5.B.5(b)).

Haemoglobin Level

Haemoglobin levels expressed in grams of haemoglobin per 100 millilitres of venous blood were determined by the cyanmethaemoglobin method. Blood samples were taken by fingerprick.

Table 5.B.6 shows that the mean haemoglobin level was low for all children The maximum mean was 9.7 and the minimum was 7.8. For children between 6 months and 6 years, and living at sea-level, anaemia is considered to exist if the haemoglobin level is below 11 grams per 100 ml of venous blood.[1] Thus, all the children examined were suffering from anaemia.

The mean haemoglobin level increased slightly with age, except during the second year which had the lowest mean. It was slightly higher among rural than among urban children. This could be attributed to the fact that in the rural area children are in the habit of helping themselves to green vegetables, dates, or nuts between meals.

No relationship existed between mean haemoglobin levels and the social

---

[1] WHO Technical Report Series, 1968, No. 405.

232

TABLE 5.B.5. MEAN WEIGHTS OF CHILDREN UNDER 5, BY RESIDENCE AND AGE AND BY FAMILY SIZE OR BIRTH ORDER

(a) By family size

Residence	Age (years)	Mean weights (kg) in families of size:							Total no. weighed in age group
		1	2	3	4	5	6 and over	All family sizes	
Rural	<1	6.0	7.4	7.4	7.0	6.5	6.6	6.7	315
	1–2	7.4	7.5	6.9	7.6	7.1	7.3	7.2	238
	2–3	9.0	9.1	9.2	8.9	8.9	8.4	8.7	363
	3–4	10.8	10.6	11.1	10.8	11.6	11.3	11.0	355
	4–5	10.7	12.3	12.4	13.5	13.3	12.9	12.5	405
Urban	<1	7.3	6.9	6.9	6.7	6.7	6.8	6.8	307
	1–2	8.8	9.1	8.4	9.8	8.4	8.7	8.8	258
	2–3	9.0	10.2	10.0	10.0	10.1	9.8	10.0	334
	3–4	12.2	11.8	12.2	11.9	11.8	11.9	11.9	361
	4–5	12.5	12.9	14.1	13.3	13.6	13.3	13.2	335

(b) By birth order

Residence	Age (years)	Mean weights (kg) of children of birth order:							Total no. weighed in age group
		1	2	3	4	5	6 and over	All birth orders	
Rural	<1	6.9	6.7	7.2	6.5	6.7	6.8	6.8	315
	1–2	8.1	7.4	7.5	6.9	6.5	7.5	7.3	238
	2–3	9.5	8.6	9.5	9.2	8.8	8.5	8.8	363
	3–4	11.4	10.9	10.5	10.4	11.0	11.2	10.7	355
	4–5	11.6	12.6	12.8	13.5	13.0	12.9	12.8	405
	Unknown								2
Urban	<1	7.3	7.2	6.5	7.3	7.2	6.7	6.9	307
	1–2	8.9	9.3	8.7	8.9	8.9	8.6	8.7	256
	2–3	9.7	10.2	9.7	10.0	10.2	9.9	9.9	333
	?–4	12.1	11.6	12.2	11.8	12.1			360
	4–5	13.2	14.1	13.5	13.2	13.0	13.5	13.4	334
	Unknown								5

status or sex of the child. Tables 5.B.7(a) and 5.B.7(b) show that there was no consistent relationship between mean haemoglobin level and either family size or birth order.

Prevalence of Infections

All types of infection diagnosed during clinical examinations were recorded. The percentages of infections in rural and urban areas were almost equal, being 48.1% and 48.5% respectively. Tables 5.B.8(a) and 5.B.8(b) show that there

TABLE 5.B.6. MEAN HAEMOGLOBIN LEVELS OF CHILDREN UNDER 5, BY RESIDENCE, SOCIAL STATUS, AGE, AND SEX

Residence and social status	Mean haemoglobin levels (g/100 ml) of male (M), female (F), and all (T) children at specified ages (years):														
	<1			1–2			2–3			3–4			4–5		
	M	F	T	M	F	T	M	F	T	M	F	T	M	F	T
Rural															
Middle	8.6	9.3	8.9	9.0	8.6	8.8	9.5	8.9	9.2	8.9	9.5	9.2	9.3	9.7	9.5
Low	9.5	8.7	9.0	7.8	8.9	8.3	8.8	8.7	8.8	8.9	8.2	8.0	9.8	9.9	9.8
Both categories	9.2	8.9	8.9	8.1	8.8	8.4	9.4	8.7	8.9	8.9	9.3	9.1	9.6	9.8	9.7
Urban															
Middle	8.9	8.2	8.5	8.7	8.7	8.7	8.7	8.7	8.7	8.7	9.2	8.9	9.2	9.0	9.1
Low	8.7	8.5	8.6	8.3	8.3	8.3	8.9	8.9	8.9	8.3	9.1	9.2	8.9	8.9	8.9
Both categories	8.8	8.3	8.3	8.5	8.5	8.5	8.8	8.8	8.8	8.9	9.1	9.0	9.0	8.9	9.0

TABLE 5.B.7. MEAN HAEMOGLOBIN LEVELS OF CHILDREN UNDER 5, BY RESIDENCE AND AGE,
AND BY FAMILY SIZE OR BIRTH ORDER*

(a) By family size

Residence	Age (years)	Mean haemoglobin levels (g/100 ml) in families of size:							Total no. investigated in age group
		1	2	3	4	5	6 and over	All family sizes	
Rural	<1	9.6	9.9	8.5	8.9	(7.7)	(8.6)	8.8	178
	1–2	8.2	(8.2)	8.7	(8.2)	(8.3)	9.1	8.5	148
	2–3	9.5	8.8	9.1	9.1	8.6	8.2	8.8	260
	3–4	(10.3)	8.5	9.3	9.3	9.2	8.9	(9.2)	292
	4–5	(10.7)	9.9	10.0	10.1	9.5	9.2	9.9	321
Urban	<1	8.8	8.2	8.9	8.3	8.7	8.2	8.4	253
	1–2	9.2	8.0	8.8	8.1	8.2	8.6	8.3	225
	2–3	9.3	8.9	9.3	8.7	8.5	8.2	8.7	289
	3–4	(9.2)	9.2	9.4	8.6	9.1	8.9	9.0	335
	4–5	(9.5)	9.2	9.2	8.8	9.2	8.8	9.0	311

(b) By birth order

Residence	Age (years)	Mean haemoglobin levels (g/100 ml) of children of birth order:							Total no. investigated in age group
		1	2	3	4	5	6 and over	All birth orders	
Rural	<1	9.9	9.0	(9.8)	(7.9)	(8.3)	8.9	8.9	177
	1–2	(7.9)	(7.6)	(9.2)	(8.4)	(8.7)	8.7	8.6	148
	2–3	9.6	8.7	8.8	9.6	(8.0)	8.6	8.8	260
	3–4	9.3	9.3	9.3	9.1	8.5	9.0	9.1	292
	4–5	9.9	9.4	10.4	10.3	10.2	9.2	9.9	317
	Unknown								5
Urban	<1	8.6	8.4	9.1	8.6	(8.0)	8.5	8.5	253
	1–2	9.1	8.5	8.1	8.4	(8.1)	8.5	8.3	223
	2–3	9.3	9.0	8.8	8.7	9.6	8.3	8.9	288
	3–4	9.3	9.5	9.6	8.6	9.3	8.7	9.1	335
	4–5	9.5	9.4	8.5	9.0	9.0	8.9	8.9	310
	Unknown								4

* Figures in parentheses refer to fewer than 25 children.

was no consistent relationship between infection and either family size or birth order. However, reported infections were slightly higher in small families (1 to 2 children) than in larger families.

Table 5.B.9 shows that children aged 1 or 2 years had more infections than older children in rural and urban areas. No consistent relationship existed between the prevalence of infection and either family size or age, except that infection among members of small families (1 or 2 children) in both the rural and urban areas decreased with increase in age.

235

TABLE 5.B.8. PREVALENCE OF INFECTIONS IN CHILDREN UNDER 5 YEARS OF AGE

(a) By residence and family size

Residence	Percentage of children with infections in families of size:				Total no. investigated
	1 & 2	3 & 4	5 and over	All family sizes	
Rural	49.8	46.2	48.2	48.1	1618
Urban	50.6	43.7	43.1	48.5	1711

(b) By residence and birth order

Residence	Percentage of children with infections for birth order:				Total no. investigated
	1 & 2	3 & 4	5 and over	All family sizes	
Rural	47.0	50.0	45.5	48.2	1618
Urban	46.2	47.0	49.8	48.5	1711

TABLE 5.B.9. PREVALENCE OF INFECTIONS IN CHILDREN UNDER 5, BY RESIDENCE, AGE, AND FAMILY SIZE

Residence	Age (years)	Percentage of children with infections in families of size:				Total no. investigated in age group
		1 & 2	3 & 4	5 & 6	All family sizes	
Rural	1–2	53.6	50.4	52.9	53.2	339
	2–3	74.1	50.0	58.4	51.6	304
	3–4	51.6	48.5	51.5	50.5	390
	4–5	48.5	38.5	36.9	38.9	465
	All ages	49.1	46.2	48.3	47.8	1597
	Unknown					120
Urban	1–2	55.4	46.2	50.5	50.9	432
	2–3	50.7	51.0	50.8	50.5	395
	3–4	47.1	46.9	43.3	45.5	435
	4–5	29.2	47.4	48.0	44.9	403
	All ages	48.0	48.1	48.0	48.0	1665
	Unknown					46

Occurrence of Fever, Diarrhoea, or Cough reported by Eligible Women in Children under 10 during the Month Preceding the Interview

Table 5.B.10(a) shows a consistent tendency for the reporting of fever or diarrhoea to decrease with increasing family size. This unexpected finding might be attributable to the fact that mothers of large families tend to pay less attention to the health of their children as compared to the mothers of small families. The prevalence of reported fever or diarrhoea was higher in rural than in urban areas for all family sizes. The reported occurrence of fever and

236

TABLE 5.B.10. REPORTED OCCURRENCE OF FEVER AND DIARRHOEA AMONG CHILDREN UNDER 10, DURING THE MONTH PRECEDING MOTHER'S INTERVIEW, BY RESIDENCE AND FAMILY SIZE OR BIRTH ORDER

(a) By residence and family size

Residence and condition	Percentage of infections reported by EW with families of:						Total no. of children in age group
	1	2	3	4	5	6 and over	
Rural							
Fever	19.9	19.7	14.7	15.6	14.5	11.6	8104
Diarrhoea	20.3	17.1	14.0	13.8	12.8	9.7	8104
Urban							
Fever	19.1	17.2	13.6	11.9	10.4	8.7	8231
Diarrhoea	20.2	15.7	11.8	9.8	7.5	7.0	8231

(b) By residence and birth order

Residence and condition	Percentage of infections reported by EW for birth order:						Total no. of children in age group
	1	2	3	4	5	6 and over	
Rural							
Fever	16.0	15.9	16.9	17.0	19.9	20.7	6775
Diarrhoea	14.5	14.2	15.9	14.9	17.3	18.7	6775
Unknown							1329
Urban							
Fever	12.2	12.2	10.9	13.6	16.4	15.4	7107
Diarrhoea	11.2	9.9	9.7	10.6	13.0	13.0	7107
Unknown							1124

diarrhoea was also higher among children of birth orders 5 and over than among those of lower birth orders.

Intestinal Parasitic Infestation

Stools of young children were examined for ancylostomes, ascarides, oxyurids, and tapeworms. History-taking for oxyuriasis was also revealing.

From Table 5.B.11 and Fig. 5.B.1 it can be observed that the prevalence of parasitic infestation was higher among rural than among urban children (66.9% and 50.1%, respectively) and the difference was significant at the 0.01 level.

There was a direct relationship between parasitic infestation and the age of the child; as age increased, the prevalence increased. This could be explained by the fact that older children run more freely out-of-doors and would have more contact with the infested environment. As age increased from 1 to 5 years, parasitic infestation increased in prevalence from 44.3% to 82.7% in the rural area and from 26.1% to 70.8% in the urban area.

TABLE 5.B.11. PREVALENCE OF PARASITIC INFESTATION IN CHILDREN UNDER 5, BY
RESIDENCE, AGE, AND FAMILY SIZE

Residence and age	Percentage of children with parasitic infestations in families of size:				Total no. of children investigated in age group
	1 & 2	3 & 4	5 and over	All family sizes	
Rural					
1–2	27.5	37.3	64.5	44.3	305
2–3	42.6	46.4	75.3	56.8	553
3–4	68.8	74.3	77.5	73.9	477
4–5	78.0	82.2	86.3	82.7	538
All ages	56.7	63.7	77.3	66.9	1873
Urban					
1–2	17.3	25.8	39.6	26.1	381
2–3	31.2	34.5	44.5	36.1	590
3–4	56.8	63.6	67.8	63.3	497
4–5	62.0	69.4	78.9	70.8	446
All ages	42.5	48.6	61.4	50.1	1914

FIG. 5.B.1. PARASITIC INFESTATION IN CHILDREN UNDER 5 BY FAMILY SIZE

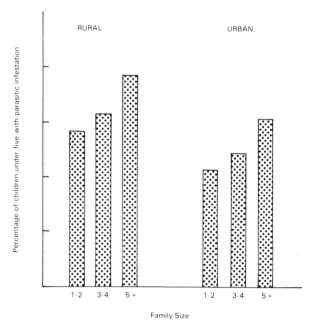

Also, there was a direct relationship between prevalence of parasitic
infestation in children under 5 years of age and the size of their families. As the
family size increased from 1 and 2 to 3 and 4 and then to 5 and more, the
prevalence of parasitic infestation increased from 56.7% to 63.7% to 77.3%,
respectively, in the rural area and from 42.5% to 48.6% to 61.4%, respectively,
in the urban area.

238

The effect of bigger family size could be important because of the increased chances of infestation due to crowding at home and lack of supervision of the outdoor activities of children in larger families compared with smaller families in the same environment.

C. PAKISTAN

Farhat Ajmal & Hafiz Zaidi

Sample for Physical and Laboratory Examination

It was originally intended to examine all the children under 5 years of age of all the eligible women, but it was later decided to examine only the children of those eligible women who had accepted physical examination. The number of such children under 5 years of age was 2558 from the semi-urban area and 2473 from the urban area. Of these, 1397 children (54.6%) from the semi-urban area and 1693 (71.4%) from the urban area actually attended for physical examination.

Height and weight measurements were performed on almost all the children who were physically examined. Blood samples could be obtained from 1072 children (77.7%) from the semi-urban area and 1362 children (80.6%) from the urban area (Table 5.C.1).

TABLE 5.C.1. CHILDREN UNDER 5 YEARS COVERED BY EACH INVESTIGATION, BY RESIDENCE

Residence	Physical examination	Height and weight		Stool investigation		Haemoglobin determination	
	No.	No.	%	No.	%	No.	%
Semi-urban	1397	1387	99.2	1252	89.6	1072	76.7
Urban	1693	1693	100.0	358	21.2	1362	80.6
Both areas	3090	3080	99.8	1610	52.2	2434	78.8

Personnel and General Procedure

Four medical officers were employed to carry out the physical examination of the children. Each had had at least 1 year's experience of working in medical departments of the teaching hospital. Two medical technologists and two laboratory technicians were also recruited. Two ayahs (nursemaids) were employed to collect stool samples from houses. The laboratory staff worked under the guidance of a highly qualified pathologist. Eight interviewers, graduates in sociology, were employed to interview eligible women and bring them and their children to the medical centre for examination.

TABLE 5.C.2. MEAN HEIGHTS OF CHILDREN UNDER 5, BY RESIDENCE, SOCIAL STATUS, AGE, AND SEX*

Mean heights (cm) of male (M), female (F), and all (T) children at specified ages (years):

Residence and social status	<1			1–2			2–3			3–4			4–5		
	M	F	T	M	F	T	M	F	T	M	F	T	M	F	T
Semi-urban															
Middle	60.8	58.3	59.6	67.7	66.5	67.1	73.5	70.2	72.8	84.1	81.6	83.0	89.2	88.9	89.0
Low	58.9	59.4	59.1	66.1	68.5	67.3	72.2	71.2	71.7	80.1	79.9	79.9	87.3	83.6	86.4
Both categories	59.8	58.9	59.3	66.8	67.6	67.2	72.8	72.0	72.4	82.0	80.5	81.3	88.2	87.0	87.6
Urban															
Middle	64.8	65.4	65.1	75.7	76.1	75.9	83.4	82.4	82.9	91.8	90.6	91.2	99.5	97.1	98.4
Low	(65.5)	(64.5)	65.0	(72.2)	(77.4)	(75.1)	(78.1)	(82.2)	80.4	(89.9)	87.8	88.7	(96.5)	(95.4)	(96.1)
Both categories	64.9	65.3	65.1	75.5	76.2	75.9	83.0	82.4	82.7	91.6	90.3	90.9	99.2	97.0	98.2

* Figures in parentheses refer to fewer than 25 children.

Two medical centres were set up for physical examinations, one in the urban and the other in a semi-urban area of Karachi.

Each medical centre had a staff of 2 medical officers, 1 medical technologist, 1 laboratory technician, 4 interviewers, and 1 ayah.

Since it was feared that a large number of women and children might not come to the clinic, an official transport vehicle was made available to collect the women from their homes. In spite of this facility, some women refused to come and bring their children to the medical centres. These women and children were visited at home by a team consisting of one medical officer, one laboratory technician, and an ayah. Clinical examinations were carried out and samples for blood and stool examinations were collected from homes.

TABLE 5.C.3. MEAN HEIGHTS OF CHILDREN UNDER 5, BY RESIDENCE AND AGE, AND BY FAMILY SIZE OR BIRTH ORDER*

(a) By family size

Residence	Age (years)	Mean heights (cm) in families of size:							Total no. measured in age group
		1	2	3	4	5	6 and over	All family sizes	
Semi-urban	0–1	59.2	59.3	59.9	60.5	57.7	59.2	59.3	288
	1–2	(67.6)	67.3	(67.4)	70.3	64.4	66.4	67.2	161
	2–3	(70.6)	73.9	71.5	71.4	73.5	72.5	72.4	305
	3–4	(78.8)	83.3	79.8	80.2	80.7	82.4	81.3	350
	4–5	(83.0)	88.8	85.3	88.3	87.0	88.0	87.6	283
Urban	0–1	65.1	68.0	64.5	65.0	64.4	61.8	65.1	386
	1–2	75.3	75.3	77.3	74.6	(75.8)	76.0	75.9	233
	2–3	84.1	82.9	83.8	81.7	84.3	80.6	82.7	352
	3–4	(93.3)	90.0	92.3	90.8	90.5	90.4	90.9	396
	4–5	(98.8)	99.4	97.6	96.9	100.2	98.2	98.2	326

(b) By birth order

Residence	Age (years)	Mean heights (cm) of children of birth order:							Total no. measured in age group
		1	2	3	4	5	6 and over	All birth orders	
Semi-urban	0–1	58.9	59.1	59.6	60.9	59.7	58.7	59.3	288
	1–2	(68.7)	(66.1)	(66.7)	(69.8)	(65.5)	66.9	67.2	161
	2–3	72.8	72.7	72.2	70.4	74.6	72.2	72.4	305
	3–4	81.2	81.8	81.1	81.2	80.8	81.6	81.3	350
	4–5	88.6	87.9	86.7	88.2	86.2	87.6	87.6	283
Urban	0–1	65.6	67.8	64.3	64.1	66.2	62.1	65.1	386
	1–2	75.9	76.5	76.0	74.9	(75.6)	75.9	75.9	233
	2–3	82.8	84.7	83.5	80.5	85.0	80.7	82.7	352
	3–4	90.9	91.8	91.4	90.9	90.9	90.1	90.9	396
	4–5	99.2	97.7	96.9	99.1	(98.6)	98.1	98.2	326

* Figures in parentheses refer to fewer than 25 children.

TABLE 5.C.4. MEAN WEIGHTS OF CHILDREN UNDER 5, BY RESIDENCE, SOCIAL STATUS, AGE, AND SEX*

Mean weights (kg) of male (M), female (F), and all (T) children at specified ages (years):

Residence and social status	<1			1–2			2–3			3–4			4–5		
	M	F	T	M	F	T	M	F	T	M	F	T	M	F	T
Semi-urban															
Middle	6.9	5.9	6.4	8.0	7.9	7.9	9.6	9.4	9.4	11.3	10.7	11.0	12.7	12.8	12.7
Low	6.1	5.9	6.1	8.1	7.8	8.0	8.9	8.6	8.7	10.6	10.3	10.4	12.0	11.8	11.9
Both categories	6.5	5.9	6.2	8.1	7.9	7.9	9.2	9.0	9.1	10.9	10.5	10.7	12.4	12.2	12.3
Urban															
Middle	7.5	7.4	7.4	9.8	9.1	9.5	11.3	10.8	10.8	12.7	12.2	12.5	14.5	14.0	14.3
Low	(7.6)	(7.4)	7.5	(8.2)	(9.2)	(8.7)	(9.8)	(10.4)	10.1	(12.6)	11.8	12.2	(13.5)	(13.2)	(13.4)
Both categories	7.5	7.4	7.4	9.7	9.1	9.4	11.2	10.7	11.0	12.7	12.2	12.4	14.4	14.0	14.2

* Figures in parentheses refer to fewer than 25 children.

Height and Weight

(a) Height

The findings indicate that male children in general were taller than female children of corresponding characteristics with one exception, age group 1–2 years where the females were taller than their male counterparts.

The children of middle social status were generally taller than those of low social status. The differences were more marked in the older age groups (Table 5.C.2).

The urban children were taller by 7–10 cm than the semi-urban children with corresponding characteristics. The difference was more pronounced in age group 4–5 years (Table 5.C.2).

The average gain in height over a period of 4 years of urban children (33.1 cm) was more than that of semi-urban children (28.3 cm).

No consistent relationship between mean height of children and family size or birth order could be established (Table 5.C.3(a) and (b)).

TABLE 5.C.5. MEAN WEIGHTS OF CHILDREN UNDER 5, BY RESIDENCE AND AGE, AND BY FAMILY SIZE OR BIRTH ORDER*

(a) By family size

Residence	Age (years)	Mean weights (kg) in families of size:							Total no. weighed in age group
		1	2	3	4	5	6 and over	All family sizes	
Semi-urban	0–1	6.1	6.1	6.2	6.6	5.9	6.3	6.3	288
	1–2	(8.1)	7.7	(8.2)	8.1	8.1	7.8	7.9	161
	2–3	(9.0)	9.0	9.3	9.1	9.5	8.9	9.1	305
	3–4	(9.8)	11.1	10.3	10.4	10.9	10.9	10.7	350
	4–5	(12.0)	12.3	12.2	11.9	12.3	12.5	12.3	283
Urban	0–1	7.4	8.0	7.1	7.1	7.3	7.3	7.4	386
	1–2	9.3	9.7	9.4	9.4	(9.4)	9.1	9.4	233
	2–3	11.4	11.3	10.9	10.9	11.1	10.4	10.1	352
	3–4	(12.6)	12.6	12.6	12.3	12.2	12.3	12.4	396
	4–5	(14.2)	14.8	14.4	13.9	14.2	14.1	14.2	326

(b) By birth order

Residence	Age (years)	Mean weights (kg) of children of birth order:							Total no. weighed in age group
		1	2	3	4	5	6 and over	All birth orders	
Semi-urban	0–1	5.9	6.3	6.2	6.5	6.4	6.3	6.3	288
	1–2	(8.4)	(7.5)	(7.7)	(8.4)	(8.5)	7.7	8.0	161
	2–3	9.2	8.9	9.4	9.5	9.5	9.8	9.4	305
	3–4	10.6	10.8	10.3	10.7	11.1	10.7	10.7	350
	4–5	12.3	12.4	11.1	12.3	12.4	12.4	12.3	283
Urban	0–1	7.4	8.0	7.1	6.9	7.4	7.3	7.4	386
	1–2	9.5	9.7	9.4	9.5	(8.9)	9.1	9.4	233
	2–3	11.4	11.2	11.0	10.4	11.5	19.4	10.1	352
	3–4	12.7	12.6	12.3	12.2	12.8	12.2	12.4	396
	4–5	14.6	14.2	14.1	14.1	(14.1)	14.1	14.2	326

* Figures in parentheses refer to fewer than 25 children.

TABLE 5.C.6. MEAN HAEMOGLOBIN LEVELS OF CHILDREN UNDER 5, BY RESIDENCE, SOCIAL STATUS, AGE, AND SEX*

Mean haemoglobin levels (g/100 ml) of male (M), female (F), and all (T) children at specified ages (years):

Residence and social status	<1			1–2			2–3			3–4			4–5		
	M	F	T	M	F	T	M	F	T	M	F	T	M	F	T
Semi-urban															
Middle	9.6	9.6	9.6	(9.7)	8.7	9.2	8.4	8.7	8.6	9.5	9.3	9.4	10.2	9.8	10.0
Low	9.2	9.8	9.4	8.9	8.8	8.8	8.2	8.2	8.2	8.2	8.8	8.6	9.8	9.9	9.9
Both categories	9.4	9.7	9.5	8.9	8.8	8.9	8.4	8.5	8.4	9.2	8.9	9.0	10.0	9.9	9.9
Urban															
Middle	9.5	9.6	9.4	9.5	9.6	9.5	9.6	9.3	9.5	9.8	9.7	9.8	10.3	10.2	10.2
Low	(9.4)	(9.2)	(9.3)	(10.2)	(9.1)	(9.5)	(8.1)	(8.5)	(8.3)	(9.6)	(9.8)	9.7	(9.9)	(9.1)	(9.5)
Both categories	9.4	9.6	9.5	9.5	9.5	9.5	9.5	9.5	9.5	9.8	9.7	9.7	10.2	10.1	10.2

* Figures in parentheses refer to fewer than 25 children.

(*b*) *Weight*

The boys were slightly heavier than the girls of corresponding characteristics. The children of middle social status were generally heavier than those of low social status. The urban children were heavier than semi-urban children. The difference was most marked in age group 4–5 years (Table 5.C.4).

No consistent relationship between weight and family size or birth order was observed (Table 5.C.5(*a*) and (*b*)).

Haemoglobin Level

Haemoglobin level was measured in grams per hundred millilitres of venous blood by the cyanmethaemoglobin method. Blood samples were taken from the heels of infants and the fingertips of older children. Haemoglobin

TABLE 5.C.7. MEAN HAEMOGLOBIN LEVELS OF CHILDREN UNDER 5, BY RESIDENCE AND AGE, AND BY FAMILY SIZE OR BIRTH ORDER*

(*a*) By family size

Residence	Age (years)	Mean haemoglobin levels (g/100 ml) in families of size:							Total no. investigated in age group
		1	2	3	4	5	6 and over	All family sizes	
Semi-urban	0–1	9.7	(9.6)	9.0	9.7	(9.5)	9.5	9.5	194
	1–2	(8.4)	(9.3)	(8.4)	(9.0)	(9.0)	9.1	8.9	120
	2–3	(7.6)	8.9	8.0	8.6	8.7	8.4	8.4	250
	3–4	(8.4)	9.3	8.6	8.9	9.0	9.2	9.0	279
	4–5	(11.5)	10.4	10.0	9.9	9.7	9.9	9.9	229
Urban	0–1	9.5	9.3	9.7	9.2	9.6	9.9	9.5	278
	1–2	9.7	9.6	9.8	9.1	(9.8)	9.3	9.5	195
	2–3	9.9	9.3	9.3	9.0	9.8	9.3	9.5	290
	3–4	(9.9)	9.7	9.7	9.8	9.9	9.7	9.7	336
	4–5	(10.9)	10.7	9.9	10.2	10.0	10.1	10.2	263

(*b*) By birth order

Residence	Age (years)	Mean haemoglobin levels (g/100 ml) of children of birth order:							Total no. investigated in age group
		1	2	3	4	5	6 and over	All birth orders	
Semi-urban	0–1	(10.0)	(9.7)	(8.8)	9.7	(9.4)	9.6	9.6	194
	1–2	(8.5)	(8.8)	(8.7)	(9.0)	(8.7)	9.2	8.9	120
	2–3	8.2	(8.6)	8.3	8.3	8.8	8.4	8.4	250
	3–4	9.2	9.0	8.7	8.8	8.8	9.2	9.0	279
	4–5	10.7	10.1	(10.0)	9.5	9.7	9.8	9.9	229
Urban	0–1	9.4	9.4	9.7	9.5	(9.5)	9.8	9.6	278
	1–2	9.9	9.5	9.3	9.2	(9.3)	9.4	9.5	195
	2–3	9.5	9.2	9.3	9.2	(9.2)	9.2	9.3	290
	3–4	9.5	10.2	9.7	9.5	10.4	9.6	9.7	336
	4–5	10.2	10.4	10.1	10.1	(10.0)	10.3	10.2	263

* Figures in parentheses refer to fewer than 25 children.

245

determination was performed on 1072 semi-urban children (41.9%) and 1362 urban children (57·5%). The average haemoglobin level of all children was fairly low, both in the semi-urban area (9.2%) and in the urban area (10.0%). There was no consistent variation with the sex of children or social status. The urban children had slightly higher haemoglobin levels than semi-urban children (Table 5.C.6). No consistent variation was found in haemoglobin levels in relation to family size or birth order (Table 5.C.7(a) and (b)).

Prevalence of Infections in Children under Five Years of Age

This category includes all infections clinically diagnosed as of bacterial, viral, fungal, or parasitic origin. It does not include parasitic infections of the intestines.

Of all the children clinically examined, 23.0% from the urban area and 31.0% from the semi-urban area were found to be suffering from different types of infection.

There was a definite rise in the prevalence of infections with increase in family size, particularly in the urban area. A higher occurrence of infections in the semi-urban (31%) than in the urban area (23.0%) was also noted (Table 5.C.8).

The infection rate was also higher in older age groups than in lower age groups for all family sizes and in both areas. The lowest infection rates in the urban area were noted in infants under 1 year of age whose mothers had small families.

TABLE 5.C.8. PREVALENCE OF INFECTIONS IN CHILDREN UNDER 5, BY RESIDENCE, AGE, AND FAMILY SIZE

| Residence | Age (years) | Percentage of children with infections in families of size: | | | | Total no. investigated in age group |
		1–2	3–4	5 and over	All family sizes	
Semi-urban	< 1	18.2	20.0	20.8	20.0	287
	1	27.4	30.2	31.5	30.1	162
	2	35.3	31.4	34.1	33.6	305
	3	32.7	33.8	37.0	35.4	350
	4	40.6	31.9	35.3	34.8	283
	All less than 5	29.4	29.6	32.5	31.0	1387
Urban	< 1	9.5	12.9	17.5	12.6	285
	1	16.3	23.0	24.3	21.0	233
	2	19.8	20.6	28.1	24.6	352
	3	25.4	27.1	28.3	27.2	396
	4	30.0	28.7	31.0	42.5	326
	All less than 5	18.0	24.1	26.5	23.0	1690

Occurrence of Fever and Diarrhoea reported by Eligible Women in Children under 10 during the Month Preceding Interview

Mothers reported that 58.6% of their children under 10 years had fever and 30.6% had diarrhoea in the month preceding the interview.

Fever was more prevalent in the urban area (65.8% compared with 51.4%), while diarrhoea occurred more often in the semi-urban area (33.8% compared with 27.4%). The reported occurrence of fever rose with increasing family size and birth order, but the reported occurrence of diarrhoea was higher for low family sizes and low birth orders (Table 5.C.9(*a*) and (*b*)).

TABLE 5.C.9. REPORTED OCCURRENCE OF FEVER AND DIARRHOEA AMONG CHILDREN UNDER 10 DURING THE MONTH PRECEDING MOTHER'S INTERVIEW, BY RESIDENCE AND FAMILY SIZE OR BIRTH ORDER

(*a*) By family size

Residence and condition	Percentage of infections reported by EW with families of:				Total no. of children in age group
	1–2	3–4	5 and over	All family sizes	
Semi-urban					
Fever	49.1	51.8	51.8	51.4	3778
Diarrhoea	37.8	36.1	31.6	33.8	3778
Urban					
Fever	57.4	68.5	69.2	65.8	2546
Diarrhoea	33.8	26.8	23.8	27.4	2546

(*b*) By birth order

Residence and condition	Percentage of infections reported by EW for birth order:				Total no. of children in age group
	1–2	3–4	5 and over	All birth orders	
Semi-urban					
Fever	51.3	51.9	51.2	51.4	3778
Diarrhoea	34.7	34.4	32.9	33.8	3778
Urban					
Fever	61.8	68.5	69.3	65.8	2546
Diarrhoea	30.7	25.3	24.3	27.4	2546

The high prevalence (58.6%) of fever in large families could be due to the fact that older children go to school and are more exposed to the infectious and viral fevers that are common in the congested areas of Karachi; in addition, older children with more siblings would be more likely to be neglected and malnourished.

D. SYRIAN ARAB REPUBLIC

M. El-Jabi

Samples for Physical and Laboratory Examination

It was originally intended to examine all children under 5 years old belonging to the eligible women, but not all such children were brought for a physical examination. Table 5.D.1 shows the numbers covered for each investigation. Of a total of 7475 children eligible for examination, 2225 (29.8%) accepted the height and weight examination and 2177 (29.1%) accepted haemoglobin determination. In addition, some information about certain diseases of children was reported by the interviewed women.

TABLE 5.D.1. CHILDREN UNDER 5 YEARS OF AGE COVERED BY EACH INVESTIGATION, BY RESIDENCE

Residence	Total no. of EW's children under 5	Physical examination		Height and weight examination		Haemoglobin determination	
		No.	%	No.	%	No.	%
Damascus	2511	415	16.5	671	26.7	661	26.3
Sweida	2124	319	15.0	601	28.3	587	27.6
Rural Aleppo	2840	689	24.3	953	33.6	929	32.7
All areas	7475	1423	19.3	2225	29.8	2177	29.1

Personnel and General Procedure

Nine lady physicians conducted the physical examination of mothers, 9 paediatricians conducted the children's examinations and 3 laboratories were used for laboratory investigations. Mothers and children were driven to the doctors' clinics and laboratories, where 62% of mothers and 27% of children in Damascus, 65% of mothers and 28% of children in Sweida, and 72% of mothers and 34% of children in Rural Aleppo were examined.

Height and Weight

(a) Height

Boys were found to be taller than girls of the same age; this difference was evident regardless of geographical area or social status (Table 5.D.2).

248

TABLE 5.D.2. MEAN HEIGHTS OF CHILDREN UNDER 5, BY RESIDENCE, SOCIAL STATUS, AND SEX*

Mean heights (cm) of male (M), female (F), and all (T) children at specified ages (years):

Residence and social status	1–2			2–3			3–4			4–5		
	M	F	T	M	F	T	M	F	T	M	F	T
Damascus												
Middle	74.5	74.7	74.6	83.9	82.0	83.0	91.4	90.6	91.0	97.9	97.9	97.9
Low	(75.4)	(72.6)	(74.3)	(81.4)	(80.3)	80.8	(89.3)	(88.9)	89.1	(96.8)	(95.0)	95.9
Both categories	74.8	74.2	74.5	83.5	81.7	82.6	91.0	90.2	90.6	97.7	97.3	97.5
Sweida												
Middle	(75.6)	(74.5)	75.2	85.2	80.8	83.0	90.6	87.5	89.1	96.2	94.3	95.4
Low	(75.2)	(65.0)	(71.4)	(81.5)	(81.6)	(81.5)	90.3	90.2	90.2	92.5	(91.1)	92.0
Both categories	75.5	(72.9)	74.4	84.6	81.0	82.8	90.5	88.3	89.4	95.4	93.7	94.7
Rural Aleppo												
Middle	77.8	72.6	74.9	82.2	82.8	82.5	88.0	88.3	88.1	95.5	92.8	94.4
Low	76.4	74.0	75.3	81.9	81.5	81.7	87.9	86.0	87.0	95.1	94.9	95.0
Both categories	76.8	73.4	75.2	82.0	82.0	82.0	87.9	86.7	87.4	95.2	94.3	94.8

* Figures in parentheses refer to fewer than 25 children.

In general, a positive relationship between height and social status was present. There was no consistent relationship between mean height and family size (Table 5.D.3(*a*)) or between mean height and birth order (Table 5.D.3(*b*)).

TABLE 5.D.3. MEAN HEIGHTS OF CHILDREN UNDER 5, BY RESIDENCE AND AGE, AND BY FAMILY SIZE OR BIRTH ORDER*

(a) By family size

Residence	Age (years)	Mean heights (cm) in families of size:							Total no. measured in age group
		1	2	3	4	5	6 and over	All sizes	
Damascus	1–2	75	(75)	(71)	(69)	(72)	(76)	74	79
	2–3	(80)	82	(79)	(86)	(82)	83	82	152
	3–4	(89)	(91)	91	91	89	91	91	191
	4–5	(101)	(98)	97	97	99	97	98	244
Sweida	1–2	(75)	(71)	(63)	(70)	(78)	(81)	74	45
	2–3	(82)	84	(78)	(78)	(78)	84	83	11
	3–4	(89)	88	(92)	88	(93)	89	89	185
	4–5	(101)	(92)	95	94	94	95	95	261
Rural Aleppo	1–2	71	72	(73)	(77)	79	78	75	157
	2–3	77	79	82	84	88	82	82	299
	3–4	(82)	87	87	85	88	89	87	263
	4–5	(96)	94	93	(95)	97	95	95	223

(b) By birth order

Residence	Age (years)	Mean heights (cm) of children of birth order:							Total no. measured in age group
		1	2	3	4	5	6 and over	All birth orders	
Damascus	1–2	76	(75)	(72)	(64)	(72)	(76)	74	79
	2–3	82	(80)	(85)	(83)	(82)	83	82	152
	3–4	91	(92)	(91)	88	(89)	91	91	191
	4–5	97	97	99	96	98	97	97	244
Sweida	1–2	(74)	(76)	(70)	(65)	(80)	(80)	74	45
	2–3	83	(85)	(86)	(81)	(81)	82	83	110
	3–4	89	(91)	(89)	(92)	(88)	89	83	185
	4–5	94	97	95	92	95	95	95	261
Rural Aleppo	1–2	71	(73)	(74)	(73)	(79)	77	75	157
	2–3	79	81	81	86	85	82	82	299
	3–4	85	88	86	(89)	(88)	88	87	263
	4–5	94	(92)	(96)	(96)	97	94	95	223

* Figures in parentheses refer to fewer than 25 children.

(b) Weight

Boys were also found to be heavier than girls of the same age; this difference was present regardless of geographical area (Table 5.D.4). The mean weight of children of middle social status was higher than that of children of low social status only in Damascus. No such relationship was present in Sweida or Rural Aleppo.

250

TABLE 5.D.4. MEAN WEIGHTS OF CHILDREN UNDER 5, BY RESIDENCE, SOCIAL STATUS, AGE, AND SEX*

Mean weights (kg) of male (M), female (F), and all (T) children at specified ages (years):

Residence and social status	1–2			2–3			3–4			4–5		
	M	F	T	M	F	T	M	F	T	M	F	T
Damascus												
Middle	10.2	9.7	9.9	12.2	11.3	11.8	13.7	13.2	13.5	15.2	15.1	15.4
Low	(9.6)	(8.6)	(9.2)	(10.3)	(10.5)	10.4	(12.8)	(12.5)	12.6	(15.0)	(14.3)	14.7
Both categories	10.0	9.5	9.7	11.9	11.2	11.6	13.5	13.0	13.3	15.2	14.9	15.1
Sweida												
Middle	(10.8)	(9.0)	10.0	12.2	11.6	11.9	14.2	13.1	13.7	15.5	14.5	15.1
Low	(9.4)	(9.3)	(9.4)	(12.3)	(11.6)	(11.9)	14.5	13.8	14.1	15.3	(14.9)	15.1
Both categories	10.6	(9.1)	10.0	12.2	11.6	11.9	14.3	13.3	13.8	15.4	14.6	15.1
Rural Aleppo												
Middle	10.4	8.4	9.5	11.5	11.2	11.4	13.2	13.0	13.1	15.2	14.2	14.8
Low	10.3	8.7	9.6	11.4	10.7	11.1	13.3	12.2	12.8	15.2	14.8	15.0
Both categories	10.3	8.6	9.5	11.5	10.9	11.2	13.2	12.5	12.9	15.2	14.6	14.9

* Figures in parentheses refer to fewer than 25 children.

No significant relationship was found between weight and family size (Table 5.D.5(*a*)) or between weight and birth order (Table 5.D.5(*b*)).

TABLE 5.D.5.   MEAN WEIGHTS OF CHILDREN UNDER 5, BY RESIDENCE AND AGE, AND BY FAMILY SIZE OR BIRTH ORDER*

(*a*) By family size

| Residence | Age (years) | Mean weights (kg) of children in families of size: | | | | | | | Total no. weighed in age group |
		1	2	3	4	5	6 and over	All family sizes	
Damascus	1–2	9.8	(9.8)	(9.2)	(10.9)	(9.3)	(9.9)	9.7	79
	2–3	(10.6)	11.6	(10.9)	(12.6)	(12.1)	11.6	11.6	154
	3–4	(12.6)	(13.6)	13.6	13.4	13.3	13.1	13.3	191
	4–5	(15.1)	(15.7)	15.1	15.5	15.3	14.6	15.2	245
Sweida	1–2	(9.9)	(9.9)	(9.5)	(8.3)	(9.5)	(10.8)	10.0	45
	2–3	(11.5)	12.0	(12.4)	(11.4)	(11.1)	12.4	11.9	11
	3–4	(13.2)	13.4	(14.4)	14.0	(14.6)	13.7	13.8	185
	4–5	(16.0)	(14.9)	15.4	14.8	14.7	15.3	15.1	261
Rural Aleppo	1–2	8.3	8.7	(8.3)	(9.9)	10.4	10.1	9.5	159
	2–3	10.0	10.5	11.3	11.5	12.7	11.2	11.2	300
	3–4	(11.3)	12.7	13.2	11.9	12.8	13.4	12.9	265
	4–5	(14.6)	14.7	14.5	(14.6)	15.3	15.1	14.9	223

(*b*) By birth order

| Residence | Age (years) | Mean weights (kg) of children of birth order: | | | | | | | Total no. weighed in age group |
		1	2	3	4	5	6 and over	All birth orders	
Damascus	1–2	9.9	(9.6)	(9.5)	(10.0)	(9.7)	(9.8)	9.7	79
	2–3	11.3	(11.1)	(12.1)	(12.2)	(11.6)	11.6	11.6	154
	3–4	13.4	(14.0)	(13.4)	13.2	(13.3)	13.1	13.3	191
	4–5	14.9	15.4	15.6	15.2	15.1	14.7	15.0	245
Sweida	1–2	(10.1)	(10.3)	(8.7)	(8.5)	(10.6)	(9.9)	10.0	45
	2–3	11.8	(11.7)	(14.1)	(11.9)	(11.6)	12.0	11.9	110
	3–4	13.3	(14.3)	(14.3)	(14.5)	(13.9)	13.7	13.8	185
	4–5	15.3	15.6	15.0	14.0	15.0	15.4	15.1	261
Rural Aleppo	1–2	8.4	(8.9)	(8.6)	(8.8)	(10.4)	10.0	9.5	159
	2–3	10.6	10.9	11.1	12.3	11.9	11.2	11.2	300
	3–4	12.1	13.1	12.7	(12.7)	(12.6)	13.3	12.9	265
	4–5	14.7	(13.9)	(15.3)	(14.9)	15.8	14.8	14.9	223

* Figures in parentheses refer to fewer than 25 children.

Haemoglobin Level

The haemoglobin level tended to decline in the second year of life in all areas and in both social status groups, but thereafter it rose with age (Table 5.D.6). In urban areas, the mean haemoglobin level was slightly higher in children of middle social status than in those of low social status.

No relationship was observed between haemoglobin level and family size or between haemoglobin level and birth order (Tables 5.D.7(*a*) and 5.D.7(*b*)).

TABLE 5.D.6. MEAN HAEMOGLOBIN LEVELS OF CHILDREN UNDER 5, BY CULTURE, SOCIAL STATUS, AND SEX*

Residence and social status	Mean haemoglobin levels (g/100/ml) of male (M), female (F), and all (T) children at specified ages (years):											
	1–2			2–3			3–4			4–5		
	M	F	T	M	F	T	M	F	T	M	F	T
Damascus												
Middle	11.3	11.1	11.2	11.0	11.8	11.4	11.8	12.1	11.9	12.2	12.0	12.1
Low	(9.9)	(10.9)	(10.3)	(10.6)	(11.4)	11.0	(11.3)	(12.0)	11.7	(12.2)	(11.8)	12.0
Both categories	10.8	11.1	10.9	11.1	11.7	11.3	11.7	12.1	11.9	12.2	12.0	12.1
Sweida												
Middle	(9.4)	(9.9)	9.7	10.4	10.4	10.4	10.8	10.3	10.5	10.5	10.8	10.7
Low	(8.7)	(9.7)	(9.1)	(9.9)	(9.5)	(9.7)	9.9	9.4	9.6	11.1	(10.6)	10.9
Both categories	9.2	(9.9)	9.5	10.3	10.2	10.3	10.5	10.0	10.3	10.6	10.8	10.7
Rural Aleppo												
Middle	9.6	9.8	9.7	10.6	10.6	10.6	10.6	10.5	10.6	10.5	10.8	10.6
Low	10.2	10.1	10.2	10.0	9.8	9.9	10.0	10.2	10.1	10.7	10.2	10.5
Both categories	10.0	10.0	10.0	10.2	10.1	10.2	10.2	10.3	10.3	10.6	10.4	10.5

* Figures in parentheses refer to fewer than 25 children.

TABLE 5.D.7. MEAN HAEMOGLOBIN LEVELS OF CHILDREN UNDER 5, BY RESIDENCE AND AGE, AND BY FAMILY SIZE AND BIRTH ORDER*

(a) By family size

Residence	Age (years)	Mean haemoglobin levels (g/100 ml) of children in families of size:							Total no. examined in age group
		1	2	3	4	5	6 and over	All family sizes	
Damascus	1–2	10.9	(10.5)	(11.8)	(10.8)	(10.2	(11.1)	10.9	79
	2–3	(11.3)	10.8	(11.6)	(11.3)	(11.4)	11.5	11.3	150
	3–4	(12.4)	(12.5)	11.6	12.1	11.5	11.8	11.9	184
	4–5	(12.7)	(12.5)	12.1	12.1	12.2	11.9	12.1	243
Sweida	1–2	(9.0)	(10.0)	(10.8)	(10.1)	(9.5)	(9.9)	9.5	44
	2–3	(10.2)	10.6	(10.7)	(9.8)	(9.7)	10.5	10.3	186
	3–4	(10.1)	10.5	(9.9)	10.4	(9.7)	10.4	10.3	186
	4–5	(12.0)	(10.8)	10.6	10.6	10.7	10.8	10.7	257
Rural Aleppo	1–2	(9.7)	(9.3)	(10.1)	(10.3)	(9.7)	10.4	10.0	145
	2–3	9.7	10.3	10.3	10.2	10.4	10.1	10.2	296
	3–4	(10.6)	9.9	10.1	10.1	10.2	10.5	10.3	261
	4–5	(9.7)	10.2	10.4	(11.0)	(10.9)	10.5	10.5	216

(b) By birth order

Residence	Age (years)	Mean haemoglobin levels (g/100 ml) of children of birth order:							Total no. examined in age group
		1	2	3	4	5	6 and over	All birth orders	
Damascus	1–2	10.9	(10.9)	(11.5)	(10.0)	(10.7)	(11.2)	10.9	79
	2–3	10.9	(10.9)	(11.5)	(11.3)	(11.6)	11.6	11.3	150
	3–4	12.7	(11.4)	(11.8)	12.1	(11.2)	11.7	11.9	184
	4–5	12.1	12.3	12.0	12.3	12.2	11.9	12.1	243
Sweida	1–2	(9.4)	(8.2)	(10.3)	(9.6)	(7.5)	(10.1)	9.5	44
	2–3	10.5	(10.3)	(10.4)	(9.5)	(10.0)	10.4	10.3	106
	3–4	10.0	(10.8)	(10.2)	(10.7)	(9.7)	10.4	10.3	180
	4–5	11.2	10.3	10.5	11.0	10.3	10.0	10.7	257
Rural Aleppo	1–2	(9.8)	(9.6)	(9.5)	(9.0)	(10.2)	10.3	10.0	145
	2–3	10.1	10.4	10.2	(10.5)	10.7	10.0	10.2	296
	3–4	10.2	10.4	9.9	(9.9)	(10.4)	10.4	10.3	261
	4–5	10.2	(10.4)	(11.1)	(10.5)	10.8	10.4	10.5	216

* Figures in parentheses refer to fewer than 25 children.

Reported Occurrence of Fever and Diarrhoea

Women were asked about the occurrence of fever and diarrhoea among their children during the month preceding the interview. Rural Aleppo had the highest reported occurrences and Sweida the lowest, with Damascus in an intermediate position (Table 5.D.8). The higher rate in Damascus compared with Sweida was unexpected. It may have been due to the fact that the area studied in this large city was a particularly depressed one. In addition, small cities do not have the acute housing problems of Damascus and sanitation in Sweida is much better than in Damascus (which is congested owing to rural–urban migration) or in Rural Aleppo.

TABLE 5.D.8 REPORTED OCCURRENCE OF FEVER AND DIARRHOEA AMONG CHILDREN UNDER 10 DURING THE MONTH PRECEDING MOTHER'S INTERVIEW, BY RESIDENCE AND FAMILY SIZE OR BIRTH ORDER

(a) By family size

Residence and condition	Percentage of infections reported by EW with families of size:							Total no. of children in age group
	1	2	3	4	5	6 and over	All family sizes	
Damascus								
Fever	46.8	43.0	46.1	42.9	43.5	45.2	44.6	939
Diarrhoea	56.5	44.9	39.0	28.6	39.7	34.5	37.7	939
Sweida								
Fever	50.0	42.3	38.2	33.7	37.9	38.3	38.8	949
Diarrhoea	48.4	39.2	28.2	32.1	34.7	32.7	34.2	948
Rural Aleppo								
Fever	75.7	55.6	53.8	40.6	45.0	46.2	49.5	1150
Diarrhoea	81.1	63.9	61.4	52.4	52.3	56.5	58.7	1150

(b) By birth order

Residence and condition	Percentage of infections reported by EW for birth order:							Total no. of children in age group
	1	2	3	4	5	6 and over	All birth orders	
Damascus								
Fever	40.4	47.0	47.2	49.1	42.2	44.6	44.6	939
Diarrhoea	38.6	50.4	46.6	29.2	38.8	34.1	37.7	939
Sweida								
Fever	42.5	36.6	33.3	40.5	32.6	40.8	38.8	949
Diarrhoea	36.5	32.1	30.2	39.7	33.7	33.3	34.2	948
Rural Aleppo								
Fever	60.5	54.7	48.1	41.8	43.7	47.2	49.5	1150
Diarrhoea	68.2	57.3	58.7	50.5	58.7	56.9	58.7	1150

There was a tendency for the number of reported cases to decrease with increases in family size and birth order. A possible explanation of this phenomenon is that a mother with many children would be less sensitive to their complaints and more experienced in handling them and would report only the more serious occurrences. In other countries, it has been shown that the rates of infection as determined by physicians showed an opposite trend, tending to increase with family size (the relevant table is not available for Syria).

255

II. INTELLIGENCE QUOTIENT

INTRODUCTION

A. R. Omran

Several studies have demonstrated a negative association between intelligence quotient and birth orders or family sizes in excess of 4 or 5; they have also shown a slight positive association with maternal age. The tests used in the different studies varied considerably from one to another.

In the present collaborative study, involving centres in different cultural areas, it would have been preferable to use a test developed, tested, and standardized locally in each area. Since no such test was available, it was decided to adopt the Cattell & Cattell Culture-Fair Test in Colombia, Pakistan, and the Syrian Arab Republic. After the data had been collected and analysed, however, several problems became obvious.

The test is designed for children 8–14 years of age who are literate and have some familiarity with figures and forms. The applicability of the test was therefore restricted to eligible women's children who were 8–14 years of age and attending school. In a number of study areas, the proportion of school enrolment was relatively low. This meant that those covered by the test were, in some areas, a selected sample.

For converting the raw scores into standard scores, initially the tables provided in the test manual were used, but unfortunately they proved unsuitable because some 10–20% of the raw scores were lower than the lowest score in the tables and some 1–2% were higher than the highest score in the tables. This should not be taken as an indication that the children in the study population were of lower intelligence than the populations among whom the test was standardized. It simply means that the test is not as culture fair as it is claimed, and that the standard conversion tables are not appropriate for our study populations.

The following method was therefore used to convert the raw scores into standard scores:

First, the mean and the standard deviation for each age group (namely, 8, 9, 10, 11, 12, 13, and 14 years) were calculated. For example, for children aged 8 years:

$$M_8 = \frac{\Sigma \chi}{n}$$

$$S_8 = \sqrt{\frac{\Sigma \chi^2 - \frac{(\Sigma \chi)^2}{n}}{n}}$$

where,

χ = any raw IQ score of children aged 8 years
n = total number of children aged 8 years who took the IQ test
M_8 = mean for children aged 8 years
S_8 = standard deviation for children aged 8 years

Then each child's raw IQ score was converted to a standard score. For example, for children aged 8 years:

$$\text{Standard score} = \frac{\chi - M_8}{S_8} (\sigma\ 8\text{--}9) + 100$$

$$= \frac{\chi - M_8}{S_8} (27.0) + 100$$

where,

σ 8–9 – 27.0 for children aged 8 and 9 years or younger
σ 10–12 = 24.4 for children aged 10, 11 and 12 years
σ 13–14 = 22.5 for children aged 13 and 14 years or older

The centre in Egypt decided, however, to use the Goodenough "Draw a Man" Performance Test, which they had applied in other studies. The test is intended for children 6–11 years of age. The statistical techniques described above were also used for the analysis of the results of the Goodenough test.

A. COLOMBIA

Angelina Gil, German Ochoa, & A. R. Omran

Coverage of the IQ Study

The Cattell & Cattell Culture-Fair Intelligence Test was administered as a group test to school-age children of the eligible women, as previously mentioned in chapter 1. During the women's interview, information was obtained about their children in regard to age, grade, and school attendance. IQ tests were given to groups of 25 children in each of the school settings. In a school situated near the health centre (headquarters of the study) tests were given to children attending schools outside the zone of residence and to children who could not attend on the first test date.

The tests were given by a team of investigators: doctors, social workers, auxiliary nurses, and assistants trained previously by a psychologist. The test was administered to a total of 2077 schoolchildren, 1072 residing in the OUZ and 1005 in the NSZ (Table 5.A.I).

TABLE 5.A.I. MEAN STANDARDIZED IQ SCORES, BY RESIDENCE, SOCIAL STATUS, AND FAMILY SIZE*

Residence and social status	Mean standardized IQ scores of children in families of:						Total no. tested
	1	2	3	4	5	6 and over	
Old urban zone							
Middle	(117.87)	114.60	114.00	110.87	110.24	107.23	1003
Low	—	(101.00)	(100.33)	(99.00)	(97.50)	95.26	69
All OUZ	(117.88)	113.37	112.76	110.54	108.38	105.13	1072
Newly settled zone							
Middle	(76.20)	(95.19)	98.35	97.52	102.80	93.13	294
Low	—	(87.62)	(91.25)	96.87	89.00	87.14	711
All NSZ	(76.20)	95.44	95.72	97.10	93.96	88.95	1005

* Figures in parentheses refer to fewer than 25 children.

IQ Scores, Residence, and Social Status

Children from the OUZ had, on the average, higher IQ scores than those from the NSZ ($P < 0.01$), and in both zones children of middle social status had, on the average, higher IQ scores than those of low social status (Table 5.A.I).

IQ Scores and Family Size

In the OUZ, the mean standardized IQ scores declined, in general, with increases in family size. The difference in mean IQ scores between children from families of 1 or 2 children and those from families of 4 or more children was statistically significant at the 0.01 level. This pattern persisted when the social status was held constant. In the NSZ, however, the relationship was not so clear (Table 5.A.I). When the two sexes were considered individually, the decline in mean IQ scores with family size persisted, with greater fluctuations in the NSZ. In both zones, the mean IQ of the boys was consistently higher than that of the girls, except for a family size of 5 in the OUZ (Table 5.A.II).

IQ and Birth Order

The mean IQ scores declined consistently ($P < 0.01$) above birth order 2 or 3 in both residential areas, even when social status was held constant (Table 5.A.III). When both social classes were combined, the mean score for first-born children in the OUZ was 112.72, and it fell progressively to 104.27 for the sixth and higher birth orders. The corresponding figures in the NSZ were 92.83 and 85.11, respectively. When social status was held constant and one sex only considered, some fluctuations were observed, but children of high birth order (6 and over) still had the lowest mean scores (Table 5.A.IV).

258

TABLE 5.A.II. MEAN STANDARDIZED IQ SCORES, BY RESIDENCE, SEX OF THE CHILD,
AND FAMILY SIZE*

Residence and sex of child	Mean standardized IQ scores of children in families of size:						Total no. tested
	1	2	3	4	5	6 and over	
Old urban zone							
Male	—	117.70	114.48	112.39	105.10	105.63	530
Female	(117.88)	(107.45)	111.27	108.64	111.07	104.60	542
Both sexes	(117.88)	113.37	112.76	110.54	108.38	105.13	1072
Newly settled zone							
Male	(91.67)	(97.54)	96.84	100.58	96.77	90.29	492
Female	(53.00)	(94.00)	(94.22)	93.95	91.25	86.89	513
Both sexes	(76.20)	95.44	95.72	97.10	93.96	88.55	1005

* Figures in parentheses refer to fewer than 25 children.

TABLE 5.A.III. MEAN STANDARDIZED IQ SCORES, BY RESIDENCE, SOCIAL STATUS,
AND BIRTH ORDER*

Residence and social status	Mean standardized IQ scores of children of birth order:						Total no. tested
	1	2	3	4	5	6 and over	
Old urban zone							
Middle	113.60	114.22	108.04	108.45	107.48	104.60	1003
Low	(94.09)	(101.50)	(98.87)	(88.92)	(87.80)	(99.92)	69
All OUZ	112.72	110.18	106.42	106.74	106.44	104.27	1072
Newly settled zone							
Middle	99.62	97.90	103.85	95.14	(88.95)	88.50	290
Low	89.72	89.27	91.41	87.07	90.20	83.70	711
All NSZ	92.83	91.82	94.97	89.22	89.94	85.11	1005

* Figures in parentheses refer to fewer than 25 children.

TABLE 5.A.IV. MEAN STANDARDIZED IQ SCORES, BY RESIDENCE, SEX OF CHILD,
AND BIRTH ORDER

Residence and sex of child	Mean standardized IQ scores of children of birth order:						Total no. tested
	1	2	3	4	5	6 and over	
Old urban zone							
Male	113.81	111.35	106.60	106.07	108.47	103.43	530
Female	111.66	109.11	106.25	107.43	104.62	105.22	542
Both sexes	112.72	110.18	106.42	106.74	106.44	104.27	1072
Newly settled zone							
Male	96.93	92.28	95.34	91.93	93.19	87.27	492
Female	88.65	91.41	94.56	87.36	86.52	83.05	513
Both sexes	92.83	91.82	94.97	89.22	89.94	85.12	1005

IQ and Maternal Age

When IQ scores were examined by residence and maternal age no clear pattern emerged. In the OUZ children born to mothers of age 30–34 had the lowest scores, but in the NSZ no pattern was evident (Table 5.A.V).

TABLE 5.A.V. MEAN STANDARDIZED IQ SCORES, BY RESIDENCE, SOCIAL STATUS, AND MATERNAL AGE*

Residence and social status	Mean standardized IQ scores of children born to mothers of age:				Total number tested
	15–19	20–24	25–29	20–34	
Old urban zone					
Middle	108.96	110.52	108.68	107.43	1004
Low	(95.83)	(95.74)	97.67	(93.57)	69
All OUZ	107.67	109.65	107.95	106.82	1073
New settled zone					
Middle	104.42	93.48	97.95	93.71	294
Low	90.50	87.26	88.30	91.40	711
All NSZ	94.65	88.96	91.28	92.09	1005

* Figures in parentheses refer to fewer than 25 children.

IQ Scores, Birth Order, and Maternal Age

Since birth order and maternal age were important correlates of IQ levels the data were cross-tabulated by both factors. When maternal age was kept constant, the previously mentioned decline in mean IQ scores with increasing birth order was evident with minor fluctuations. In other words, for each of the different maternal age groups (< 20, 20–24, 25–29, and 30 +), children of low birth order (1–3) had on the average higher mean scores than children of higher birth order.

B. EGYPT

H. M. Hammam, A. Guinena, A. H. Zarzour & M. Elarkan

Coverage of the IQ Study

The Goodenough Draw-a-Man Performance Test was administered to children aged 6–11 years who were attending school. Although the Cattell and Cattell Culture-Fair Test was recommended by WHO, it was not used since it had not been tried before in Egypt. The Goodenough test had been used and standardized in Egypt. The IQ scoring was conducted by an experienced psychologist, and the scoring result of each pupil was entered on his family origin sheet before it was analysed. The standardization of the raw scores was done according to the method described by WHO (see page 256). Table 5.B.I gives standardized IQ scores of children living in the rural area (548 children) and in the urban area (1172 children).

TABLE 5.B.I. MEAN STANDARDIZED IQ SCORES BY RESIDENCE, SOCIAL STATUS
AND FAMILY SIZE*

Residence and social status	Mean standardized IQ scores of children in families of:						Total no. tested
	1	2	3	4	5	6 and over	
Rural							
Middle	(110.91)	(86.03)	95.68	104.87	102.42	97.74	210
Low	(81.13)	94.63	94.74	95.55	101.82	97.66	338
Both categories	(98.99)	92.05	95.11	99.09	102.05	97.69	548
Urban							
Middle	(116.70)	104.92	102.87	105.53	102.05	102.17	678
Low	(92.60)	100.30	101.59	96.89	99.24	100.58	494
Both categories	(104.65)	102.80	102.36	101.91	100.98	101.46	1172

* Figures in parentheses refer to fewer than 25 children.

IQ and Family Size

Table 5.B.I shows an inconsistent relationship between IQ and family size in
the rural and urban areas. The IQ score of the rural child was lower than that
of the urban. Children whose parents were of middle social status had higher
IQs than those whose parents were of low social status, irrespective of family
size in both the urban and rural areas. In the rural area, boys had higher IQs
than girls in families of all sizes except 5, while the reverse was true in the urban
area (Table 5.B.II). The preference of parents for boys rather than girls in rural
areas may be partly responsible for this difference.

TABLE 5.B.II. MEAN STANDARDIZED IQ SCORES BY RESIDENCE, SEX OF CHILD,
AND FAMILY SIZE*

Residence and sex of child	Mean standardized IQ scores of children in families of:						Total no. tested
	1	2	3	4	5	6 and over	
Rural							
Male	(101.09)	93.12	95.91	99.86	101.06	99.75	336
Female	(90.64)	(89.77)	94.12	97.04	103.84	94.81	212
Both sexes	(98.99)	92.05	95.11	99.10	102.05	97.70	548
Urban							
Male	(103.85)	91.15	101.68	101.29	102.43	99.15	631
Female	(115.04)	114.09	103.18	102.65	99.22	103.89	541
Both sexes	(104.65)	102.82	102.31	101.45	100.43	101.89	1172

261

IQ and Birth Order

Table 5.B.III shows that there was no consistent relationship between IQ and birth order in the rural and urban areas. This was true for both social status groups. However, slightly higher IQ scores were observed among children of higher birth orders in the rural area and the reverse was found in the urban area.

No special trend in IQ was observed in either area (Table 5.B.IV) in relation to the sex of the child. In the urban area girls had higher IQs than boys for all birth orders except for birth order 4.

TABLE 5.B.III. MEAN STANDARDIZED IQ SCORES BY RESIDENCE, SOCIAL STATUS, AND BIRTH ORDER*

Residence and social status	Mean standardized IQ scores of children of birth order:						Total no. tested
	1	2	3	4	5	6 and over	
Rural							
Middle	92.63	103.51	103.85	(104.49)	(103.24)	95.41	210
Low	93.68	91.48	98.35	94.60	99.24	101.64	338
Both categories	93.21	95.67	100.40	98.14	100.66	99.20	548
Urban							
Middle	105.01	102.26	106.56	102.41	103.05	101.64	678
Low	100.45	99.42	98.09	96.63	95.39	101.78	494
Both categories	103.39	101.12	103.05	100.36	99.41	101.70	1172

* Figures in parentheses refer to fewer than 25 children.

TABLE 5.B.IV. MEAN STANDARDIZED IQ SCORES BY RESIDENCE, SEX OF CHILD, AND BIRTH ORDER

Residence and sex of child	Mean standardized IQ scores of children of birth order:						Total no. tested
	1	2	3	4	5	6 and over	
Rural							
Male	88.85	100.49	109.69	96.85	101.91	98.61	336
Female	101.26	90.73	87.23	100.33	98.23	100.25	212
Both sexes	93.21	95.67	100.40	98.14	100.65	99.19	548
Urban							
Male	101.93	99.60	102.82	101.89	97.76	99.67	631
Female	105.18	103.04	103.28	98.42	101.82	103.95	541
Both sexes	103.32	101.10	103.05	100.35	99.44	101.71	1172

IQ and Maternal Age

As shown in Table 5.B.V, no special relationship existed between IQ and maternal age in either the rural or the urban area. However, in both areas and both social status groups, the highest IQs were observed among children whose mothers were aged 30–34 years. Also, children of middle social status had higher IQ's than children of low social status. In the urban area, the highest standardized IQ scores were 106.98 among children of middle social status and 102.05 among children of low social status. In the rural area the corresponding scores were 100.04 and 103.04. In the urban area, the lowest IQ scores were among children born to mothers aged 35–39 years, while in the rural area the lowest IQ scores were among children born to mothers aged 15–19 years.

TABLE 5.B.V. MEAN STANDARDIZED IQ SCORES BY RESIDENCE, SOCIAL STATUS, AND MATERNAL AGE*

Residence and social status	Mean standardized IQ scores of children born to mothers aged:					Total no. tested
	15–19	20–24	25–29	30–34	35–39	
Rural						
Middle	90.98	104.93	99.09	100.04	(94.92)	210
Low	92.53	96.67	94.54	103.04	(104.95)	338
Both categories	91.89	100.18	96.09	101.91	101.50	548
Urban						
Middle	102.63	103.91	102.04	106.98	98.08	678
Low	101.49	96.06	101.11	102.05	96.27	494
Both categories	102.21	100.85	101.56	104.74	97.23	1172

* Figures in parentheses refer to fewer than 25 children.

Industrial Area

In a parallel study among schoolchildren in the industrial area, analysis of standardized IQ scores of 1330 children aged 6–15 years revealed correlations with both social and biological characteristics. Higher IQ scores were associated with lower birth orders (below 7), younger maternal age at the birth of the child, primary education (as opposed to no education) of the parents, and middle (as opposed to low) social status. Standardized IQ scores also decreased grdually with increase in family size (Table 5.B.VI).

TABLE 5.B.VI. MEAN STANDARDIZED IQ SCORES OF SCHOOLCHILDREN IN THE INDUSTRIAL AREA BY FAMILY SIZE AND BIRTH ORDER

Family size	Mean standardized IQ scores of children	Birth order	Mean standardized IQ scores of children
3–5	103.5	1–2	101.2
6–7	101.3	3–4	101.3
8	100.4	5–6	101.2
9 and over	100.1	7 and over	99.8

263

C. PAKISTAN

Farhat Ajmal & Hafiz Zaidi

Coverage of the IQ Study

The Cattell & Cattell Culture-Fair Test was administered as a group intelligence test to school-going children (8–14 years of age) of the eligible women included in the study (selection of children depended upon the eligibility of their mothers). The children tested came from families that, in terms of local socioeconomic criteria, could be designated as belonging to middle and lower socioeconomic classes. The test was administered to the school-going children in groups of 10–15. For children in the higher grades, however, the groups of children were larger. In all, 3393 children were tested.

IQ Scores, Residence, and Social Status

The average IQ scores in the urban area were higher than those in the semi-urban area ($P < 0.01$). In both zones, children of middle social status had, on the average, higher IQ scores than those of low social status.

IQ and Family Size

In the urban area, the mean standardized IQ scores declined with increases in family size. The difference in mean IQ scores between children from families of 1–3 children and those from families of 4 or more children was statistically significant at the 0.05 level for the total population and for both social status groups (Table 5.C.I). In the semi-urban area, there was no apparent pattern of

TABLE 5.C.I. MEAN STANDARDIZED IQ SCORES, BY RESIDENCE, SOCIAL STATUS, AND FAMILY SIZE*

Residence and social status	Mean standardized IQ scores of children in families of:						Total no. tested
	1	2	3	4	5	6 and over	
Urban							
Middle	(118.85)	110.49	106.37	107.11	104.34	103.76	1913
Low	(97.00)	(95.00)	(116.80)	(96.60)	94.63	96.57	154
Both categories	(114.00)	110.21	106.69	106.73	103.53	103.14	2067
Semi-urban							
Middle	(110.00)	(90.89)	98.05	97.81	100.09	95.68	609
Low	(90.60)	(87.64)	88.83	94.92	90.60	91.35	717
Both categories	(96.14)	89.51	92.85	96.39	95.82	92.52	1326
Both areas							
Middle	(116.88)	105.45	104.82	104.70	103.04	101.63	2522
Low	(92.43)	(88.13)	91.47	95.09	91.42	92.36	871
Both categories	(106.19)	102.54	102.00	102.61	100.26	99.04	3393

* Figures in parentheses refer to fewer than 25 children.

differences by family size. For children of the same sex, the decline in mean IQ scores with increase in family size persisted in the urban area. In the semi-urban area, no pattern was evident (Table 5.C.II). There were no significant differences in IQ scores by sex.

TABLE 5.C.II. MEAN STANDARDIZED IQ SCORES, BY RESIDENCE, SEX OF THE CHILD, AND FAMILY SIZE*

Residence, social status, and sex of child	Mean standardized IQ scores of children in families of:						Total no. tested
	1	2	3	4	5	6 and over	
Urban							
Middle							
Male	124.25	105.96	106.63	107.53	102.71	104.55	952
Female	(111.66)	(116.33)	106.05	106.63	106.09	103.06	961
Both sexes	(118.85)	110.49	106.37	107.11	104.34	103.76	1913
Low							
Male	(99.00)	—	(111.67)	(99.50)	(97.25)	98.17	73
Female	—	(95.00)	(124.50)	(92.25)	(91.64)	95.35	81
Both sexes	(97.00)	(95.00)	(116.80)	(96.60)	94.63	96.57	154
Semi-urban							
Middle							
Male	(121.00)	(92.44)	(104.76)	98.66	103.88	95.20	300
Female	(100.00)	(89.50)	(94.41)	97.00	96.50	93.05	309
Both sexes	(110.00)	(90.89)	98.05	97.81	100.09	95.68	609
Low							
Male	(91.5)	(85.40)	94.72	95.14	89.19	92.07	356
Female	(87.00)	(88.89)	(82.43)	94.65	92.22	90.07	361
Both sexes	(90.60)	(87.64)	88.93	94.92	90.60	91.45	717
Both areas							
Male	(107.00)	100.98	104.29	103.16	100.02	99.81	1681
Female	(104.40)	104.14	99.50	101.99	100.51	98.33	1712
Both sexes	(106.19)	102.54	102.00	102.61	100.26	99.04	3393

* Figures in parentheses refer to fewer than 25 children.

IQ and Birth Order

The data revealed only small variations in the mean IQ scores by birth order. In both social classes and for both residential areas there was a tendency for children of birth orders 1–3 to score higher on the tests than children of higher birth orders. This pattern was found for both boys and girls. Again, there was little variation in IQ scores by sex (Tables 5.C.III and 5.C.IV).

TABLE 5.C.III. MEAN STANDARDIZED IQ SCORES, BY RESIDENCE, SOCIAL STATUS, AND BIRTH ORDER*

Residence, social status, and sex of child	Mean standardized IQ scores of children of birth order:							Total no. tested
	1	2	3	4	5	6 and over	All birth orders	
Urban								
Middle								
Male	104.39	105.57	105.20	103.87	103.74	106.23	104.99	952
Female	106.74	104.96	104.50	102.78	107.73	102.71	104.59	961
Both sexes	105.46	105.25	104.87	103.31	105.70	104.36	104.79	1913
Low								
Male	(93.09)	(102.80)	(103.80)	(106.00)	(99.64)	(95.58)	98.60	73
Female	(104.00)	(100.67)	(101.67)	(94.17)	(90.57)	88.11	95.27	81
Both sexes	(96.94)	(101.64)	102.11	(97.65)	(96.62)	91.70	96.85	154
Semi-urban								
Middle								
Male	96.27	104.43	97.66	93.93	94.78	100.55	98.16	300
Female	97.51	94.69	92.94	92.59	95.57	93.67	94.49	309
Both sexes	96.90	99.32	95.15	93.26	95.11	97.06	96.30	609
Low								
Male	92.36	93.15	94.73	88.56	92.65	91.42	92.07	356
Female	88.40	92.29	95.66	92.60	86.13	89.31	90.78	361
Both sexes	90.49	92.69	95.24	90.15	89.39	90.35	91.42	717
Both areas								
Male	100.08	102.50	101.73	98.33	99.38	101.71	100.76	1681
Female	100.82	100.19	100.03	98.42	99.84	97.94	99.42	1712
Both sexes	100.42	101.27	100.87	98.38	99.59	99.74	100.08	3393

* Figures in parentheses refer to fewer than 25 children.

TABLE 5.C.IV. MEAN STANDARDIZED IQ SCORES, BY RESIDENCE, SEX OF THE CHILD, AND BIRTH ORDER

Residence and sex of the child	Mean standardized IQ scores for children of birth order:							Total no. tested
	1	2	3	4	5	6 and over	All birth orders	
Urban								
Male	103.78	105.40	105.08	103.95	103.28	105.21	104.54	1025
Female	106.64	104.68	104.17	102.10	106.66	101.36	103.87	1042
Both sexes	105.07	105.02	104.63	102.97	104.89	103.17	104.20	2067
Semi-urban								
Male	94.15	98.17	96.14	91.04	93.60	95.60	94.86	656
Female	92.89	93.35	94.40	92.60	89.91	91.32	92.50	670
Both sexes	93.53	95.62	95.20	91.79	91.82	93.44	93.66	1326

IQ and Maternal Age

When IQ scores were examined by residence and maternal age, no clear pattern emerged. In the urban area, children born to mothers aged 35–40 had the lowest scores, but in the semi-urban area no such relationship was apparent (Table 5.C.V).

TABLE 5.C.V. MEAN STANDARDIZED IQ SCORES, BY RESIDENCE, SOCIAL STATUS, AND MATERNAL AGE*

Residence and social status	Mean standardized IQ scores of children born to mothers of age:					Total no. tested
	<20	20–24	25–29	30–34	35–40	
Urban						
Middle	103.52	104.89	105.24	105.70	99.44	1913
Low	97.00	101.13	92.73	94.44	(96.00)	154
Both sexes	103.00	104.60	104.39	104.91	99.07	2267
Semi-urban						
Middle	98.11	94.94	97.14	96.25	(82.33)	609
Low	88.92	95.27	89.62	88.03	(104.17)	717
Both sexes	92.92	95.12	93.27	92.04	(93.25)	1326

* Figures in parentheses refer to fewer than 25 children.

D. SYRIAN ARAB REPUBLIC

M. El-Jabi

Coverage of the IQ Study

IQ testing, using the Cattell & Cattell Culture-Fair Test, was administered as a group test to eligible women's children aged 8–14 years who were attending schools. The children covered by the study totalled 3468, distributed as follows: 1541 from Damascus, 1244 from Sweida, and 683 from Rural Aleppo.

IQ and Family Formation

By residence and social status

Standardized IQ scores for children 8–14 decreased progressively from Damascus (large city) to Sweida (small towns) to Rural Aleppo ($P < 0.01$). In each residential area, children of middle social status had, on the average, higher IQ scores than those of low social status (Table 5.D.I).

TABLE 5.D.I. MEAN STANDARDIZED IQ SCORES BY RESIDENCE, SOCIAL STATUS, AND FAMILY SIZE*

Residence and social status	Mean standardized IQ scores of children in families of:					
	1	2	3	4	5	6 and over
Damascus						
Middle	(135.0)	(128.0)	117.3	109.2	109.4	106.0
Low	(80.0)	(136.0)	(93.8)	107.6	101.4	104.2
Both categories	(116.7)	(129.4)	110.7	108.9	107.8	105.5
Sweida						
Middle	(89.6)	(104.6)	102.2	102.8	103.2	103.7
Low	(83.5)	(95.5)	(98.9)	101.2	99.6	99.1
Both categories	(87.9)	(102.5)	101.2	102.4	102.2	102.5
Rural Aleppo						
Middle	—	(107.0)	(83.3)	(90.5)	83.5	87.8
Low	—	(67.7)	(74.3)	74.6	80.0	84.2
Both categories	—	(77.5)	77.1	80.0	81.5	85.6

* Figures in parentheses refer to fewer than 25 children. Dashes indicate that there were no cases for the family size and category in question.

By family size

No consistent relationship was observed between family size and IQ scores. Whereas in Damascus IQ scores tended to decrease with increases in family size, the reverse was true for Sweida and Rural Aleppo (Tables 5.D.I and 5.D.II).

TABLE 5.D.II. MEAN STANDARDIZED IQ SCORES, BY RESIDENCE, SEX OF CHILD, AND FAMILY SIZE*

Residence and sex of child	Mean standardized IQ scores of children in families of:					
	1	2	3	4	5	6 and over
Damascus						
Male	(105.0)	(118.2)	115.0	108.5	106.9	105.9
Female	(140.0)	(143.5)	104.3	109.5	108.5	105.2
Both sexes	(116.7)	(129.4)	110.7	108.9	107.8	105.5
Sweida						
Male	(87.8)	(99.5)	101.2	102.8	103.5	102.3
Female	(88.0)	(108.0)	101.2	101.8	100.8	102.7
Both sexes	(87.9)	(102.5)	101.2	102.4	102.2	102.5
Rural Aleppo						
Male	—	(84.7)	(77.1)	79.9	83.9	86.7
Female	—	(56.0)	(77.1)	80.2	75.9	83.5
Both sexes	—	(77.5)	77.1	80.0	81.5	85.6

* Figures in parentheses refer to fewer than 25 children. Dashes indicate that there were no cases for the family size and category in question.

By sex

Girls in Damascus tended to have the same IQ scores as boys or higher ones. No consistent pattern was found in the other two areas (Table 5.D.II).

By birth order

The IQ scores declined with birth order only in Damascus (especially among middle class children). In the other two areas, the relationship was not consistent (Tables 5.D.III and 5.D.IV).

TABLE 5.D.III. MEAN STANDARDIZED IQ SCORES, BY RESIDENCE, SOCIAL STATUS, AND BIRTH ORDER

Residence and social status	Mean standardized IQ scores of children of birth order:						Total no. tested
	1	2	3	4	5	6 and over	
Damascus							
Middle	110.5	108.5	108.4	108.9	103.4	106.1	1155
Low	103.3	105.6	103.2	106.3	100.4	103.0	370
Both categories	109.1	107.9	106.5	108.3	102.4	105.2	1525
Sweida							
Middle	103.1	101.1	104.0	104.0	105.5	103.2	915
Low	100.5	100.6	103.8	95.9	95.1	99.2	322
Both categories	102.7	101.0	103.9	102.5	102.3	101.7	1237
Rural Aleppo							
Middle	90.3	88.8	85.7	84.0	85.9	88.2	247
Low	80.3	80.3	80.9	84.6	83.6	81.3	388
Both categories	84.7	83.7	82.8	84.4	84.4	84.0	635

TABLE 5.D.IV. MEAN STANDARDIZED IQ SCORES, BY RESIDENCE, SEX OF CHILD, AND BIRTH ORDER

Residence and sex of child	Mean standardized IQ scores of children of birth order:						Total tested
	1	2	3	4	5	6 and over	
Damascus							
Male	107.92	111.02	108.75	111.36	101.21	102.91	737
Female	110.19	105.17	104.07	106.12	103.73	107.38	788
Both sexes	109.05	107.89	106.47	108.28	102.43	105.20	1525
Sweida							
Male	103.71	101.82	104.34	102.75	101.16	100.46	660
Female	101.29	100.18	103.42	102.17	103.45	103.31	577
Both sexes	102.66	101.00	103.91	102.46	102.30	101.69	1237
Rural Aleppo							
Male	86.899	84.182	81.419	85.324	86.625	86.304	424
Female	79.800	82.618	85.786	82.194	80.212	80.255	211
Both sexes	84.747	83.650	82.778	84.373	84.443	84.041	635

By maternal age

Only small differences were observed when children's IQ was analysed by maternal age, except in Damascus where there was a tendency for the IQ to increase with the maturity of the mother (Table not shown).

General comment

It seems that the results obtained with children from Damascus were more reliable than for other areas because in developing countries the IQ test used is more applicable to "urbanized" than to rural children.

Chapter Six

FAMILY FORMATION
AND MATERNAL HEALTH

INTRODUCTION

M. R. Bone

The effects of family formation patterns on child health have been investigated more often than have the effects on maternal health, which cover a wide range of conditions. In the present enquiry it was decided to concentrate on one main theme. Since many obstetric complications increase with parity, it seemed possible that gynaecological conditions, blood pressure changes, and anaemia might behave similarly. This chapter is therefore devoted mainly to a discussion of data on gynaecological examinations of eligible women, measurement of blood pressure, and laboratory investigation of haemoglobin level.

The women were also weighed and measured and their ponderal index (height, measured in inches, divided by the cube root of weight, measured in pounds) was calculated. By definition, the higher the index, the lighter is the subject in relation to her height.

Interest in the ponderal index stems from the literature on the "maternal depletion syndromes", including protein-energy malnutrition, one of the signs of which is decreasing weight with increasing age and parity. The condition has been observed but not thoroughly investigated in areas where a combination of frequent pregnancies, prolonged lactation, heavy work, and local food customs produces a "continuous cumulative nutritional drain" on married women.[1] Although it was not expected that a reduction in body weight with age and parity would necessarily be found in all the participating areas—or, indeed, in any of them—the possibility appeared to be worth investigation.

The haemoglobin level, measured in grams per 100 millilitres of venous blood, was used to determine the presence of anaemia. Anaemia is considered

---

[1] JELLIFFE, D. B. (1966) The assessment of the nutritional status of the community, Geneva, World Health Organization, pp. 210–211.

to exist in adult non-pregnant women if the haemoglobin level is below 12 g/100 ml, and in pregnant women if it is below 11 g/100 ml. These figures hold at sea level; at greater altitudes higher limiting values apply.[1]

The data on gynaecological diseases were derived from clinical examination alone and attempts to standardize the procedure were unsuccessful. Some information on the methods adopted in each area is given in the reports of the relevant centres.

All conditions diagnosed were classified according to the International Classification of Diseases (1965 Revision).[2] The prevalence of each condition in the 4 areas shows considerable differences. It is possible, however, that different areas used different criteria in assigning conditions to ICD categories. The standard coding form permitted the recording of up to 5 conditions for each woman.

In each participating area it was intended that all the women interviewed, or a representative sample, should be gynaecologically examined. The data for Egypt, however, are not available. The response rates varied from 70% in the Syrian Arab Republic to 42% in Colombia and 40% in Pakistan. The response rates in the Syrian Arab Republic and Pakistan were high, since these are traditional societies. However, these rates are not high enough to exclude the possibility of a selection bias that might obscure the relationships under study.

For these reasons no comparison of prevalence rates between areas is possible nor should it be attempted.

All eligible women were asked at interview whether they had experienced any of a list of gynaecological symptoms during the 3 months preceding interview. Most of the items on the list concern menstrual disorders. The remaining 3 (discharge, itching, and prolapse) might be expected to bear some relationship to some of the conditions sought at clinical examination. In fact, there were considerable differences between the proportions found to have the conditions and those reporting them, even in the case of prolapse. These differences could be due to: the differing time periods covered (although not in the case of prolapse); differences between the subsamples of women gynaecologically examined and the women who were interviewed; or to the more subjective nature of the interview questions in comparison with the clinical examination.

The last topic covered in the present chapter is breast feeding. It was presupposed that inability to breast feed because of lack of milk would increase with parity and maternal age; and that the duration of lactation would decline with parity and maternal age. In order to minimize memory errors, only the breast feeding of the last-born child was considered.

The proportion of women breast feeding their last child ranged from 70% to 96% in the different centres. Under these circumstances no analysis is presented for the relatively small numbers who had not breast fed because of a reported insufficiency of milk. An additional reason for omitting this analysis

---

[1] WHO Scientific Group on Nutritional Anaemias (1968) Report, Geneva, World Health Organization (WHO Technical Report Series No. 405).
[2] *Manual of the International Statistical Classification of Diseases, Injuries, and Causes of Death*, 1965 Revision, vol. 1, Geneva, World Health Organization, 1967.

272

is the lack of information on the extent of full, as opposed to partial, breast feeding.

The analysis of duration of lactation was also abandoned, when it was found that considerable proportions of the women were still breast feeding their last-born child. Calculation of the mean length of breast feeding from the numbers of those who were no longer doing so would have produced a spuriously low figure; other things being equal, the women who were still breast feeding were doing so for longer than those who had stopped. It was not possible to show the percentages of mothers breast feeding at stated intervals following birth, since neither the month of birth of the child nor the month of interview were recorded.

The family formation variable used throughout this chapter is parity, except in the case of breast feeding, for which birth order and maternal age are used.

Parity was considered to be more reliable than gravidity and more relevant than family size. Initially, analyses were made of the relationships between some of the health variables and gravidity and family size, but in no case did the results differ from those between parity and the health indicators.

A. COLOMBIA

G. Ochoa & A. Gil

Sample for Medical Examinations

Selection procedures

At the beginning of the study it was decided that about 4 out of every 10 women could be examined. The selection procedure for physical examination was based on a systematic probability sampling of households. The physical examination consisted of measurement of weight and height, haemoglobin determination, gynaecological examination, and cervical cytology. Of the 2581 eligible women selected to be examined, 2210 (85.6%) were actually given physical examinations. These women represent 41.9% of the total number of eligible women interviewed (Table 6.A.1(a)). Tables 6.A.1(b) and (c) indicate that in respect of age and family size there was little difference between the women interviewed and those examined gynaecologically.

Professional Personnel and General Procedure

Two general medical doctors (one male and one female), previously trained and supervised by a gynaecologist, conducted an interview and a physical examination that included a gynaecological examination and the taking of a cervical sample for cytology.

273

The examinations took place in an official public health centre situated in each of the zones. An auxiliary nurse took the blood pressure and measured the weight and height before the gynaecological examination. Women were weighed, using a beam balance, wearing light clothes and without shoes. If the women broke their appointments, they were visited by an outreach worker to establish the most convenient time for a physical examination. A woman who broke 3 appointments was considered to have refused the examination. All clinical histories were reviewed by the two doctors and the gynaecologist working together, and results were coded according to the ICD (8th revision)[1] by a hospital statistician/coder.

---

[1] *Manual of the International Statistical Classification of Diseases, Injuries, and Causes of Death*, 8th revision, vol. 1, Geneva, World Health Organization, 1967.

TABLE 6.A.1. ELIGIBLE WOMEN INTERVIEWED COMPARED WITH THOSE EXAMINED

(a) Coverage for each type of investigation, by residence

Procedure	Old urban zone			Newly settled zone			Total		
	No. of EW inter-viewed	No. of EW examined		No. of EW inter-viewed	No. of EW examined		No. of EW inter-viewed	No. of EW examined	
		No.	%		No.	%		No.	%
Gynaecological examination	2669	1063	39.8	2601	1147	44.1	5270	2210	41.9
Weight and height measurement	2669	1062	40.0	2601	1146	44.1	5270	2208	41.9
Haemoglobin determination	2669	1050	39.3	2601	1146	44.1	5270	2196	41.7

(b) Breakdown by age group and residence of eligible women interviewed and of those gynaeco-logically examined

Age group	Old urban zone				Newly settled zone			
	EW interviewed		EW gynaecologically examined		EW interviewed		EW gynaecologically examined	
	No.	%	No.	%	No.	%	No.	%
<20	66	2.5	24	2.3	98	3.8	34	3.0
20–24	398	14.9	145	13.6	424	16.3	189	16.5
25–29	666	25.0	273	25.7	614	23.6	267	23.3
30–34	590	22.1	227	21.4	602	23.1	266	23.2
35–39	529	19.8	238	22.4	483	18.6	218	19.0
40–44	420	15.7	156	14.7	380	14.6	173	15.1
Total	2669	100.0	1063	100.0	2601	100.0	1147	100.0

TABLE 6.A.1 (*continued*)

(*c*) Breakdown by family size and residence of eligible women interviewed and of those gynaecologically examined

Family size	Old urban zone				Newly settled zone			
	EW interviewed		EW gynaecologically examined		EW interviewed		EW gynaecologically examined	
	No.	%	No.	%	No.	%	No.	%
0	294	11.0	90	8.5	187	7.2	68	5.9
1	500	18.7	202	19.0	339	13.0	125	10.9
2	587	22.0	240	22.6	427	16.4	192	16.7
3	386	14.5	157	14.8	345	13.3	155	13.5
4	281	10.5	120	11.3	304	11.7	135	11.8
5	211	7.9	90	8.5	246	9.5	130	11.3
6 and over	410	15.4	164	15.4	753	28.9	342	29.8
Total	2669	100.0	1063	100.0	2601	100.0	1142	100.0

TABLE 6.A.2. MEAN PONDERAL INDEX OF ELIGIBLE WOMEN

(*a*) By residence and parity

Residence	Mean ponderal index at parity:							Total no. investigated
	0	1	2	3	4	5	6 and over	
Old urban zone	12.4	12.3	12.2	12.2	12.1	12.1	12.0	1060
Newly settled zone	12.2	12.3	12.2	12.1	12.1	12.0	12.0	1145

(*b*) By residence and age

Residence	Mean ponderal index at age:						Total no. investigated
	< 20	20–24	25–29	30–34	35–39	40–44	
Old urban zone	(12.7)[a]	12.5	12.3	12.2	12.1	12.0	1060
Newly settled zone	12.3	12.2	12.1	12.1	12.0	12.0	1145

[a] Refers to fewer than 25 eligible women.

Ponderal Index

On the whole, there was no difference in the ponderal index of the women in the two zones. There is a slight tendency for the index to decrease with age, i.e., the older women were a little heavier (Tables 6.A.2(*a*) and (*b*)).

Haemoglobin Level

Blood samples were taken from fingers (using fingerpricks) and the level of haemoglobin was determined immediately by a laboratory technician using an electric haemoglobinometer with an optical system. No clear relationship was observed between the level of haemoglobin and parity or age in either of the zones of residence (Tables 6.A.3(a) and (b)).

TABLE 6.A.3. MEAN HAEMOGLOBIN LEVELS OF ELIGIBLE WOMEN

(a) By residence and parity

Residence	Mean haemoglobin level (g/100 ml) at parity:							Total no. investi- gated
	0	1	2	3	4	5	6 and over	
Old urban zone	12.63	12.88	12.90	12.68	12.56	12.57	12.34	1050
Newly settled zone	12.42	12.83	12.89	12.75	12.78	12.79	12.47	1146

(b) By residence and age

Residence	Mean haemoglobin level (g/100 ml) at age:						Total no. investi- gated
	< 20	20–24	25–29	30–34	35–39	40–44	
Old urban zone	(12.69)[a]	12.70	12.74	12.85	12.66	12.31	1050
Newly settled zone	12.57	12.63	12.89	12.86	12.46	12.38	1146

[a] Refers to fewer than 25 eligible women.

Blood Pressure

Blood pressure was taken after a prescribed rest period of 15–20 minutes. It was taken on the left arm with the woman seated. A calibrated mercury sphygmomanometer was used. The systolic pressure was recorded upon hearing the first sound, and the diastolic pressure was recorded when the sound suddenly diminished.

No significant differences were found with age or parity (Table 6.A.4).

Gynaecological Findings

The gynaecological findings are listed in Table 6.A.5 according to ICD categories. It is apparent that the prevalence of gynaecological morbidity was quite high in both zones, considering all diagnoses combined. In the majority

TABLE 6.A.4. MEAN BLOOD PRESSURE, BY RESIDENCE, AGE, AND PARITY*

(a) Systolic

Residence and age	Mean systolic blood pressure (mmHg) at parity:						Total no. investigated
	<0	1 & 2	3 & 4	5 & 6	7 and over	All parities	
Old urban zone							
<20	(108.5)	(108.2)	—	—	—	(108.3)	24
20–24	111.6	113.5	110.0	—	—	112.9	145
25–29	(113.9)	113.0	114.3	(112.5)	(125.0)	113.4	273
30–34	(106.0)	114.4	114.2	115.3	(118.3)	114.4	227
35–39	(118.2)	120.9	117.7	116.2	120.0	118.3	238
40–44	(120.0)	(127.8)	(120.8)	123.5	129.1	125.4	157
Newly settled zone							
<20	(113.1)	(112.4)	—	—	—	112.7	34
20–24	113.8	113.3	(113.0)	(108.0)		113.2	190
25–29	(116.0)	113.5	113.0	113.3	(116.2)	113.4	267
30–34	(115.0)	114.2	114.8	115.3	115.6	115.0	266
35–39	(107.5)	(112.7)	117.6	121.4	117.0	117.8	218
40–44	(145.7)	(124.3)	118.5	125.3	124.8	124.4	173

(b) Diastolic

Residence and age	Mean diastolic blood pressure (mmHg) at parity:						Total no. investigated
	<0	1 & 2	3 & 4	5 & 6	7 and over	All parities	
Old urban zone							
<20	(67.7)	(70.9)	—	—	—	(69.2)	24
20–24	75.0	76.0	(75.0)	—	—	75.7	145
25–29	(75.0)	75.3	76.6	(73.3)	(70.0)	75.4	273
30–34	(74.0)	76.4	76.9	78.3	(76.7)	76.9	227
35–39	(79.1)	77.8	79.1	78.0	80.2	78.9	237
40–44	(75.0)	(83.0)	80.6	82.3	83.0	82.0	157
Newly settled zone							
<20	(77.7)	(77.6)	—	—	—	77.6	34
20–24	78.6	76.1	75.9	(70.0)	—	76.3	190
25–29	(80.0)	78.2	29.2	78.5	(80.0)	78.8	267
30–34	(80.0)	78.5	79.3	80.2	80.2	79.6	266
35–39	(77.5)	(78.7)	80.3	82.8	80.8	81.0	218
40–44	85.0	(82.9)	(81.5)	82.6	83.7	83.2	173

* Figures in parentheses refer to fewer than 25 eligible women.

of cases, the findings were placed in category ICD 629 (Other Diseases of Female Genital Organs); such findings were present in over 60% of the women. Where more specific diagnoses were reached, the following patterns were found:

TABLE 6.A.5. ELIGIBLE WOMEN FOUND TO HAVE SPECIFIED GYNAECOLOGICAL DISEASES, BY RESIDENCE, AGE, AND PARITY*

(a) Old urban zone

Age	Percentage of EW diagnosed as having disease at parity:						Total no. investigated
	<0	1 & 2	3 & 4	5 & 6	7 and over	All parities	
	ICD 620	Infective diseases of cervix					
<25	0.0	2.5	(0.0)	—	—	2.0	169
25–34	0.0	1.0	2.5	7.5	(0.0)	2.0	500
35–44	(0.0)	1.5	3.5	6.0	5.5	4.5	394
All ages	0.0	1.5	3.6	6.5	5.5	3.0	1063
	ICD 621	Other diseases of cervix					
<25	6.5	16.0	16.5	—	—	13.5	169
25–34	3.5	17.5	20.0	13.5	(25.0)	17.0	500
35–44	(13.5)	22.0	18.5	12.0	22.0	18.0	394
All ages	7.0	18.0	19.0	12.5	22.0	17.0	1063
	ICD 622	Infective diseases of uterus, vagina, and vulva					
<25	2.0	1.0	(0.0)	—	—	1.0	169
25–34	(0.0)	0.0	0.0	0.0	(0.0)	—	500
35–44	(0.0)	0.0	0.0	1.0	—	0.5	394
All ages	1.0	0.0	0.0	0.5	—	0.5	1063
	ICD 623	Uterovaginal prolapse					
<25	0.0	0.0	(0.0)	—	—	—	169
25–34	3.5	2.0	5.5	11.5	37.5	5.0	500
35–44	(6.5)	5.0	11.5	20.0	24.0	15.5	394
All ages	2.5	2.0	8.0	17.0	25.0	8.0	1063
	ICD 624	Malposition of uterus					
<25	9.0	2.5	(33.5)	—	—	5.5	169
25–34	3.5	5.0	7.0	4.0	(0.0)	5.5	500
35–44	(6.5)	5.0	3.5	5.0	4.0	4.5	394
All ages	7.0	4.0	6.0	4.5	3.5	5.0	1063
	ICD 629	Other diseases of female genital organs					
<25	44.5	54.0	(83.5)	—	—	52.5	169
25–34	64.5	58.5	71.5	79.0	(137.5)	66.5	500
35–44	(40.0)	52.5	68.5	72.0	69.5	66.0	394
All ages	50.0	56.5	70.5	74.5	74.5	64.0	1063

TABLE 6.A.5 (continued)

(b) Newly settled zone

Age	Percentage of EW diagnosed as having disease at parity:						Total no. investigated
	<0	1 & 2	3 & 4	5 & 6	7 and over	All parities	
	ICD 620	Infective diseases of cervix					
<25	2.5	4.5	2.5	(0.0)	—	3.5	223
25–34	(0.0)	7.5	5.0	9.5	9.0	7.0	533
35–44	(0.0)	(13.5)	4.0	7.5	14.5	11.5	391
All ages	1.5	6.5	4.5	13.0	8.0		1147
	ICD 621	Other diseases of cervix					
<25	5.0	22.5	11.0	(40.0)	—	17.5	223
25–34	(11.0)	20.5	24.0	24.5	15.5	25.5	533
35–44	(0.0)	(15.5)	16.5	16.5	16.5	16.0	391
All ages	6.0	21.0	21.0	21.5	16.5	19.0	1147
	ICD 622	Infective diseases of uterus, vagina, and vulva					
<25	0.0	0.0	0.0	(0.0)	—	0.0	223
25–34	(0.0)	1.0	2.0	1.0	2.5	1.5	533
35–44	(0.0)	(0.0)	6.0	2.0	0.0	1.5	391
All ages	—	0.5	2.5	1.5	0.5	1.0	1147
	ICD 623	Uterovaginal prolapse					
<25	0.0	1.5	8.0	(20.0)	—	2.5	223
25–34	(0.0)	7.0	12.0	17.0	27.5	13.5	533
35–44	(0.0)	(18.0)	20.5	38.5	41.5	36.0	391
All ages	—	5.0	13.0	26.5	37.5	19.0	1147
	ICD 624	Malposition of uterus					
<25	5.0	4.5	0.0	(0.0)	—	3.2	223
25–34	(5.5)	4.5	3.5	3.0	5.0	4.0	533
35–44	(0.0)	(9.0)	2.0	7.5	4.0	5.0	391
All ages	4.5	5.0	3.0	5.0	4.5	4.0	1147
	ICD 629	Other diseases of female genital organs					
<25	26.0	48.0	59.5	(60.0)	—	46.5	223
25–34	(39.0)	48.5	54.5	62.5	79.0	57.5	533
35–44	(66.5)	(63.5)	71.5	68.0	75.5	72.5	391
All ages	33.5	50.0	58.0	65.0	76.5	60.5	1147

* Figures in parentheses refer to fewer than 25 eligible women.

1. *Infectious diseases of the cervix*

The frequency of these conditions was higher in the NSZ than in the OUZ, the rates being 8% and 3%, respectively. There was a tendency for the incidence of cervical infection to increase with increases in age and parity. This pattern was not as clear when the relationship was examined in each age group and parity group.

2. *Other diseases of the cervix*

The relationship between disease rates, parity, and age was less distinct for other diseases of the cervix than for infectious diseases. However, in the OUZ there was a tendency for the rates to increase for higher parities and older ages.

3. *Infectious diseases of uterus, vagina, and vulva*

These rates were too low to be analysed by age or parity.

4. *Uterovaginal prolapse*

This is one of the more serious conditions that affect women of reproductive age. It was present in 8% of the women in the OUZ and 19% of those in the NSZ. In both zones, there was a sharp increase in the prevalence of prolapse with increasing parity. Likewise, with one or two exceptions, there was a sharp increase in prolapse among women aged 35 and over. When the data are cross-tabulated, as in Table 6.A.5, it is seen that the higher prevalence occurred among older women of high parity.

Malposition of the uterus

This condition showed no consistent pattern in relation to age and parity.

Other diseases of female genital organs

As already mentioned, these conditions were highly prevalent in both regions with a clear tendency to increase with age and parity. For any given parity group, however, the relationship was less pronouced. There was a slight drop in the rates for the higher ages in each parity group. However, there was an increase in rates with increases in parity for each age group.

Gynaecological Complaints Reported by Eligible Women at Interview

The frequency of gynaecological symptoms (based on the complaints made by the women at the time of the interview) was greater in the NSZ than in the OUZ, except for "irregular periods" (Table 6.A.6). The relation between gynaecological symptoms and parity differed from one symptom to another. In both zones, higher parity was associated with an increased frequency of excessive bleeding, itching, and prolapse. On the other hand, pain characteristically decreased in frequency with increasing parity, while the other complaints showed no consistent pattern.

TABLE 6.A.6. GYNAECOLOGICAL SYMPTOMS REPORTED BY ELIGIBLE WOMEN, BY RESIDENCE AND PARITY

Residence and symptoms	Percentage of EW reporting symptoms at parity:								Total no. of women replying[a]
	0	1	2	3	4	5	6 and over	All parities	
Old urban zone									
Irregular period	83.6	83.7	85.3	85.8	76.9	85.7	81.1	83.3	2669
Excessive bleeding	15.3	16.3	17.5	18.9	22.4	22.4	23.4	19.2	2669
Bleeding between periods	5.9	6.9	8.0	7.4	14.2	12.9	12.2	9.2	2667
Pain	50.5	40.3	45.1	44.1	39.0	43.3	33.8	42.0	2669
Discharge	32.9	41.6	42.6	40.9	40.0	37.1	33.8	38.9	2668
Itching	23.1	22.8	22.4	27.4	27.6	26.7	26.6	24.9	2667
Prolapse	0.4	2.2	2.5	2.1	2.4	3.8	3.8	2.5	2667
Newly settled zone									
Irregular period	71.8	15.9	80.2	78.5	76.3	72.3	75.6	76.2	2597
Excessive bleeding	22.8	18.5	21.9	21.8	34.5	31.5	32.6	27.2	2595
Bleeding between periods	11.6	10.5	17.3	19.1	16.7	20.4	19.0	17.0	2596
Pain	61.9	53.1	51.3	57.4	54.0	54.3	47.0	52.2	2598
Discharge	38.1	48.3	52.3	49.4	55.2	54.5	40.6	40.4	2598
Itching	28.2	27.1	32.1	30.1	37.7	34.9	38.6	34.0	2601
Prolapse	2.8	2.8	4.0	5.4	4.7	6.8	5.2	4.7	2597

[a] The figures in this column represent the total number of women answering either "Yes" or "No" to each question. Women who answered "Unknown" are not included.

TABLE 6.A.7. ELIGIBLE WOMEN WHO BREAST FED THEIR LAST CHILD

(a) By residence and age

Residence	Percentage of EW reporting breast feeding last child at age:							Total no. of EW
	<20	20–24	25–29	30–34	35–39	40–44	All ages	
Old urban zone	80.3	80.7	76.7	76.5	76.5	74.8	77.8	2102
Newly settled zone	87.6	86.4	84.0	84.6	77.2	71.7	83.9	2124

(b) By residence and birth order

Residence	Percentage of EW who breast fed last child of birth order:						All birth orders	Total no. of EW
	1	2	3	4	5	6		
Old urban zone	78.0	75.1	79.5	76.7	76.1	81.1	77.8	2100
Newly settled zone	83.7	84.2	83.6	87.5	85.9	83.9	83.8	2123

Breast Feeding

In order to establish the pattern of breast feeding and its relation to age and parity, women were asked whether they had breast fed their last child. Approximately 78% in the OUZ and 84% in the NSZ, replied that they had breast fed their last child. The proportion giving a positive reply diminished somewhat over age 25 in the OUZ and over age 35 in the NSZ (Table 6.A.7(*a*)). There was no clear relation between birth order and breast feeding (Table 6.A.7(*b*)).

B. EGYPT

M. Fathalla, H. M. Hammam, A. F. El-Sherbini &
M. Yassin

Coverage

It was hoped that it would be possible to perform the following examinations on all the eligible women interviewed: (*a*) physical examination, including measurement of height and weight and of systolic and diastolic blood pressure; (*b*) laboratory determination of haemoglobin level by the photometric oxyhaemoglobin method (using a 1 g/litre sodium carbonate solution) on a blood sample obtained by fingerprick; (*c*) a gynaecological examination by a gynaecologist. However, while a high response rate was achieved for the physical examination and the haemoglobin estimation (70% in the rural area and 88% in the urban area, as shown in Table 6.B.1), it was clear from the beginning that the response rate for the gynaecological examination would be very low, even when the examination was performed by an experienced female physician who had been the woman's family doctor for years before the study. Only when the women were suffering from specific complaints did they submit to gynaecological examination, and in those cases they asked for it. For this reason, no analysis was made of the gynaecological findings.

TABLE 6.B.1. ELIGIBLE WOMEN INTERVIEWED COMPARED WITH THOSE EXAMINED, BY RESIDENCE

Residence	Total no. of EW interviewed	Height and weight		Haemoglobin determination		Blood pressure	
		No.	%	No.	%	No.	%
Rural	2145	1504	70.1	1504	70.1	1504	70.1
Urban	2097	1848	88.1	1848	88.1	1848	88.1

Ponderal Index

Table 6.B.2 shows that on the whole urban women were heavier (had a lower ponderal index) than rural women for almost all parities. Age and parity seem to have little effect on the ponderal index.

TABLE 6.B.2. MEAN PONDERAL INDEX OF ELIGIBLE WOMEN

(a) By residence and parity

| Residence | Mean ponderal index at parity: | | | | | | | Total no. investigated | Unknown |
	0	1	2	3	4	5	6 and over		
Rural	12.6	12.7	12.8	13.0	12.9	13.0	12.7	1421	83
Urban	12.4	13.5	12.6	12.3	12.4	12.4	12.7	1839	9

(b) By residence and age

| Residence | Mean ponderal index at age: | | | | | | Total no. investigated |
	<20	20–24	25–29	30–34	35–39	40–44	
Rural	12.7	13.4	13.6	12.6	12.9	12.5	1504
Urban	12.3	13.3	12.5	12.4	12.5	12.7	1848

Haemoglobin Level

Table 6.B.3 shows that the rural women did not suffer from anaemia at any level of parity (taking 12 g/100 ml as the cut-off point for adult nonpregnant women); the levels ranged from 12 to 13.9 g/100 ml. In contrast, urban women were anaemic most of the time and sometimes borderline anaemic, the levels ranging between 11.0 and 12.2 g/100 ml. No significant differences were found with age or parity.

Blood Pressure

Blood pressure was measured while the women were seated and the diastolic pressure was noted when the sound of the heartbeat suddenly diminished.

It can be seen from Table 6.B.4(a) that the highest mean systolic blood pressure was found among women in the industrial area, followed by urban women and then rural women. Ranges for the 3 areas were: 121–131 mmHg, 117–124 mmHg, and 116–121 mmHg respectively.

It can also be observed in Table 6.B.4(a) that for the 3 areas of residence there was a consistent direct relationship between age and mean systolic blood pressure. In other words, for all parities mean systolic blood pressure increased with increase in age.

TABLE 6.B.3. MEAN HAEMOGLOBIN LEVELS OF ELIGIBLE WOMEN

(a) By residence and parity

Residence	Mean haemoglobin level (g/100 ml) at parity:							Total no. investigated
	0	1	2	3	4	5	6 and over	
Rural	12	13.3	13.5	12.8	13.3	12.4	13.9	1504
Urban	12.2	11.9	12.0	11.7	11.0	12.2	11.6	1848

(b) By residence and age

Residence	Mean haemoglobin levels (g/100 ml) at age:						Total no. investigated
	<20	20–24	25–29	30–34	35–39	40–44	
Rural	12.9	13.4	12.6	13.2	13.0	13.0	1504
Urban	12.5	11.6	12.1	11.8	11.8	11.8	1848

TABLE 6.B.4. MEAN BLOOD PRESSURE BY RESIDENCE, AGE, AND PARITY*

(a) Systolic

Residence and age	Mean systolic blood pressure (mmHg) at parity:						Total no. investigated
	0	1–2	3–4	5–6	7 and over	All parities	
Rural							
<20	120.0	(113.0)	(115.0)	—	—	116.0	143
20–24	122.0	(117.0)	118.0	(117.0)	—	118.0	289
25–29	(128.0)	(118.0)	119.0	116.0	115.0	119.0	332
30–34	(130.0)	(119.0)	118.0	116.0	116.0	120.0	272
35–39	(115.0)	(121.0)	123.0	120.0	117.0	119.0	265
40–44	—	(123.0)	(119.0)	121.0	121.0	121.0	193
Unknown							10
Urban							
<20	117.0	120.0	(118.0)	—	—	118.0	127
20–24	121.0	114.0	(118.0)	117.0	—	117.0	369
25–29	(122.0)	118.0	118.0	(119.0)	115.0	118.0	361
30–34	(128.0)	(119.0)	(118.0)	120.0	(117.0)	120.0	368
35–39	(134.0)	(119.0)	120.0	120.0	120.0	123.0	343
40–44	—	(121.0)	(122.0)	124.0	122.0	124.0	273
Unknown							7
Industrial							
<20	(127.0)	(115.0)	—	—	—	(121.0)	20
20–24	(113.0)	116.0	126.0	—	—	127.0	140
25–29	(118.0)	(117.0)	126.0	—	—	128.0	60
30–34	—	(125.0)	133.0	—	—	129.0	66
35–39	—	137.0	(126.0)	(117.0)	113.0	130.0	38
40–44	—	—	—	(130.0)	(131.0)	(131.0)	14

TABLE 6.B.4 (continued)

(b) Diastolic

Residence and age	Mean diastolic blood pressure (mmHg) at parity:						Total no. investigated
	0	1–2	3–4	5–6	7 and over	All parities	
Rural							
<20	73.0	(73.0)	(70.0)	—		72.0	143
20–24	74.0	(74.0)	72.0	(73.0)	—	73.0	289
25–29	(75.0)	(75.0)	74.0	72.0	70.0	73.0	332
30–34	(76.0)	(78.0)	74.0	73.0	73.0	74.0	272
35–39	(85.0)	(80.0)	75.0	73.0	75.0	75.0	265
40–44	—	(69.0)	(73.0)	74.0	76.0	75.0	193
Unknown							10
Urban							
<20	73.0	74.0	(72.0)	—	—	73.0	127
20–24	75.0	75.0	(73.0)	71.0	—	73.0	369
25–29	(74.0)	76.0	75.0	(73.0)	75.0	75.0	361
30–34	(77.0)	(75.0)	76.0	73.0	(78.0)	74.0	368
35–39	(81.0)	(67.0)	76.0	75.0	75.0	75.0	343
40–44	—	(69.0)	(78.0)	76.0	76.0	76.0	273
Unknown							7
Industrial							
<20	(77.0)	(75.0)	—	—	—	(76.0)	20
20–24	(80.0)	79.0	79.0	—	—	79.0	140
25–29	(82.0)	(79.0)	80.0	—	—	80.0	60
30–34	—	(80.0)	80.0	—	—	80.0	66
35–39	—	82.0	(80.0)	(86.0)	83.0	82.0	38
40–44	—	—	—	(89.0)	(83.0)	(84.0)	14

* Figures in parentheses refer to fewer than 25 eligible women.

The highest mean systolic pressures were observed mainly among nulliparous women in both the rural and the urban areas. Otherwise, no consistent pattern was observed for mean systolic blood pressure in relation to parity. In fact, if any conclusion can be drawn regarding the rural area, it is that there was no increase of mean systolic blood pressure with parity, but rather the reverse. In the industrial area, some high values were noticed for mean systolic blood pressure with parities 3–4 at ages from 20 up to 34 years.

From Table 6.B.4(b) it may be observed that the lowest mean diastolic blood pressures were among rural women (range 72–75 mmHg), followed closely by urban women (range 73–76 mmHg), and the highest mean diastolic blood pressures were among women in the industrial area (range between 76 and 84 mmHg).

A direct relationship between age and the mean diastolic blood pressure was observed in the 3 areas of residence, i.e. as age increased, the mean diastolic blood pressure increased.

By parity, again the highest mean diastolic blood pressures in the rural area were observed among nulliparous women in all age groups. In the rural area, the trend throughout the range of age groups from less than 20 up to 34 years was an inverse relationship between parity and mean diastolic blood pressure (the latter decreased as the parity increased); but, beyond 35 years of age, parity of 6 and more showed an increased mean diastolic blood pressure; and beyond 40 years of age, parity of 4 or more showed an increased mean diastolic blood pressure.

On the other hand, in neither the urban nor the industrial area, was a consistent trend observed between parity and mean diastolic blood pressure.

Breast Feeding of the Last Child

Table 6.B.7(a) shows that women in the rural area more often breast fed their last child than did urban women (72.3% compared with 67.5%).

Also, it is clear from the same table that for both the rural and the urban areas, breast feeding of last children increased with increasing age of the mother. The increase in the rural area was from 51.6% for mothers aged less than 20 years to 78.4% for mothers aged 40–44 years; in the urban area there was an even greater differential—from 38.4% for mothers aged less than 20 years to 80.3% for mothers aged 40–44 years.

The change in the number of mothers breast feeding their last children could be the result of a new trend among women of the younger generations— perhaps partly due to increasing pressure of propaganda by multinational corporations selling milk powders. Also, larger numbers of women are now leaving their homes (and babies) to go to work. Such a trend, if it continues to be observed in future studies and in different parts of the country, should be counteracted by health education through home-visit programmes, and by encouraging working mothers to take paid holidays to breast feed their babies.

TABLE 6.B.5. ELIGIBLE WOMEN WHO BREAST FED THEIR LAST CHILD

(a) By residence and age

Residence	Percentage of EW who breast fed last child at age:							Total no. investigated	Unknown
	<20	20–24	25–29	30–34	35–39	40–44	All ages		
Rural	51.6	64.5	73.0	75.5	78.3	78.4	72.3	1968	177
Urban	38.4	61.2	63.3	71.9	70.1	80.3	67.5	1945	152

(b) By residence and birth order

Residence	Percentage of EW who breast fed last child of birth order:							Total no. investigated	Unknown
	1	2	3	4	5	6 and over	All birth orders		
Rural	64.6	72.3	76.2	79.8	69.7	74.5	73.4	1930	215
Urban	53.2	67.1	68.9	70.0	68.0	73.0	69.1	1900	197

Table 6.B.7(*b*) shows the percentage of women who breast fed their last child by residence and birth order.

Breast feeding is more popular among rural than among urban women, the percentages being 73.4% and 69.1%, respectively.

C. PAKISTAN

Talat Khan

Sample for Physical Examination

It was intended that all the 4861 women included in the study should be submitted to a medical examination, including a pelvic examination and a Papanicolaou smear test. All the women were informed about the examination at the time of the interview. The purpose of the interview and medical examination was explained to them with the request to visit the clinic for medical check-up. Transportation was provided to bring the women to the clinic and to take them back home after the examination. In spite of this service some women did not agree to the vaginal examination. In such instances, a lady doctor, along with the interviewer and a technician, was sent to the woman's residence to attempt further persuasion and to perform the vaginal examination. In spite of all these efforts, the number of women who submitted to examination was not satisfactory. Therefore, an attempt to increase the number of medical check-ups was made by sending male staff of the Institute to the area in the evening to contact the husbands of the women who refused examination, requesting them to seek the co-operation of their wives in agreeing to a medical check-up. As a result of these strenuous efforts the response rate for the medical check-up increased. Even so, only 40% of the interviewed population submitted themselves for the gynaecological examination.

Table 6.C.1 gives the breakdown of all the examinations. Of the total number of women interviewed, a physical examination, i.e., measurement of height, weight, and blood pressure, and haemoglobin determination, was carried out on about 78%. The findings indicate that in both urban and semi-urban localities, women who submitted themselves for medical examination and those who refused the examination did not differ in respect of age and family size distribution.

There is a slight indication that older women in both groups were more ready to co-operate in the examination than younger women, especially in the semi-urban area.

TABLE 6.C.1. ELIGIBLE WOMEN INTERVIEWED COMPARED WITH THOSE EXAMINED

(a) Coverage for each type of investigation, by residence

Residence	Total EW interviewed	Blood pressure, height and weight		Haemoglobin determination		Gynaecological examination	
		No.	%	No.	%	No.	%
Semi-urban	2388	1753	73.1	1457	61.0	809	33.9
Urban	2473	2050	82.9	1805	73.0	1142	46.2

(b) Breakdown by residence and age group of eligible women interviewed and of those gynaecologically examined

Age group	Semi-urban				Urban			
	All eligible women		Eligible women examined		All eligible women		Eligible women examined	
	No.	%	No.	%	No.	%	No.	%
<20	118	4.9	28	3.5	96	3.9	30	2.6
20–24	395	16.6	106	13.1	423	17.1	160	14.0
25–29	527	22.1	180	22.2	662	26.8	292	25.6
30–34	523	21.9	183	22.6	466	18.8	233	20.4
35–39	430	18.0	164	20.3	385	15.6	206	18.0
40–44	395	16.5	148	18.3	441	17.8	221	19.4
All age groups	2388	100.00	809	100.00	2473	100.00	1142	100.00

(c) Breakdown by residence and family size of eligible women interviewed and of those gynaecologically examined

Family size	Semi-urban				Urban			
	All eligible women		Eligible women examined		All eligible women		Eligible women examined	
	No.	%	No.	%	No.	%	No.	%
0	232	9.7	78	9.6	276	11.2	105	9.2
1	209	8.7	55	6.8	276	11.2	104	9.2
2	278	11.6	86	10.6	388	15.7	160	14.0
3	278	11.7	86	10.6	358	14.5	178	15.6
4	345	14.5	111	13.7	313	12.7	149	13.0
5	315	13.2	117	14.5	265	10.6	128	11.2
6 and over	731	30.6	276	34.2	297	24.1	318	27.8
All family sizes	2388	100.00	809	100.00	2473	100.00	1142	100.00

Professional Personnel and General Procedure

In the initial stages of the survey of the selected localities a temporary accommodation for the clinic and laboratory was acquired and equipped. Four lady doctors with experience in obstetrics, gynaecology, and general medicine were engaged. Two medical technologists, 4 technicians and some other ancillary staff were also employed to work in the field laboratory, mobile clinics, and the laboratory of the Institute. Urine and stool specimens were examined in the temporary laboratories at the site, but blood for haemoglobin tests, and cervical cytology smears were sent to the main laboratory at the National Research Institute of Fertility Control, where the examinations were carried out by trained medical technologists under the supervision of a senior pathologist.

Ponderal Index

Women were weighed wearing their normal light clothing on bathroom scales.

No difference was found in the ponderal index of urban and semi-urban women, nor was a difference by parity seen. However, there was a clear tendency for the ponderal index to decrease with age (Table 6.C.2(a) and (b)).

TABLE 6.C.2. MEAN PONDERAL INDEX OF ELIGIBLE WOMEN

(a) By residence and parity

Residence	Mean ponderal index at parity:							Total no. investigated
	0	1	2	3	4	5	6 and over	
Semi-urban	12.6	12.6	12.6	12.7	12.5	12.2	12.5	1753
Urban	12.6	12.5	12.5	12.5	12.3	12.2	12.2	2050

(b) By residence and age

Residence	Mean ponderal index at age:						Total no. investigated
	<20	20–24	25–29	30–34	35–39	40–44	
Semi-urban	12.9	12.7	12.6	12.5	12.4	12.4	1753
Urban	12.7	12.6	12.5	12.3	12.2	12.1	2050

Haemoglobin Level

Haemoglobin was determined by the cyanmethaemoglobin method. Blood samples were extracted by fingerprick and taken to the main laboratory for examination. The mean haemoglobin level was low for all women. No association was observed between haemoglobin level and either age or parity.

A slight difference was noted in haemoglobin value between urban and semi-urban areas. Women in the semi-urban area had comparatively lower haemoglobin levels in all age groups than women in the urban area (Table 6.C.3(*a*) and (*b*)).

TABLE 6.C.3. MEAN HAEMOGLOBIN LEVELS OF ELIGIBLE WOMEN

(*a*) By residence and parity:

Residence	Mean haemoglobin level (g/100 ml) at parity:							Total no. investigated
	0	1	2	3	4	5	6 and over	
Semi-urban	10.9	10.7	10.7	10.7	10.7	10.6	10.8	1457
Urban	11.4	11.3	11.2	11.2	11.1	11.2	11.2	1805

(*b*) By residence and age

Residence	Mean haemoglobin level (g/100 ml) at age:						Total no. investigated
	<20	20–24	25–29	30–34	35–39	40–44	
Semi-urban	10.3	10.6	10.7	10.8	10.8	10.9	1457
Urban	11.3	11.1	11.1	11.2	11.4	11.3	1805

Blood Pressure

Blood pressure was recorded in the sitting position, either in the clinic or at the woman's residence after the interview schedule had been filled in.

Mean blood pressure readings seemed to be within normal limits in both the groups. An increase in blood pressure level with an increase in age was noticed in both urban and semi-urban populations, but there was no apparent change with increased parity (Table 6.C.4).

Gynaecological Disease

The gynaecological examination was performed on 1951 women. Although this number constitutes only about 40% of the eligible women, it was quite an achievement to persuade almost 2000 women to submit to a gynaecological examination in such a conservative, modesty-conscious community. Admittedly, there is a risk of selection bias in that women with gynaecological problems are more likely to submit to the examination than those without such problems. Apparently, a substantial number of women were free of problems, but the prevalence of gynaecological conditions was relatively high. Fortunately, all parities and age groups were represented. In fact, the parity distribution of those examined was not very different from that of the total sample population. This is important when considering the pattern of distribution of gynaecological disorders by age and parity.

TABLE 6.C.4. MEAN BLOOD PRESSURE BY RESIDENCE, AGE, AND PARITY*

(a) Systolic

Residence and age group	Mean systolic blood pressure (mmHg) at parity:						Total no. investigated
	0	1 & 2	3 & 4	5 & 6	7 and over	All parities	
Semi-urban							
<20	117.3	112.7	(130.0)	—	—	115.6	73
20–24	120.4	115.3	114.7	(117.5)	(120.0)	116.7	276
25–29	121.8	118.9	118.3	117.4	118.8	118.2	399
30–34	(125.0)	(120.0)	118.6	117.0	119.4	118.5	372
35–39	(134.7)	(127.4)	124.3	124.8	120.1	122.7	329
40–44	(128.7)	(129.8)	133.5	125.0	126.7	127.3	302
Urban							
<20	114.6	116.5	(117.5)	—	—	115.6	76
20–24	116.1	113.6	114.9	(113.3)	—	114.4	335
25–29	114.0	115.4	115.0	113.4	(117.3)	114.9	540
30–34	(125.8)	120.7	119.2	118.7	118.5	119.5	391
35–39	(125.7)	127.5	123.4	121.3	121.3	122.5	326
40–44	(120.0)	(130.0)	128.0	128.0	127.8	127.8	385

(b) Diastolic

Residence and age group	Mean diastolic blood pressure (mmHg) at parity:						Total no. investigated
	0	1 & 2	3 & 4	5 & 6	7 and over	All parities	
Semi-urban							
<20	82.1	78.9	(95.0)	—	—	81.2	73
20–24	82.2	79.9	79.9	(83.6)	(90.0)	80.5	276
25–29	83.1	81.6	83.5	81.3	82.5	82.4	399
30–34	(84.4)	(85.6)	82.7	80.9	83.4	82.5	372
35–39	(91.7)	(92.5)	86.4	87.3	84.2	86.0	329
40–44	(93.3)	(89.6)	92.8	88.2	87.4	88.3	302
Urban							
<20	78.2	80.9	(77.5)	—	—	79.5	76
20–24	80.2	77.7	79.0	(74.2)	—	78.5	335
25–29	78.2	79.2	79.0	77.8	(80.9)	78.9	540
30–34	(86.3)	83.6	82.8	81.5	82.7	82.7	391
35–39	(85.0)	86.8	84.2	84.9	82.1	83.9	326
40–44	(85.5)	(88.6)	88.3	86.8	87.9	87.6	385

The diseases diagnosed on the basis of the pelvic examination were assigned to the 5 categories of the ICD[1] (Table 6.C.5).

Gynaecological disorders were quite prevalent in the study population. The prevalence was higher in the semi-urban area. Infective diseases of the cervix, such as chronic cervicitis, cervical catarrh, and endocervicitis resulting in

---

[1] *Manual of the International Statistical Classification of Diseases, Injuries, and Causes of Death*, 8th revision, vol. 1, Geneva, World Health Organization, 1967.

TABLE 6.C.5. ELIGIBLE WOMEN FOUND TO HAVE SPECIFIED GYNAECOLOGICAL DISEASES, BY RESIDENCE, AGE, AND PARITY*

(a) Semi-urban

Age	Percentage of EW diagnosed as having disease at parity:						Total no. investigated
	0	1 & 2	3 & 4	5 & 6	7 and over	All parities	
ICD 620 Infective diseases of cervix uteri							
<25	25.3	55.3	48.3	(66.7)	(0.0)	37.3	134
25–34	(16.7)	36.6	45.3	38.3	45.3	39.4	363
35–44	(45.5)	(33.3)	39.1	34.9	44.1	41.0	312
All ages	24.6	35.5	44.1	38.1	43.9	39.7	809
ICD 621 Other diseases of cervix							
<25	26.7	38.2	37.9	(50.0)	(0.0)	35.8	134
25–34	(29.2)	31.7	46.3	49.2	56.0	46.6	363
35–44	(27.3)	(60.0)	43.5	73.0	60.5	59.5	312
All ages	27.7	38.7	44.1	56.9	58.9	49.7	809
ICD 622 Infective diseases of uterus, vagina, and vulva							
<25	3.3	10.3	6.9	(0.0)	(0.0)	7.5	134
25–34	(4.2)	7.3	9.5	7.8	6.7	7.7	363
35–44	(20.0)	(0.0)	4.3	7.9	9.0	8.0	312
All ages	6.2	8.6	7.6	7.6	8.5	7.8	809
ICD 623 Uterovaginal prolapse							
<25	0.0	5.9	17.2	(16.7)	(0.0)	7.5	134
25–34	(0.0)	19.5	22.1	24.2	30.7	22.9	363
35–44	(0.0)	(20.0)	23.9	31.7	40.1	33.7	312
All ages	0.0	12.1	21.8	26.4	37.2	24.5	809
ICD 629 Other diseases of female genital organs							
<25	50.0	50.0	58.6	(66.7)	(0.0)	53.0	134
25–34	(33.3)	14.7	50.5	54.7	50.7	49.0	363
35–44	(9.1)	(46.7)	41.3	44.4	51.4	46.8	312
All ages	36.9	44.4	49.4	51.8	51.4	48.8	809

292

TABLE 6.C.5 (*continued*)

(*b*) Urban

| Age | Percentage of EW diagnosed as having disease at parity: | | | | | | Total no. investigated |
	0	1 & 2	3 & 4	5 & 6	7 and over	All parities	
	ICD 620	Infective diseases of cervix uteri					
<25	11.8	23.5	24.3	(50.0)	—	21.6	190
25–34	22.6	23.4	25.0	24.3	23.6	24.2	525
35–44	(18.8)	6.3	26.3	20.0	23.2	21.5	427
All ages	13.3	21.5	25.2	22.7	23.3	22.7	1142
	ICD 621	Other diseases of cervix					
<25	3.9	11.2	18.9	(0.0)	—	10.5	190
25–34	3.2	18.0	17.5	19.8	15.3	17.0	525
35–44	(0.0)	9.4	14.5	18.1	26.3	19.9	427
All ages	3.06	14.1	16.9	18.6	23.3	17.1	1142
	ICD 622	Infective diseases of uterus, vagina, and vulva					
<25	3.9	3.1	8.1	(0.0)	—	4.2	190
25–34	0.0	7.2	2.5	4.5	0.0	17.1	525
35–44	(0.0)	6.3	7.9	6.7	5.1	5.9	427
All ages	2.0	5.4	4.5	5.5	3.7	4.5	1142
	ICD 623	Uterovaginal prolapse					
<25	0.0	8.2	5.4	(0.0)	—	9.5	190
25–34	0.0	5.4	11.0	18.0	19.4	2.4	525
35–44	(6.3)	3.1	14.5	13.3	12.6	12.2	427
All ages	1.0	6.2	11.2	15.5	14.4	10.9	1142
	ICD 629	Other diseases of female genital organs					
<25	23.5	18.4	21.6	(25.0)	—	20.5	190
25–34	9.7	17.1	20.0	24.3	16.7	19.2	525
35–44	(12.5)	21.9	27.6	21.0	24.8	23.7	427
All ages	17.3	18.3	22.0	18.2	22.6	21.1	1142

* Figures in parentheses refer to fewer than 25 eligible women.

unpleasant vaginal discharges, were found to be highly prevalent, affecting 23% of the urban women and 40% of the semi-urban women. It is evident from Table 6.C.5 that infective diseases of the cervix increased steadily with both age and parity. In the semi-urban area, the prevalence of cervical infection increased from 24.6% in nulliparous women to 43.9% in grand multiparas with 7 or more live births. The increase with age was from 37.3% in women under 25 years of age to 41.0% in women aged 35–44. The condition was thus

293

independently associated with age and parity. A similar pattern was evident in the urban area.

There was also a high prevalence of other diseases of the cervix (including chronic erosion and ulceration), especially in the semi-urban area where almost 50% of the women were affected, compared with 17% in the urban area. These conditions increased steadily with age and parity.

Uterovaginal prolapse, a serious gynaecological condition often requiring surgical repair, was highly prevalent, affecting 10.9% of the urban women and 34.5% of the semi-urban women. A definite increase with parity and age is apparent in Table 6.C.5. In the semi-urban area, prolapse was absent in nulliparous women, but increased from 12.1% in women of low parity (1–2), to 21.8% in women of parity 3–4 and 26.4% in those of parity 5–6; in grand multiparas of parity 7 or more, it reached the very high figure of 37.2%. Prolapse increased also with age from 7.5% in those aged under 25 to 33.7% in those aged 35–44. The prevalence of prolapse was much lower in the urban area, although a similar pattern of increasing with both age and parity was noted.[1]

Other gynaecological disorders were also prevalent, more so in the semi-urban than in the urban area, and demonstrated a definite increase with age and parity.

Gynaecological Complaints During 3 Months Preceding Interview

The frequency of gynaecological disorders as reported by women was higher in the semi-urban area than in the urban area. However, the frequencies reported by the urban women were closer to the findings of physicians during pelvic examinations than were the frequencies reported by the semi-urban women. Many women in both areas complained of irregular or excessive bleeding, pain, discharge, itching and prolapse. There was some association of several of these complaints with parity. While pain decreased with parity in both areas (as expected), discharge and itching increased with parity in both areas. The most interesting finding was that 12–14% of the women complained of having prolapse. This was lower than the actual prevalence detected by physicians. One explanation might be that some forms of prolapse can only be detected by medical examination. Another could be that the sample of women reporting complaints was much larger than that of women actually examined. Women with prolapse might have come preferentially to the gynaecological examination.

Breast Feeding

85% of the urban women and 92% of semi-urban women reported that they had breast fed their last child. No consistent relation was found between breast feeding and age or parity (Table 6.C.7).

---

[1] One explanation of the unduly high prevalence of prolapse in women from the semi-urban area is the likelihood that most of the women who overcame their objections to the gynaecological examination were those with gynaecological complaints, including prolapse.

294

TABLE 6.C.6. GYNAECOLOGICAL SYMPTOMS REPORTED BY ELIGIBLE WOMEN, BY
RESIDENCE AND PARITY

Residence and symptoms	Percentage of EW reporting symptoms at parity:								Number of EW responding
	0	1	2	3	4	5	6 and over	All parities	
Semi-urban									
Irregular period	37.4	21.5	22.7	23.8	22.2	23.0	38.4	25.9	2255
Excessive bleeding	15.3	13.2	12.5	11.9	14.7	16.9	23.8	16.2	2256
Bleeding between periods	15.9	12.7	10.7	9.0	7.4	12.3	17.9	13.2	2184
Pain	56.8	39.5	43.6	43.3	36.1	37.4	53.4	39.2	2284
Discharge	49.7	48.0	60.8	60.2	53.1	57.2	81.3	55.8	2367
Itching	15.9	16.8	12.8	17.4	19.6	20.0	29.9	19.5	2369
Prolapse	7.7	11.2	9.6	12.9	12.2	17.2	18.4	13.5	2372
Urban									
Irregular period	23.0	18.9	19.0	21.3	19.9	18.9	24.5	20.7	2334
Excessive bleeding	11.0	12.7	15.0	15.8	17.1	17.4	27.5	16.4	2388
Bleeding between periods	8.2	9.2	9.0	8.8	10.3	8.7	14.5	9.8	2388
Pain	44.0	43.7	41.0	37.3	41.5	35.0	50.3	38.5	2390
Discharge	39.6	39.4	48.0	52.6	46.6	51.3	48.6	47.5	2452
Itching	11.3	12.4	16.4	17.8	15.9	18.9	22.1	16.3	2455
Prolapse	2.4	7.9	8.4	12.5	15.5	15.7	14.9	11.7	2455

TABLE 6.C.7. ELIGIBLE WOMEN WHO BREAST FED THEIR LAST CHILD, BY RESIDENCE AND
AGE OR BIRTH ORDER

(a) By residence and age

Residence	Percentage of EW reporting breast feeding last children at age:					
	<20	20–24	25–29	30–34	35–40	40 and over
Semi-urban	90.4	91.5	90.5	92.0	90.5	85.3
Urban	87.1	89.2	83.8	84.7	87.9	92.3

(b) By residence and birth order

Residence	Percentage of EW who breast fed last children of birth order:					
	1	2	3	4	5	6 and over
Semi-urban	85.9	93.3	93.8	91.8	93.2	90.4
Urban	83.3	85.6	85.2	86.8	83.9	89.0

295

D. SYRIAN ARAB REPUBLIC

A. Dahman, M. Gharib & A. R. Omran

Sample for Physical Examination

This project was very ambitious in aiming to persuade 100% of the eligible women to submit to physical examination. Considerable effort was expended to achieve this target and a high degree of success was attained, considering that the women are highly conservative and do not submit easily to medical examinations unless they are very sick. An important factor in overcoming the women's resistance was the employment of 9 lady physicians to perform the examination. Even in the rural areas, where the society is more traditional, 72% of the women interviewed could be gynaecologically examined. This makes the Syrian study unique, not only in the Middle East but in the entire Muslim world.

Blood samples for haemoglobin determination were taken from 3953 or 70.3% of the interviewed women, while height and weight were measured for 4000 or 71.2% of the interviewed women. Physical examinations were accepted by 3724 women out of the 5621 women interviewed. This gives a response rate of 66.3%, which is a record for developing countries. The results of this examination may therefore be considered highly reliable.

TABLE 6.D.1. ELIGIBLE WOMEN INTERVIEWED COMPARED WITH THOSE EXAMINED: COVERAGE FOR EACH TYPE OF EXAMINATION, BY RESIDENCE

Residence	Total EW inter-viewed	Weight and height		Haemoglobin determination		Physical examination[a]	
		No.	%	No.	%	No.	%
Damascus	1975	1199	60.7	1207	61.1	1214	61.5
Sweida	1711	1293	75.6	1267	74.0	1116	65.2
Rural Aleppo	1935	1508	77.9	1479	76.4	1394	72.0

[a] Including those examined gynaecologically.

Ponderal Index

No differences were detected when ponderal index was analysed by residence. In general, the index decreased with age (older women were heavier) in all three areas. The mean ponderal index of eligible women in Damascus decreased from 12.3 for the first age category (under 20 years) to 11.5 for the last category (40–44 years). The corresponding figures for Sweida were 12.4 and 11.7, while for Rural Aleppo they were 12.4 and 11.8, respectively.

There was also some evidence of a slight decline in mean ponderal index at parities 5 and 6 and over (as shown in Table 6.D.2(a)). This study confirms the clinical observation that older women as well as grand multiparas tend to be slightly heavier than younger ones and those of lower parity.

296

TABLE 6.D.2. MEAN PONDERAL INDEX OF ELIGIBLE WOMEN, BY RESIDENCE AND
PARITY OR MATERNAL AGE

(a) By parity

Residence	Mean ponderal index at parity:							Total no. investigated
	0	1	2	3	4	5	6 and over	
Damascus	12.1	12.0	12.0	12.0	11.8	11.8	11.6	1199
Sweida	11.9	12.1	12.1	12.0	12.0	12.0	11.7	1293
Rural Aleppo	12.1	12.2	12.3	12.1	12.0	12.0	11.9	1508

(b) By maternal age

Residence	Mean ponderal index at age:						Total no. investigated
	<20	20–24	25–29	30–34	35–39	40–44	
Damascus	12.3	12.1	11.9	11.8	11.5	11.5	1199
Sweida	12.4	12.1	12.0	11.9	11.7	11.7	1293
Rural Aleppo	12.4	12.2	12.1	11.9	11.8	11.8	1508

Haemoglobin Level

Blood samples were taken by fingerprick and the haemoglobin level
determined by the cyanmethaemoglobin method.

At most parities and ages, rural women had a marginally lower haemoglobin
level than women in Damascus. No consistent relationship was observed
between mean haemoglobin level and either age or parity (Table 6.D.3). The
low haemoglobin level found in Rural Aleppo was probably due to a lower iron
supply, higher parity, and less medical care.

Blood Pressure

Both mean systolic and mean diastolic blood pressure increased with age,
but there was no evidence that either pressure increased with parity when age
was held constant (Table 6.D.4).

Gynaecological Disease

The frequency of gynaecological disease or complaints received particular
attention in this study as it provided an indicator of the relationship between
women's health and family formation. The findings were based on two sets of
data:

(a) Gynaecological complaints reported by the women. Such data were
obtained from 5621 women.

TABLE 6.D.3. MEAN HAEMOGLOBIN LEVELS OF ELIGIBLE WOMEN, BY RESIDENCE AND PARITY OR AGE

(a) By residence and parity

Residence	Mean haemoglobin level (g/100 ml) at parity:							Total no. investigated
	0	1	2	3	4	5	6 and over	
Damascus	12.9	12.5	12.4	12.6	12.8	12.4	12.4	1207
Sweida	11.6	11.2	11.2	10.8	10.8	10.9	11.1	1267
Rural Aleppo	11.2	11.0	10.7	10.9	10.8	10.9	11.1	1479

(b) By residence and age

Residence	Mean haemoglobin level (g/100 ml) at age:						Total no. investigated
	<20	20–24	25–29	30–34	35–39	40–44	
Damascus	12.7	12.4	12.6	12.5	11.5	12.5	1207
Sweida	11.2	10.9	11.2	10.9	11.1	11.3	1267
Rural Aleppo	11.2	10.9	10.8	11.1	11.2	11.1	1479

(b) Gynaecological disease detected by physicians during physical examinations of 3724 women. The diseases were classified according to the ICD.[1]

Both sets represent the three residential areas. Surprisingly the representation of rural women was even higher than the representation of women from the other areas, reaching 72% of rural women compared with 65% representation of women in Sweida and 62% coverage in Damascus.

The gynaecological examination was carried out by a group of 9 specialists and general practitioners, all of whom were lady physicians who had been in practice for several years. They agreed to concentrate on infections of the cervix, uterus and other genital organs, grouped together as one condition, and on uterovaginal prolapse. All these conditions are of special relevance in Syria especially prolapse, which requires either medical or surgical treatment.

Gynaecological complaints reported by eligible women

The symptoms reported by the women are listed in Table 6.D.5 according to parity. In general, the reported prevalence of gynaecological conditions was relatively high in all three areas. The conditions most frequently reported in the three areas were pelvic pain, irregular periods, discharge, and itching. It is very interesting that the reported prevalence of prolapse was relatively high, ranging from 8.8% in Damascus to 10.3% in Sweida and 15.4% in Rural Aleppo. Thus, it must have been symptomatic or otherwise detectable by the women. It is also interesting that the rates reported by the women in Sweida and Rural Aleppo are much higher than those found by the examining physicians.

---

[1] *Manual of the International Statistical Classification of Diseases, Injuries, and Causes of Death.* 8th revision, vol. 1. Geneva, World Health Organization, 1967.

298

TABLE 6.D.4. MEAN BLOOD PRESSURE BY RESIDENCE, AGE, AND PARITY*

(a) Systolic

Residence	Age group	Mean systolic blood pressure (mmHg) at parity:					All parities	Total no. investigated
		0	1–2	3–4	5–6	7 and over		
Damascus	<20	117	121	(123)	—	—	119	83
	20–24	(123)	119	118	(119)	(130)	119	218
	25–29	(123)	118	123	121	(119)	121	239
	30–34	(122)	(116)	122	122	123	122	252
	35–39	(135)	(121)	(126)	127	124	125	221
	40–44	(137)	(130)	(128)	140	131	133	200
Sweida	<20	(120)	121	(120)	—	—	120	54
	20–24	(123)	121	124	(124)	—	122	190
	25–29	(120)	123	123	125	(122)	123	281
	30–34	(133)	127	124	120	128	127	273
	35–39	(123)	(127)	135	129	132	131	219
	40–44	(141)	(122)	(150)	137	137	138	268
Rural Aleppo	<20	124	124	(111)	—	—	124	125
	20–24	120	124	124	(125)	(120)	123	295
	25–29	(135)	122	120	123	120	122	269
	30–34	(120)	(123)	124	124	126	125	276
	35–39	(120)	(129)	(125)	125	126	126	251
	40–44	(125)	(126)	(125)	127	127	127	278

(b) Diastolic

Residence	Age group	Mean diastolic blood pressure (mmHg) at parity:					All parities	Total no. investigated
		0	1–2	3–4	5–6	7 and over		
Damascus	<20	67	71	(72)	—	—	69	83
	20–24	(74)	70	70	(69)	(75)	70	218
	25–29	(70)	72	74	70	(70)	70	239
	30–34	(70)	(73)	75	76	75	75	252
	35–39	(83)	(71)	(77)	78	76	76	221
	40–44	(84)	(80)	(83)	86	80	82	200
Sweida	<20	(67)	75	(60)	—	—	71	54
	20–24	(66)	70	73	(71)	—	71	190
	25–29	(75)	75	73	74	(75)	74	281
	30–34	(83)	78	74	78	76	77	273
	35–39	(76)	(74)	81	76	79	78	219
	40–44	(85)	(73)	(86)	83	81	81	268
Rural Aleppo	<20	69	72	(60)	—	—	70	125
	20–24	72	72	72	(71)	(80)	72	295
	25–29	(75)	69	69	74	74	72	269
	30–34	(69)	(70)	75	71	75	73	276
	35–39	(72)	(72)	(74)	73	73	73	251
	40–44	(67)	(67)	(71)	70	74	73	278

* Figures in parentheses refer to fewer than 25 eligible women.

TABLE 6.D.5. GYNAECOLOGICAL SYMPTOMS REPORTED BY ELIGIBLE WOMEN, BY RESIDENCE AND PARITY

Residence and symptoms	Percentage of EW reporting symptoms at parity:								No. of EW responding
	0	1	2	3	4	5	6 and over	All parities	
Damascus									
Irregular periods	30.6	20.8	25.8	22.5	20.3	15.4	22.4	22.1	1964
Excessive bleeding	9.7	7.1	3.9	8.1	6.5	6.6	9.8	8.0	1965
Bleeding between periods	16.3	4.4	3.3	4.5	3.0	4.9	6.4	5.0	1977
Pain	61.8	47.5	40.1	37.8	29.6	32.6	7.5	39.0	1967
Discharge	22.9	19.7	21.3	20.6	20.1	17.2	20.6	20.3	1974
Itching	13.2	13.7	14.2	13.5	12.0	14.5	15.6	14.3	1974
Prolapse	5.5	4.4	6.6	9.4	9.0	7.9	11.0	8.8	1974
Sweida									
Irregular periods	32.2	33.1	27.8	29.4	27.4	23.4	29.6	28.8	1699
Excessive bleeding	7.8	10.5	12.1	8.8	6.7	13.5	12.8	11.1	1707
Bleeding between periods	7.8	8.3	5.8	4.7	8.0	7.8	10.2	8.3	1707
Pain	40.5	38.4	35.8	30.6	29.3	25.9	30.5	31.7	1708
Discharge	17.2	16.4	18.5	14.7	16.4	14.5	17.2	16.6	1710
Itching	17.2	21.6	12.1	18.8	13.8	12.4	15.7	15.6	1710
Prolapse	3.5	6.1	11.2	8.3	7.6	14.8	12.2	10.3	1688
Rural Aleppo									
Irregular periods	21.9	15.0	18.4	21.4	21.2	26.0	20.0	20.3	1865
Excessive bleeding	6.5	4.9	6.1	9.5	9.8	11.7	11.7	9.6	1875
Bleeding between periods	6.0	2.8	6.1	7.7	4.6	7.8	9.8	7.7	1873
Pain	39.1	37.0	27.8	30.4	31.8	27.9	28.8	30.7	1874
Discharge	15.8	17.3	14.7	14.3	15.2	22.1	17.4	16.9	1881
Itching	18.5	22.9	16.2	19.1	13.6	22.7	16.9	17.9	1878
Prolapse	11.0	10.5	11.2	15.2	15.5	18.2	16.7	15.4	1842

The reported prevalence of prolapse decidedly increased with parity in all three residential areas. It should be noted that 3.5–11% of nulliparous women reported having prolapse.

On the other hand, pelvic pain decreased consistently with parity in all three residential areas, a finding that may be attributable either to an increased tolerance of pain following experience of the birth process or to a lessening of tension with repeated births.

The other conditions did not show consistent patterns in relation to parity when the three areas were compared.

Gynaecological disease found by physicians

The prevalence of infective diseases of the cervix and other genital organs was higher in Damascus than in the other two areas. The frequency of these infections increased with parity in each of the three areas. There was also an increase with age when parity was held constant (Table 6.D.6).

TABLE 6.D.6. ELIGIBLE WOMEN FOUND TO HAVE GYNAECOLOGICAL DISEASES, BY RESIDENCE, AGE, AND PARITY*

Residence	Age	Percentage of EW diagnosed as having disease at parity:						Total no. investigated
		0	1–2	3–4	5–6	7 and over	All parities	
		ICD 620 & 629	Infective diseases of cervix and other genital organs					
Damascus	<25	4.4	11.2	16.2	16.0	(20.0)	11.7	299
	25–34	1.3	12.5	14.1	15.5	15.5	14.3	492
	35–44	6.0	7.8	15.0	15.7	15.6	15.0	423
	All ages	4.0	11.2	14.9	15.6	15.6	13.9	1214
Sweida	<25	2.2	6.5	11.0	6.7	—	7.0	214
	25–34	7.5	6.6	10.5	11.9	11.7	10.5	493
	35–44	8.6	12.1	9.0	9.6	11.1	10.6	409
	All ages	4.8	7.3	10.4	11.0	11.3	9.9	1116
Rural Aleppo	<25	4.4	6.6	5.6	8.9	(0.0)	6.0	369
	25–34	4.2	5.1	6.8	7.4	8.3	7.2	512
	35–44	3.7	8.6	5.2	8.7	8.0	7.8	513
	All ages	4.2	6.4	6.2	7.9	8.0	7.1	1394
		ICD 623	Uterovaginal prolapse					
Damascus	<25	0.3	5.0	9.1	6.7	(0.0)	5.4	299
	25–34	0.0	5.9	10.0	9.8	10.7	9.3	492
	35–44	0.0	3.3	12.0	12.6	14.1	12.8	423
	All ages	0.2	5.1	10.0	10.6	13.0	9.5	1214
Sweida	<25	0.0	0.4	1.7	(0.0)	—	0.7	214
	25–34	0.0	2.0	1.1	2.8	4.2	2.2	493
	35–44	0.0	3.6	3.8	4.5	7.8	6.3	409
	All ages	0.0	1.3	1.6	3.2	7.0	3.4	1116
Rural Aleppo	<25	0.5	4.7	4.9	7.8	(20.0)	4.1	369
	25–34	0.0	5.9	7.2	8.0	10.7	8.0	512
	35–44	3.7	14.3	6.1	11.0	9.5	9.5	513
	All ages	0.9	5.5	6.2	8.9	9.7	7.5	1394

* Figures in parentheses refer to fewer than 25 eligible women.

Uterovaginal prolapse was more frequent in Sweida than in the other two areas. Within each area, there was a consistent and progressive increase of prolapse with parity. The difference became more evident when women who had borne 3 or more children were compared with women of lower parity. To illustrate, the prevalence of uterovaginal prolapse increased from 5.1% at parity 1–2 to 13.0% at parity 7 and over in Damascus; the corresponding figures were 1.3% to 7.0% in Sweida and 5.5% to 9.7% in Rural Aleppo. There was also an increase of prolapse with age when parity was held constant (Table 6.D.6).

These findings suggest that in all three areas, having more than three children was associated with serious health risks to the mother. Likewise, having children at a later reproductive age (over 35) was associated with similar risks. To put it more positively, family planning aimed at ensuring that not more than 3 children were born to a mother of less than 35 years of age would considerably reduce the health risks to the mothers.

Breast Feeding

The overwhelming majority of women reported that they had breast fed their last-born child. There was little difference between the three residential areas in this regard (Sweida, 97.1%; Rural Aleppo, 96.1%; and Damascus, 95%). No consistent pattern of breast feeding with age was found (Table 6.D.7(a)), but there was a slight increase in breast feeding in children of the higher birth orders.

TABLE 6.D.7. ELIGIBLE WOMEN WHO BREAST FED THEIR LAST CHILD

(a) By residence and age

Residence	Percentage of EW reporting breast feeding last child at age:							Total no. of EW responding
	<20	20–24	25–29	30–34	35–39	40–44	All ages	
Damascus	93.7	96.0	94.6	94.4	95.7	95.1	95.0	1610
Sweida	100.0	96.6	97.6	96.7	96.7	96.6	97.1	1431
Rural Aleppo	94.3	95.2	97.0	94.6	98.0	97.5	96.1	1570

(b) By residence and birth order

Residence	Percentage of EW reporting breast feeding last child of birth order:							Total no. of EW responding
	1	2	3	4	5	6 and over	All birth orders	
Damascus	93.3	94.6	94.5	95.1	95.0	95.7	95.0	1610
Sweida	94.3	96.8	96.8	99.0	97.7	97.1	97.1	1431
Rural Aleppo	92.7	96.8	94.9	95.1	97.1	98.8	96.1	1570

Chapter Seven

CHILD LOSS AND FAMILY FORMATION

INTRODUCTION

A. R. Omran

It is tempting to assume that family formation ideals and performance are influenced, at least to some extent, by child loss experience. This chapter examines the hypothesis that a woman who loses one or more of her live-born children will have, on the average, higher gravidity, higher parity, and a larger actual and ideal family size than a woman who loses no children, and that the higher the child loss, the greater will be the differences. The suggestion is that women attempt to replace lost children in the course of their reproductive lives. It is also postulated that the inter-pregnancy interval following a surviving child is longer than the one following a live-born child who was lost.

The pregnancy history and opinion data of each woman provide the basis for analysis. Child loss refers to the mortality of a live-born child under 5 years in all analyses except that for birth interval, in which case it indicates the death of a live-born child within the first year of life.

Each study area report begins by presenting data on the following 4 measurements of family formation in relation to total child loss: (*a*) mean gravidity or mean number of pregnancies per woman; (*b*) mean parity or mean number of live births per woman; (*c*) mean family size or mean number of living children per woman; (*d*) mean ideal family size.

Total child loss information is valuable, but poses problems. In retrospective history data, it is possible to have a two-way interaction between child loss and fertility, whereby child loss may either cause or result from higher gravidity and higher parity, since excess pregnancies and live births raise the probability of death for high birth order children. Thus, because the total child loss figure includes all birth orders, it is important to consider child mortality in relation to birth order.

The analysis presented here considers also child loss among the first 3 live births for those women who had achieved a parity of at least 3; the tables in the second part of each report therefore exclude deaths for birth orders higher than 3 and for women who have borne fewer than 3 children.

The extent to which the sex of the lost child influences fertility is a subject of interest in many cultures. It was difficult to calculate this influence because many women who lost male children also lost children of the opposite sex. As the numbers were small, it was not possible to concentrate on women whose losses were all males or all females.

In order to examine the biological influence of child survival on the birth interval, the length of the interval succeeding a live birth was considered in relation to whether the live-born child died within or survived the first year of life. The assumption is that the duration of post-partum amenorrhoea and the period of infertility are prolonged by lactation and/or by practices such as abstinence from intercourse or infrequent intercourse. The samples in the study relate to communities in which breast feeding is prevalent.

A. COLOMBIA

G. Ochoa, A. Gil & A. R. Omran

The loss of children under 5 was deduced from information given by the eligible women as a part of their pregnancy history. In this chapter, a distinction will be made between total child loss (i.e., the total number of children lost throughout the preceding reproductive life span of the woman) and child losses among the first 3 live births. The rationale for the use of the latter criterion will become apparent later in the chapter.

Total Child Loss and Family Formation

Table 7.A.1 shows the percentage distribution of the eligible women by total child loss. Approximately 15% of all of the women had lost one or more of their live-born children. The percentage for the women residing in the NSZ was approximately double that for those residing in the OUZ, i.e., 19.8% and 9.6% respectively.

TABLE 7.A.1. DISTRIBUTION OF ELIGIBLE WOMEN BY RESIDENCE AND CHILD LOSS EXPERIENCE

Residence	Percentage of EW with child loss of:			Total no. of EW interviewed
	0	1–2	3 and over	
Old urban zone	90.5	9.1	0.4	2669
Newly settled zone	80.2	18.4	1.4	2601
Both zones	85.4	13.7	0.9	5270

Total child loss and mean ideal family size

Most of the women in the study preferred a family size of 3 or 4 children, with more preferring the former than the latter. The ideal family size was unaffected by child loss. In the OUZ, the ideal family size for women with no loss was 3.2, while for those with losses of 3 or more children it was 3.5. In the NSZ, the numbers were 3.2 and 3.4, respectively. Since the differences were so small, it appears that child loss had little influence on ideal family size. In the OUZ, this also applied to the actual size of the family, but this was not the case in the NSZ. There was a direct relation between ideal family size and actual family size in all the categories of child loss experience (Table 7.A.2).

TABLE 7.A.2. MEAN IDEAL FAMILY SIZE BY RESIDENCE, ACTUAL FAMILY SIZE, AND TOTAL CHILD LOSS EXPERIENCE*

Residence and actual family size	Mean ideal family size of EW with child loss of:		
	0	1–2	3 and over
Old urban zone			
0–3	3.0	3.2	(4.5)
4–5	3.6	3.5	(2.0)
6 and over	3.6	3.6	(3.7)
All family sizes	3.2	3.4	(3.5)
Newly settled zone			
0–3	3.1	3.0	(3.3)
4–5	3.4	3.2	(1.8)
6 and over	3.4	3.2	(4.0)
All family sizes	3.2	3.2	3.4

* Figures in parentheses refer to fewer than 25 eligible women.

Total child loss and mean gravidity

The mean number of pregnancies per woman was shown to be directly related to the total child loss experience of the family (Table 7.A.3). This relation applied in both zones and for each age group of the eligible women. For the age group 40–44, by which time most women will have completed their reproductive span, the pattern was clearly established. In this age group, for example, women in the OUZ who had lost none of their children had had an average of 6.3 pregnancies, compared with 9.4 pregnancies for those who had lost 1 or 2 children and 10.8 pregnancies for those who had lost 3 or more children. The corresponding mean numbers of pregnancies for the NSZ were higher: 8.3, 11.2, and 12.7, respectively.

Total child loss and mean parity

The pattern for parity by age and zone of residence was similar to that found for gravidity (Table 7.4). In the age group 40–44, women in the OUZ

TABLE 7.A.3. MEAN NUMBER OF PREGNANCIES, BY RESIDENCE, TOTAL CHILD LOSS
EXPERIENCE, AND AGE OF ELIGIBLE WOMEN*

Residence and child loss	Mean number of pregnancies of EW aged:					
	15–19	20–24	25–29	30–34	35–39	40–44
Old urban zone						
0	0.5	1.2	2.2	3.6	5.1	6.3
1–2	—	(2.8)	4.1	5.7	7.8	9.4
3 and over	—	—	—	—	(13.2)	(10.8)
Newly settled zone						
0	0.8	1.7	3.3	5.0	6.9	8.3
1–2	(1.8)	(2.9)	5.4	7.2	9.5	11.2
3 and over	—	—	(8.0)	(9.2)	(12.6)	(12.7)

* Figures in parentheses refer to fewer than 25 eligible women.

TABLE 7.A.4. MEAN PARITY BY RESIDENCE, TOTAL CHILD LOSS EXPERIENCE, AND
AGE OF ELIGIBLE WOMEN*

Residence and child loss	Mean parity of EW aged:						All EW
	15–19	20–24	25–29	30–34	35–39	40–44	
Old urban zone							
0	0.4	1.1	1.9	3.0	4.1	4.9	2.8
1–2	—	(2.5)	3.6	5.0	6.4	7.8	6.2
3 and over	—	—	—	—	(11.2)	(9.7)	(10.3)
Newly settled zone							
0	0.7	1.5	2.8	4.2	5.7	6.6	3.7
1–2	(1.6)	(2.6)	4.5	6.2	7.9	9.0	7.0
3 and over	—	—	(7.0)	(8.8)	(10.2)	(10.5)	10.1

* Figures in parentheses refer to fewer than 25 eligible women.

without child loss experience had had an average of 4.9 live births, compared
with 7.8 for those who had lost 1 or 2 children and 9.7 for those who had lost
3 or more children. The corresponding mean numbers of live births, for the
NSZ were again higher: 6.6, 9.0, and 10.5, respectively.

Total child loss and mean family size

There was a positive association between family size and child loss
experience in both zones and in each age group (Table 7.A.5). It is noteworthy
that the family size achieved at the age of 40–44 years surpassed by more
than one child the ideal family size shown in Table 7.A.2.

306

TABLE 7.A.5. MEAN FAMILY SIZE, BY RESIDENCE, TOTAL CHILD LOSS EXPERIENCE, AND
AGE OF ELIGIBLE WOMEN*

Residence and child loss	Mean family size of EW aged:						All EW
	15–19	20–24	25–29	30–34	35–39	40–44	
Old urban zone							
0	0.4	1.1	1.9	3.0	4.1	4.9	2.8
1–2	—	(1.5)	2.6	3.8	5.2	6.7	5.0
3 and over	—	—	—	—	(5.6)	(6.1)	(5.9)
Newly settled zone							
0	0.7	1.5	2.8	4.2	5.7	6.6	3.7
1–2	(0.6)	(1.5)	3.4	5.0	6.7	7.8	5.8
3 and over	—	—	(4.0)	(5.3)	(6.8)	(7.0)	6.6

* Figures in parentheses refer to fewer than 25 eligible women.

Child Loss Among the First Three Live Births

The birth order of children lost is important in examining the relationship between child loss and family formation. High child loss can be either a determinant or a consequence of high fertility (measured by gravidity and parity). An attempt to isolate the impact of child loss is made here by restricting the analysis to child loss early in reproductive life. Family formation is thus examined here in relation to the loss of children under 5 years of age among the first 3 live births only, for each woman who had achieved this parity. Data relating to women who had fewer than 3 live births are therefore excluded from Tables 7.A.6 to 7.A.10. The same family formation variables, including mean ideal family size, mean gravidity, mean parity and mean family size, will now be examined in relation to this new criterion. In addition, contraceptive behaviour and subsequent birth interval will also be considered.

Child loss among the first three live births and mean ideal family size

When the data were confined to child loss experience among the first 3 live births (Table 7.A.6), little difference was found in the mean ideal family sizes preferred by women with different child loss experience.

TABLE 7.A.6. MEAN IDEAL FAMILY SIZE BY RESIDENCE AND CHILD LOSS AMONG THE
FIRST THREE LIVE BIRTHS*

Residence	Mean ideal family size of EW with child loss of:			No. of EW in sample
	0	1	2–3	
Old urban zone	3.6	3.4	3.6	1325
Newly settled zone	3.4	3.2	3.2	1697
Both zones	3.4	3.3	3.3	3022

* The data exclude women who had had fewer than 3 live births.

Child loss among the first three live births and mean gravidity

The mean gravidity specific for age was positively associated with child loss among the first 3 live births in both residential areas (Table 7.A.7). Within each residential area, the mean gravidity specific for age was higher among women who had lost at least one child than among those who had lost none. Women in the OUZ, aged 40–44 at the interview, who had had 0, 1, and 2–3 losses averaged 7.6, 8.8, and 10.0 pregnancies, respectively. The corresponding figures for women in the NSZ were 9.5, 10.7, and 9.2 pregnancies (Table 7.A.7(a)).

The results of t-tests run for the differences in mean gravidity at ages 40–44 in the two zones showed that the difference in the mean number of pregnancies for women who had lost one child and for those who had lost none was statistically significant in both areas at the 0.05 level (in the OUZ, $t = 2.31$ ($df = 341$), $P < 0.05$, and in the NSZ, $t = 2.49$ ($df = 344$), $P < 0.05$) (Table

TABLE 7.A.7. MEAN NUMBER OF PREGNANCIES AND CHILD LOSS AMONG FIRST THREE LIVE BIRTHS*

(a) By age of EW and residence

| Age of EW | Mean no. of pregnancies of EW in each residential area with child loss of: | | | | | | | |
| | Old urban zone | | | | Newly settled zone | | | |
	0	1	2–3	N[a]	0	1	2–3	N[a]
<20	—	—	—	—	(3.5)	—	—	2
20–24	(3.5)	(3.5)	—	23	3.7	(3.4)	(5.0)	78
25–29	4.0	(4.3)	(5.0)	178	4.8	5.0	(4.7)	350
30–34	4.8	5.6	(5.0)	364	6.1	6.5	(6.7)	480
35–39	6.1	7.5	(9.0)	413	7.8	9.5	(10.4)	435
40–44	7.6	8.8	(10.0)	347	9.5	10.7	(9.2)	352
All ages	5.8	7.1	(7.3)	1325	6.8	8.0	8.6	1697

* Figures in parentheses refer to fewer than 25 eligible women.
[a] N = total number of eligible women in the sample (excludes women with fewer than 3 live births).

(b) Statistical tests for the 40–44 age group

| | Significance of differences in mean gravidity between child loss categories of EW aged 40–44: | | | | | |
| | Old urban zone | | | Newly settled zone | | |
	0 versus 1	0 versus 2+3	1 versus 2+3	0 versus 1	0 versus 2+3	1 versus 2+3
t-values	2.31[a]	1.15	0.53	2.49[a]	0.21	1.03
df (degrees of freedom	341	295	52	344	273	81

[a] $P < 0.05$.

308

7.A.7(b)). The differences in the mean number of pregnancies for other categories of child loss experience at this age were not statistically significant (for 0 versus 2 + 3 losses and 1 versus 2 + 3 losses, $P > 0.10$). The differences in mean gravidity between women with no child loss experience among the first 3 live births and those with some child loss experience (1–3) was also statistically significant at the 0.05 level.

Child loss among the first three live births and mean parity

A positive association was also observed between mean parity and child loss among the first 3 live births. In general, mean parity was positively associated with child loss in both zones. In most cases, there was concomitant variation with the magnitude of child loss. In a few cases, mean parity for those who lost one child was somewhat higher than for those who lost none and those who lost 2–3.

Women at age 40–44 in the OUZ with 0, 1, and 2–3 child losses reported on the average 6.4, 7.4, and 8.0 live births. The corresponding figures for women in the NSZ were 8.0, 8.7, and 7.7 (Table 7.A.8(a)). The results of t-tests showed the difference in the mean parity for women who had lost one child and for women who had lost none to be statistically significant ($P < 0.05$, $t = 2.06$ ($df = 341$)). The difference in mean parity between those with no child loss experience and those with some child loss (1–3) among the first 3 live births was also significant at the 0.05 level. For other categories of child loss experience the differences were not statistically significant ($P > 0.10$) (Table 7.A.8(b)). The differences among child loss categories in the NSZ were also not significant at the 0.05 level.

Child loss among the first three live births and mean family size

The association between family size and child loss among the first 3 live births was generally negative. There were a few exceptions in the OUZ, while in the NSZ, mean family size declined fairly consistently with increases in child loss. At age 40–44 in the NSZ, the mean family sizes were 7.7, 7.0, and 5.2 for women with 0, 1, and 2.3 losses, respectively. In the OUZ, the negative association was present in most age groups. At age 40–44, however, the difference was very small, with means of 6.2, 5.9, and 6.0 for women with 0, 1, and 2–3 losses, respectively (Tables 7.A.9(a) and (b)). The results of t-tests confirmed these findings and indicated that the observed differences were not statistically significant.

Approval and ever-use of birth control in relation to child loss among the first three live births

Rates of approval and ever-use of birth control, shown in Table 7.A.10, were extremely high in both zones. At least 4 of every 5 women claimed to have used birth control. It should be remembered, however, that these women were all of high parity and had had at least 3 live births. Both approval and use

TABLE 7.A.8. MEAN PARITY AND CHILD LOSS AMONG FIRST THREE LIVE BIRTHS*

(a) By age of EW and residence

| | Mean parity of EW in each residential area with child loss of: | | | | | | | |
| | Old urban zone | | | | Newly settled zone | | | |
Age of EW	0	1	2–3	N[a]	0	1	2–3	N[a]
<20	—	—	—	—	(3.0)	—	—	2
20–24	(3.2)	(3.2)	—	23	3.4	(3.4)	(4.0)	78
25–29	3.6	(3.8)	(5.0)	178	4.2	4.1	(4.3)	350
30–34	4.2	5.1	(4.6)	364	5.4	5.7	(6.2)	480
35–39	5.2	6.6	(5.0)	413	6.7	7.9	(8.6)	435
40–44	6.4	7.4	(8.0)	347	8.0	8.7	(7.7)	352
All ages	5.0	6.1	(5.8)	1325	5.9	6.7	7.3	1697

* Figures in parentheses refer to fewer than 25 eligible women.
[a] N = total number of eligible women in sample (excludes women with fewer than 3 live births).

(b) Statistical tests for the 40–44 age group

| | Significance of differences in mean parity between child loss categories of EW aged 40–44: | | | | | |
| | Old urban zone | | | Newly settled zone | | |
	0 versus 1	0 versus 2+3	1 versus 2+3	0 versus 1	0 versus 2+3	1 versus 2+3
t-values	2.06[a]	1.17	0.45	1.56	0.26	0.71
df (degrees of freedom)	341	295	52	344	273	81

[a] $P < 0.05$.

of birth control were negatively associated with child loss. This could mean that a woman who had lost one or more of her first 3 live-born children was more likely to desire other pregnancies and less likely to express approval of birth control.

Child Loss and Subsequent Birth Interval

The interval that follows a live birth, especially when it occurs early in the reproductive span, is assumed to be longer than that following the death of a child. This difference exists because of a biological mechanism (post-partum amenorrhoea, which may be prolonged by lactation) and/or absence of replacement motivation. It must be emphasized that the present data came from a lactating community and that biological mechanisms may have been involved, at least partly, in prolonging the interval after a live-born child who was breast fed.

310

TABLE 7.A.9. MEAN FAMILY SIZE AND CHILD LOSS AMONG FIRST THREE LIVE BIRTHS*

(a) By age of EW and residence

| | Mean family size of EW in each residential area with child loss of: | | | | | | | |
| Age of EW | Old urban zone | | | | Newly settled zone | | | |
	0	1	2–3	N[a]	0	1	2–3	N[a]
<20	—	—	—	—	(3.0)	—	—	2
20–24	(3.2)	(2.2)	—	23	3.4	(2.4)	(2.0)	78
25–29	3.6	(2.8)	(3.0)	178	4.2	3.1	(2.0)	350
30–34	4.1	4.0	(2.6)	364	5.3	4.5	(3.7)	480
35–39	5.1	5.2	(3.0)	413	6.5	6.5	(6.1)	435
40–44	6.2	5.9	(6.0)	347	7.7	7.0	(5.2)	352
All ages	4.9	4.8	(3.8)	1325	5.8	5.3	4.9	1697

* Figures in parentheses refer to fewer than 25 eligible women.
[a] N = total number of eligible women in sample (excludes women with fewer than 3 live births).

(b) Statistical tests for the 40–44 age group

| | Significance of differences in mean family size between child loss categories of EW aged 40–44. | | | | | |
| | Old urban zone | | | Newly settled zone | | |
	0 versus 1	0 versus 2 + 3	1 versus 2 + 3	0 versus 1	0 versus 2 + 3	1 versus 2 + 3
t-values	0.68	0.17	0.04	1.79	1.67	1.19
df (degrees of freedom)	341	295	52	344	273	81

TABLE 7.A.10. APPROVAL AND EVER-USE OF BIRTH CONTROL BY RESIDENCE AND CHILD LOSS AMONG FIRST THREE LIVE BIRTHS

| Residence | Percentage approval of birth control among EW with child loss of: | | | Percentage ever-use of birth control among EW with child loss of: | | | Total no. of EW in sample[a] |
	0	1	2 & 3	0	1	2 & 3	
Old urban zone	96.6	94.6	91.7	93.2	94.0	91.7	1270/1230
Newly settled zone	94.1	92.4	83.3	88.6	81.9	80.0	1589/1482

[a] First figure refers to approval of birth control, second figure to ever-use of birth control; both figures exclude women with fewer than 3 live births.

In the present data, the interval between the end of two successive pregnancies was calculated both for a live-born child who had survived the first year and for one who had died in infancy (during the first year). The results are presented in Table 7.A.11.

TABLE 7.A.11. MEAN SUBSEQUENT BIRTH INTERVAL BY RESIDENCE, CHILD SURVIVAL, AND BIRTH ORDER

Residence and child survival	Mean subsequent birth interval (months) for birth order:							Reported no. live births
	1	2	3	4	5	6 and over	All birth orders	
Old urban zone (both sexes)								
Child alive at age 1	21.8	25.9	27.4	26.7	27.0	27.1	25.2	5988
Child died at age < 1	17.5	19.6	24.0	15.3	16.9	20.1	19.1	213
Newly settled zone (both sexes)								
Child alive at age 1	18.9	21.0	21.7	22.1	22.6	21.6	21.1	8783
Child died at age < 1	16.3	17.5	17.3	21.4	18.4	18.3	18.1	425

The average interval between the birth of a child who survived the first year of life and the end of the subsequent pregnancy was about 25 months in the OUZ and about 21 months in the NSZ. When the child died during the first year, the interval was shortened by about 6 months in the OUZ and 3 months in the NSZ. Although no clear pattern was seen in either area in relation to birth order, for all birth orders the interval succeeding a live birth was longer than the interval for a child who died in infancy.

B. EGYPT

A. F. El-Sherbini, A. F. Moustafa, H. M. Hammam, F. S. Hassanein & A. R. Omran

Total Child Loss and Family Formation

Table 7.B.1 shows that there was a high level of child loss among the 3 groups of eligible women. Of the total of 4861 women, 46.2% had lost 1 or more of their live-born children: 29.7% had lost 1–2 children, and 16.5% had lost 3 or more. Total child loss was high in the 3 areas; the highest percentage was 51.7% in the rural area, followed by 45.1% in the urban area, and 30.8% in the industrial area. The percentage of women who had had 3 or more child losses was about half that of those who had had 1–2 losses in the rural and urban areas, while the ratio dropped to about one-fourth in the industrial area. The better social and medical services in the industrial area were definitely partly responsible for this difference.

312

TABLE 7.B.1. DISTRIBUTION OF ELIGIBLE WOMEN BY RESIDENCE AND CHILD LOSS EXPERIENCE

Residence	Percentage of EW with child loss of:			Unknown	Total no. of EW interviewed
	0	1–2	3 and over		
Rural	29.2	31.8	19.9	19.1	2145
Urban	33.0	29.0	16.1	21.9	2097
Industrial	40.3	25.0	5.8	28.9	619

Total child loss and mean ideal family size

Of the 4861 women, only 44.2% gave a numerical reply to the question about ideal family size. A high percentage gave nonspecific answers, such as "Up to God" or "I do not know". It is evident, therefore, that many of the women had no clear concept of ideal family size that would be reflected in actual family size.

Table 7.B.2 shows that the reported mean ideal family size was directly associated with actual family size, whether the mother had lost a child or not. This was true in all three residential areas. While the mean ideal family size was lower for women who had not lost any children, there was no direct association between ideal family size and number of child deaths. In the urban area, the mean ideal family size for mothers who had lost 1–2 children was 4.2,

TABLE 7.B.2. MEAN IDEAL FAMILY SIZE BY RESIDENCE, ACTUAL FAMILY SIZE, AND TOTAL CHILD LOSS EXPERIENCE*

Residence and actual family size	Mean ideal family size of EW with child loss of:			Total no. of EW interviewed
	0	1–2	3 and over	
Rural				
0–3	3.3	3.5	3.1	213
4–5	4.4	4.5	4.9	137
6 and over	5.5	5.7	(5.6)	83
All family sizes	3.9	4.2	4.2	433
Urban				
0–3	3.1	3.2	2.9	317
4–5	3.8	4.0	4.2	184
6 and over	5.1	4.6	4.9	138
All family sizes	3.6	4.2	4.1	639
Industrial				
0–3	3.0	3.4	(3.5)	63
4–5	3.8	3.6	(3.9)	104
6 and over	4.0	4.0	(3.9)	160
All family sizes	3.7	3.8	3.9	327

* Figures in parentheses refer to fewer than 25 eligible women.

compared with 4.1 for mothers who had lost 3 or more children and 3.6 for mothers with no child losses. In the rural area, the mean ideal family size was 4.2 both for women who had lost 1–2 children and for those who had lost 3 or more children. Women in the industrial area were the only group who showed a slight increase in mean ideal family size with an increase in the number of children lost. The mean was 3.7 for mothers with no child loss, 3.8 for those with 1–2 child losses, and 3.9 for mothers with 3 or more losses. Therefore, it can be concluded that the mean ideal family size was relatively higher among women with child losses as opposed to those without losses, but that an increase in child loss was not associated with a further increase in family size.

Total child loss and mean gravidity

Table 7.B.3 shows that mean gravidity was directly related to child loss. This relationship was observed within each age group in all 3 residential areas. Women with no child losses had a mean of 5.6 pregnancies in the rural and urban areas, and 6.4 in the industrial area. The comparable figures for women with 1–2 child losses were 6.5, 6.9, and 7.4, respectively; mean gravidity for women with 3 or more losses was 8.9 for the rural and 10.0 for both the urban and the industrial areas.

TABLE 7.B.3. MEAN NUMBER OF PREGNANCIES BY RESIDENCE, TOTAL CHILD LOSS EXPERIENCE, AND AGE OF ELIGIBLE WOMEN*

Residence and child loss	Mean number of pregnancies of EW aged:							Total no. of EW interviewed
	15–19	20–24	25–29	30–34	35–39	40–44	All EW	
Rural								
0	3.3	4.0	4.3	5.7	7.1	7.5	5.6	425
1–2	5.0	4.3	5.2	6.5	7.9	8.6	6.5	620
3 and over	6.5	(5.0)	6.7	8.7	9.2	10.9	8.9	417
Urban								
0	(3.0)	3.6	4.6	5.9	7.3	8.1	5.6	469
1–2	4.2	4.4	5.3	6.5	8.2	9.4	6.9	561
3 and over	—	(5.1)	(6.7)	8.4	10.3	11.4	10.0	337
Industrial								
0	—	(3.4)	4.2	5.6	6.9	8.7	6.4	188
1–2	—	(3.1)	(4.1)	(6.4)	8.0	9.6	7.4	140
3 and over	—	—	—	(7.5)	(9.8)	(11.1)	10.0	34

* Figures in parentheses refer to fewer than 25 eligible women.

Urban women had the highest mean gravidity in most of the specified age groups. At age 40–44 years, which is close to the end of the reproductive period, the highest mean gravidity for women with 3 or more losses was 11.4 in the urban area, 11.1 in the industrial area, and 10.9 in the rural area.

Total child loss and mean parity

Table 7.B.4 shows that mean parity had a direct relationship with the number of child losses in all 3 residential areas and in most age groups. This

TABLE 7.B.4. MEAN PARITY BY RESIDENCE, SOCIAL STATUS, TOTAL CHILD LOSS
EXPERIENCE, AND AGE OF ELIGIBLE WOMEN*

Residence, social status, and child loss	Mean parity of EW aged:							Total no. of EW interviewed
	15–19	20–24	25–29	30–34	35–39	40–44	All EW	
RURAL								
Middle								
0	(3.0)	3.7	4.1	4.7	6.1	7.0	4.9	332
1–2	(5.2)	3.9	4.8	5.9	7.2	7.9	5.9	520
3 and over	(6.5)	(4.4)	6.3	7.8	8.4	9.6	8.2	360
Low								
0	—	(3.5)	3.9	(5.3)	6.9	(7.2)	5.4	89
1–2	(4.0)	(4.5)	(4.6)	6.2	(7.0)	(7.9)	6.3	99
3 and over	—	(4.5)	(5.5)	(6.9)	(7.5)	(9.5)	7.2	57
Both categories								
0	(3.0)	3.7	4.8	4.7	6.3	7.1	5.0	421
1–2	(5.0)	3.9	4.8	6.0	7.1	7.9	5.8	619
3 and over	(6.5)	4.4	6.1	7.7	8.2	9.5	8.1	417
URBAN								
Middle								
0	(3.0)	3.3	4.1	4.9	6.3	6.9	4.8	440
1–2	(3.6)	4.1	4.7	5.9	7.1	8.2	6.1	512
3 and over	—	(4.4)	(5.6)	(7.3)	9.4	10.5	9.0	307
Low								
0	—	(3.0)	(3.9)	(5.8)	(6.7)	(7.7)	5.3	26
1–2	—	(4.0)	(3.7)	(5.8)	(8.2)	(8.6)	6.8	52
3 and over	—	—	(6.0)	(8.6)	(8.8)	(10.1)	9.3	30
Both categories								
0	(3.0)	3.3	4.0	5.0	6.4	7.0	5.0	466
1–2	(3.6)	4.1	4.4	5.8	7.1	8.2	6.3	564
3 and over		(4.4)	5.0	7.4	0.0	10.1	0.0	007
INDUSTRIAL								
Middle								
0	—	(3.2)	4.0	5.0	6.0	8.4	5.7	144
1–2	—	(3.2)	(4.1)	(5.9)	7.4	8.7	6.8	122
3 and over	—	—	—	(7.3)	(9.5)	(10.1)	6.0	34
Low								
0	—	(4.0)	(5.5)	(5.8)	(7.5)	(7.8)	7.8	34
1–2	—	(3.0)	(4.0)	(7.0)	(7.3)	(8.2)	6.8	22
3 and over	—	—	—	—	(9.0)	—	(9.0)	2
Both categories								
0	—	3.3	4.2	5.1	6.2	8.2	6.7	178
1–2	—	(3.2)	(4.1)	(6.0)	7.4	(8.6)	6.8	144
3 and over	—	—	—	(7.3)	(9.5)	(10.1)	6.2	36

* Figures in parentheses refer to fewer than 25 eligible women.

picture was similar to the pattern shown by mean gravidity and child loss. The total mean parity was generally higher among women of low social status than among those of middle status.

At age 40–44 years, women with 3 or more child losses had a mean parity of 10.4 in the urban area, 10.1 in the industrial area, and 9.5 in the rural area (Table 7.B.4).

Total child loss and mean family size

Table 7.B.5 shows that among urban women mean family size increased with an increase in the number of child losses. Women with no child losses had a mean family size of 4.6, compared with 4.7 for women who had lost 1–2 children, and 5.0 for women with 3 or more losses. The corresponding means for industrial women were 5.5 both for those with no child loss and for those who had lost 1–2 children, and 6.6 for those with 3 or more losses. On the other hand, in the rural area the total mean family size decreased with an increase in the number of children lost: 4.8 for women with no child loss and 4.2 both for women with 1–2 losses and for those with 3 or more losses. However, in each of the areas when age group was held constant a decrease in mean family size with increase in child loss was observed.

By age 40–44 years, women who had lost children must have tried to replace them to achieve the family size attained by women with no child losses. In the rural area, the mean family size for all women in this age group was high (6.0 for both women with no child loss and women with 1–2 child losses, decreasing to 5.3 for women with 3 or more child losses). The degree of compensation of child loss was higher among women with 1–2 child losses than among women who had lost 3 or more children, as shown by the figures. The same pattern was observed in the urban and industrial groups; while the women who had lost 1–2 children could make up for the loss, those with a loss of 3 or more children were unable to do so.

The mean family sizes were generally higher than the mean ideal family size reported by the eligible women, except in the case of rural women with some child loss who had attained, on the average, just their ideal family size (Table 7.B.2).

Child Loss among the First Three Live Births

Tables 7.B.6, 7.B.8, and 7.B.9 exclude the influence of higher parity on child loss, in order to give information on family formation in relation to loss of children under 5 years of age among the first 3 live births. The data relating to women who had had fewer than 3 live births are excluded from these tables.

Child loss among the first three live births and mean ideal family size

Table 7.B.6 shows that rural women expressed a higher mean ideal family size than women in the urban and industrial areas. Child loss had no striking effect on mean ideal family size except among rural families where an increase

316

TABLE 7.B.5. MEAN FAMILY SIZE BY RESIDENCE, SOCIAL STATUS, TOTAL CHILD LOSS
EXPERIENCE, AND AGE OF ELIGIBLE WOMEN*

Residence, social status, and child loss	Mean family size of EW aged:							Total no. of EW interviewed
	15–19	20–24	25–29	30–34	35–39	40–44	All EW	
RURAL								
Middle								
0	(3.0)	3.6	3.9	4.4	5.5	5.8	4.6	299
1–2	(4.0)	2.5	3.1	4.1	5.4	6.0	4.1	518
3 and over	(3.0)	(2.1)	2.9	3.8	4.5	5.3	4.2	357
Low								
0	—	(3.2)	(3.6)	(4.7)	(5.2)	(6.4)	5.4	82
1–2	(3.0)	(2.5)	(3.1)	4.0	(4.8)	(6.0)	4.4	98
3 and over	—	(2.0)	(2.3)	(3.9)	(4.1)	(5.3)	3.6	57
Both categories								
0	(3.0)	3.6	3.8	4.5	5.4	6.0	4.8	381
1–2	(3.8)	2.5	3.1	4.1	5.3	6.0	4.2	616
3 and over	(3.0)	2.1	2.7	3.8	4.3	5.3	4.2	414
URBAN								
Middle								
0	(3.0)	3.3	3.9	4.4	5.8	6.5	4.6	416
1–2	(2.6)	2.6	3.3	4.2	5.4	6.5	4.5	511
3 and over	—	(1.7)	(2.6)	3.8	5.1	5.8	4.9	307
Low								
0	—	(3.0)	(3.4)	(5.1)	(6.3)	(7.3)	5.2	25
1–2	—	(2.0)	(2.6)	(4.1)	(6.9)	(6.9)	5.3	52
3 and over	—	—	(3.0)	(4.4)	(4.7)	(5.9)	5.2	30
Both categories								
0	(3.0)	3.3	3.9	4.4	5.9	6.5	4.6	441
1–2	(2.6)	2.6	3.3	4.2	5.5	6.6	4.7	563
3 and over	—	(1.7)	(2.6)	3.8	5.1	5.8	5.0	337
INDUSTRIAL								
Middle								
0	—	(3.1)	3.8	4.8	5.9	7.3	5.3	141
1–2	—	(2.0)	(2.0)	(4.9)	6.0	7.2	5.5	120
3 and over	—	—	—	(4.2)	(6.1)	(6.5)	6.6	33
Low								
0	—	(3.0)	(4.5)	(5.5)	(6.8)	(6.4)	6.1	33
1–2	—	(2.0)	(3.0)	(6.5)	(6.9)	(6.8)	5.7	22
3 and over	—	—	—	—	(12.0)	—	6.0	2
Both categories								
0	—	3.1	3.8	5.0	6.1	7.1	5.5	174
1–2	—	(2.0)	(2.9)	5.0	6.5	7.1	5.5	142
3 and over	—	—	—	(4.2)	(6.1)	(6.5)	6.6	35

* Figures in parentheses refer to fewer than 25 eligible women.

occurred from 3.8 for women with no child loss to 4.0 for 1 loss and 4.2 for 2–3 losses among the first 3 live births. In the urban area, the mean ideal family size was the same (3.7) for women with or without child loss.

TABLE 7.B.6. MEAN IDEAL FAMILY SIZE BY RESIDENCE AND CHILD LOSS AMONG THE FIRST THREE LIVE BIRTHS

| Residence | Mean ideal family size of EW with child loss of: | | | No. of EW in sample[a] |
	0	1	2–3	
Rural	3.8	4.0	4.2	457
Urban	3.7	3.7	3.7	648
Industrial	3.6	3.5	(3.8)[b]	323

[a] Excludes women with fewer than 3 live births.
[b] Refers to fewer than 25 eligible women.

Child loss among the first three live births and mean gravidity

Table 7.B.7 shows that there was a systematic difference in mean gravidity between rural and urban women. Mean gravidity was higher among rural women up to the age of 35 years, after which the balance changed in favour of the urban group for all 3 categories of child loss.

As expected, mean gravidity increased with age and no exception was observed to his pattern. Mean gravidity also increased with increasing child loss in all 3 residential areas. The mean gravidity specific for age was generally highest among women who had lost 2–3 children, followed by those who had lost 1 child and then those with no child losses.

Child loss among the first three live births and mean parity

Table 7.B.8 shows that there was a direct relationship between mean parity and child loss in the different age groups in all 3 residential areas. In the age group 20–34 years, the mean parity of urban women was generally lower than that of rural women, while in higher age groups (35–44 years) urban women had a higher mean parity than rural women.

As expected, mean parity in the rural and urban areas increased with age for the 3 categories of child loss among the first 3 live births. This is an indication that the women wanted to compensate for child losses by replacing them with live births, thus leading to a high mean parity. In the case of women with no child loss, giving birth to more children than the "wanted" number may be considered an insurance against the threat of child death. It is worth mentioning that mean parity was high among women aged 40–44 without child loss: 8.0, 8.3, and 8.4 in the rural, urban, and industrial areas, respectively. The compensatory reaction was more evident among the urban than among the rural group; among urban women in the 40–44 age group women with no child loss, 1 child loss, and 2–3 child losses had mean parities of 8.3, 9.6, and

318

Age of EW	Rural				Urban				Industrial			
	0	1	2–3	N^a	0	1	2–3	N^a	0	1	2–3	N^a
<20	(5.7)	(3.8)	(6.0)	12	(4.2)	(3.3)	(4.7)	7				
20–24	4.1	4.2	4.9	135	3.7	4.4	5.3	124	(3.4)	(3.2)	(3.0)	25
25–29	5.0	5.3	5.7	354	4.8	5.3	8.0	302	4.2	3.8	4.2	55
30–34	6.7	7.4	7.3	364	6.3	6.6	9.6	335	5.7	6.8	5.0	65
35–39	7.9	8.2	8.6	353	7.9	9.1	9.6	328	7.7	7.9	10.9	117
40–44	8.8	9.3	10.1	241	9.3	10.8	10.5	269	9.1	10.0	8.8	96
All ages	6.6	7.2	7.7	1459	6.4	7.8	8.5	1365	6.8	7.5	7.6	358

* Figures in parentheses refer to fewer than 25 eligible women.
[a] N = total number of women in sample (excludes women with fewer than 3 live births).

TABLE 7.B.8. MEAN PARITY AND CHILD LOSS AMONG THE FIRST THREE LIVE BIRTHS, BY AGE OF ELIGIBLE WOMEN AND RESIDENCE*

	Mean parity of EW in each area with child loss of:											
	Rural				Urban				Industrial			
Age of EW	0	1	2–3	N^a	0	1	2–3	N^a	0	1	2–3	N^a
<20	(6.0)	(4.0)	(6.0)	10	(3.5)	(3.3)	—	7	—	—	—	—
20–24	3.7	3.8	4.6	135	3.4	4.0	(4.2)	125	(3.3)	(3.2)	(3.0)	21
25–29	4.6	4.9	5.5	354	4.3	4.5	5.1	303	4.1	3.7	4.2	56
30–34	6.3	6.5	6.7	364	5.4	5.9	7.4	335	5.4	6.3	5.0	65
35–39	7.0	7.6	7.9	353	7.1	8.1	8.7	328	7.0	7.9	9.1	119
40–44	8.0	8.6	9.4	241	8.3	9.6	9.7	269	8.4	9.0	8.6	96
All ages	5.9	6.5	7.1	1457	5.7	6.9	7.8	1367	6.4	7.0	7.0	357

* Figures in parentheses refer to fewer than 25 eligible women.
^{a} N = total number of women in sample (excludes women with fewer than 3 live births).

TABLE 7.B.9. MEAN FAMILY SIZE AND CHILD LOSS AMONG THE FIRST THREE LIVE BIRTHS, BY AGE OF ELIGIBLE WOMEN AND RESIDENCE*

Mean family size in each area with child loss of:

Age of EW	Rural				Urban				Industrial			
	0	1	2–3	N^a	0	1	2–3	N^a	0	1	2–3	N^a
<20	(4.3)	(2.5)	(2.0)	11	(2.8)	(2.3)	—	7	—	—	—	—
20–24	3.0	2.4	2.2	133	3.1	2.7	(1.8)	124	(3.1)	(2.0)	(1.5)	19
25–29	3.5	2.9	2.8	354	3.8	3.2	2.8	303	3.8	2.7	2.8	56
30–34	4.5	3.9	2.9	363	4.5	3.9	3.8	335	5.1	5.0	2.0	63
35–39	5.3	4.8	4.5	353	5.9	5.3	4.7	328	6.2	5.7	6.4	118
40–44	6.0	5.7	5.0	241	6.7	6.4	4.9	269	7.3	6.7	5.3	95
All ages	4.5	4.3	3.7	1455	4.7	4.6	4.0	1366	5.7	5.3	4.8	351

*Figures in parentheses refer to fewer than 25 eligible women.
[a] N = number of women in sample (excludes women with fewer than 3 live births).

9.7, respectively. The corresponding figures for rural women were 8.0, 8.6, and 9.4.

Child loss among the first three live births and mean family size

Table 7.B.9 shows that mean family size bore an inverse relationship to child loss among the first 3 live births, in contrast to the direct relationship between ideal family size and child loss (Table 7.B.6). This inverse relationship was present in all the specified age groups among women in the 3 residential areas.

Taking all age groups into consideration, rural women had 4.5, 4.3, and 3.7 living children in families with no child loss, 1 loss, and 2–3 losses, respectively, among the first 3 live births. The corresponding figures for urban women were 4.7, 4.6, and 4.0, and for women in the industrial area, 5.7, 5.3, and 4.8. When these mean actual family sizes are compared with the mean ideal family sizes (Table 7.B.6), it is found that women in all 3 residential areas (whether they had child losses or not) exceeded their desired ideal family size, except for the group of rural women with 2–3 losses who had a lower mean family size (3.7) than the mean ideal size (4.2). The excess of actual family size over the ideal family size was greatest among the industrial area women.

C. PAKISTAN

Batul Raza & A. R. Omran

Total Child Loss and Family Formation

Table 7.C.1 gives the distribution of eligible women in the two study areas according to their total child loss. In the semi-urban areas, every third woman (34.2%) had experienced a loss of one or more of her live-born children, whereas in the urban area every fifth woman (21.4%) had experienced such a loss. Of the total women interviewed (4861), 27.6% had lost one or more of their live-born children; of these, 22.3% had lost 1 or 2 children while 5.3% had lost 3 or more of their children.

TABLE 7.C.1. DISTRIBUTION OF ELIGIBLE WOMEN BY RESIDENCE AND CHILD LOSS EXPERIENCE

Residence	Percentage of EW with child loss of:			Total no. of EW interviewed
	0	1 & 2	3 and over	
Semi–urban	65.8	26.0	8.2	2388
Urban	78.6	18.8	2.6	2473
Both areas	72.3	22.3	5.3	4861

The findings further indicate that the child loss experience had been consistently higher among semi-urban than among urban women. In the semi-urban area, 26% of the women had had 1 or 2 child losses and 8.2% had had 3 or more child losses, whereas in the urban area 18.8% of the women had had 1 or 2 child losses and 2.6% had had 3 or more losses.

Total child loss and mean ideal family size

Table 7.C.2 shows the total child loss experience and mean ideal family size. The reported mean ideal family size ranged between 3.3 and 4.2. No difference in ideal family size was observed between semi-urban and urban women. The figures were low in both areas compared with those reported for Muslim women in some other countries.[1]

TABLE 7.C.2. MEAN IDEAL FAMILY SIZE BY RESIDENCE, ACTUAL FAMILY SIZE, AND TOTAL CHILD LOSS EXPERIENCE*

Residence and actual family size	Mean ideal family size of EW with child loss of:		
	0	1–2	3 or more
Semi-urban			
0–3	3.5	3.5	4.1
4–5	4.0	4.1	3.9
6 or more	4.2	4.2	4.2
All family sizes	3.8	3.9	4.1
Urban			
0–3	3.3	3.6	(3.6)
4–5	3.8	3.9	(4.2)
6 or more	4.2	4.2	(4.2)
All family sizes	3.6	3.9	4.1

* Figures in parentheses refer to fewer than 25 eligible women.

The findings also showed that the mean ideal family size increased slightly with the degree of child loss. Women with no child loss preferred 3.8 and 3.6 children in semi-urban and urban areas, respectively. Women with 1 or 2 child losses preferred to have 3.9 children, whereas women who had lost 3 or more children preferred 4.1 children in both areas.

The association between achieved family size and ideal family size is direct, with the group having an actual family size of 6 or more having the highest ideal family size in both areas. It is important to note, however, that women with 6 or more children preferred about the same ideal family size (4.2) regardless of child loss.

[1] OMRAN, A. R. & STANDLEY, C. C. *Family formation patterns and health*, Geneva, World Health Organization, 1976.

Total child loss and mean gravidity

In both study areas, mean gravidity was directly associated with total child loss. This trend was also observed for each age group of the eligible women (Table 7.C.3).

TABLE 7.C.3. MEAN NUMBER OF PREGNANCIES, BY RESIDENCE, TOTAL CHILD LOSS EXPERIENCE AND AGE OF ELIGIBLE WOMEN*

Residence and child loss	Mean number of pregnancies of EW aged:						All EW
	15–19	20–24	25–29	30–34	35–39	40–44	
Semi-urban							
0	0.8	2.0	4.1	5.8	6.6	7.2	4.6
1–2	(1.3)	3.2	5.6	7.3	8.4	8.7	7.3
3 or more	—	(6.5)	(7.7)	8.9	11.0	10.2	9.9
Urban							
0	0.8	1.8	3.2	4.9	5.8	6.9	4.0
1–2	(2.0)	(2.4)	4.9	6.9	7.9	8.7	7.2
3 or more	—	—	(7.5)	(9.2)	(9.5)	9.9	9.7

* Figures in parentheses refer to fewer than 25 eligible women.

Women with no child loss had experienced, on the average, 4.6 pregnancies in the semi-urban area and 4.0 pregnancies in the urban area. This can be compared with 7.3 and 7.2 pregnancies for those women who had experienced 1 or 2 child losses, respectively, up to the time of the survey. The corresponding pregnancies for women with 3 or more losses were 9.9 for the semi-urban area and 9.7 for the urban area.

By age 40–44 years, which is close to the end of the reproductive age span, the pattern was also well established. The mean numbers of pregnancies for women in this age group were 7.2, 8.7, and 10.2 for 0, 1–2, and 3 or more child loss, respectively, in the semi-urban area. In the urban area the corresponding mean numbers of pregnancies were 6.9, 8.7, and 9.9.

Total child loss and mean parity

Table 7.C.4 indicates that in the semi-urban area those women who had experienced no child loss ended up with 3.8 live births up to the time of the survey. The figures were 6.1 live births for women who had lost fewer than 2 children and 8.8 live births for those with 3 or more child losses. This indicates that, like mean gravidity, mean parity is also directly associated with total child loss. The same trend was noted for the urban area. A similar pattern was also observed for each age group and was well established for the age group 40–44.

324

TABLE 7.C.4. MEAN PARITY BY RESIDENCE, TOTAL CHILD LOSS EXPERIENCE, AND AGE OF ELIGIBLE WOMEN*

Residence and child loss	Mean parity of EW aged:						
	15–19	20–24	25–29	30–34	35–39	40–44	All EW
Semi-urban							
0	0.7	1.7	3.5	5.1	5.3	6.1	3.8
1–2	(1.3)	2.7	4.8	6.3	7.3	7.3	6.1
3 or more	—	(6.0)	(6.9)	8.4	9.3	9.1	8.8
Urban							
0	0.5	1.6	2.8	4.2	4.9	5.8	3.4
1–2	(2.0)	(2.3)	4.3	5.8	5.8	7.6	6.1
3 or more	—	—	(6.7)	(8.9)	(8.6)	8.7	8.6

* Figures in parentheses refer to fewer than 25 eligible women.

Total child loss and mean family size

With increasing child loss experience, an increase in mean family size specific for age was generally observed within each study area and social status group (Table 7.C.5). The achieved family size at age 40–44 years was greater than the ideal family size reported in Table 7.C.2.

In the age group 40–44 in the urban area, women who had lost children had been successful in replacing the dead children and had achieved the family size of those who had experienced no child loss. This group had a mean family size of 5.8 in the case of no child loss and 5.3 with a loss of 3 or more children. However, in the semi-urban area, the compensation had not been as great. The mean family size for no child loss was 6.0 as compared with 5.0 for the group experiencing losses of 3 or more children.

Child Loss among the First Three Live Births

The correlation between total child loss and fertility discussed above can be due either to the impact of high fertility on child loss or to the effect of child loss on fertility. To differentiate these two effects, analysis was restricted to child loss in the early reproductive span (i.e., among the first 3 live births). The data presented in subsequent tables give information on family formation in relation to the loss of children under 5 among the first 3 live births for women who had achieved this parity.

Child loss among the first three live births and mean ideal family size

Table 7.C.6 indicates that in both study areas the mean ideal family size showed only a small increase with increasing child losses among the first 3 live births. The table does not show any considerable difference between the semi-urban and urban areas.

325

TABLE 7.C.5. MEAN FAMILY SIZE BY RESIDENCE, SOCIAL STATUS, TOTAL CHILD LOSS
EXPERIENCE, AND AGE OF ELIGIBLE WOMEN*

Residence, social status, and child loss	Mean family size of EW aged:							No. of EW in sample
	15–19	20–24	25–29	30–34	35–39	40–44	All EW	
SEMI-URBAN								
Middle								
0	0.7	1.6	3.3	4.7	5.0	5.7	3.4	851
1–2	(0.7)	1.3	3.5	4.7	5.6	5.6	3.4	370
3 or more	—	(2.0)	(3.4)	(4.0)	(5.4)	4.6	4.5	68
Low								
0	0.7	1.9	3.7	5.3	5.6	6.3	4.2	772
1–2	(0.0)	1.9	3.7	5.1	6.2	6.1	5.0	350
3 or more	—	(1.0)	(3.4)	5.0	5.5	5.2	5.0	127
All semi-urban								
0	0.7	1.7	3.5	5.0	5.3	6.0	3.8	1573
1–2	(0.3)	1.6	3.6	5.0	6.0	5.8	4.8	620
3 or more	—	(1.5)	(3.4)	4.7	5.5	5.0	4.9	195
URBAN								
Middle								
0	0.5	1.5	2.7	4.1	4.8	5.7	3.3	1823
1–2	(1.0)	(1.2)	3.1	4.5	5.4	6.2	4.8	417
3 or more	—	—	(3.7)	(4.6)	5.2	5.2	5.1	54
Low								
0	(1.0)	2.2	3.9	5.7	(6.4)	(6.1)	4.4	122
1–2	—	(0.0)	(3.6)	(5.6)	(6.9)	(7.1)	5.9	47
3 or more	—	—	—	(7.0)	(5.7)	(5.7)	(5.7)	10
All urban								
0	0.5	1.6	2.8	4.2	4.9	5.8	3.4	1945
1–2	(1.0)	(1.2)	3.1	4.7	5.5	6.3	4.9	464
3 or more	—	—	(3.7)	(5.3)	(5.2)	5.3	5.2	64

* Figures in parentheses refer to fewer than 25 eligible women.

TABLE 7.C.6. MEAN IDEAL FAMILY SIZE BY RESIDENCE AND CHILD LOSS AMONG
THE FIRST THREE LIVE BIRTHS

Residence	Mean ideal family size of EW with child loss of:			No. of EW in sample[a]
	0	1	2–3	
Semi-urban	4.03	3.98	4.03	1373
Urban	3.87	3.86	4.12	1422
Both areas	3.94	3.93	4.05	2795

[a] Excludes women with fewer than 3 live births.

Child loss among the first three live births and mean gravidity

Table 7.C.7(a) shows that the mean age-specific gravidity was directly related to child loss in both urban and semi-urban women.

TABLE 7.C.7. MEAN NUMBER OF PREGNANCIES AND CHILD LOSS AMONG FIRST THREE LIVE BIRTHS*

(a) By age of EW and residence

| Age of EW | Mean no. of pregnancies of EW in each residential area with child loss of: | | | | | | | |
| | Semi-urban area | | | | Urban area | | | |
	0	1	2–3	N[a]	0	1	2–3	N[a]
<20	(3.0)	(3.0)	—	4	(3.5)	—	—	2
20–24	3.8	(4.1)	(4.1)	117	3.7	(3,2)	—	92
25–29	5.0	5.6	(6.9)	412	4.6	4.8	(6.0)	389
30–34	6.5	7.1	7.9	474	5.9	6.7	(9.6)	376
35–39	7.3	8.5	9.4	391	6.8	7.2	(8.4)	327
40–44	8.2	8.7	9.0	368	7.8	8.6	(9.1)	404
All ages	6.3	7.4	8.4	1760	6.2	7.1	8.5	1590

* Figures in parentheses refer to fewer than 25 eligible women.
[a] N = total number of eligible women in the sample (excludes women with fewer than 3 live births).

(b) Statistical tests for the 40–44 age group

| | Significance of differences in mean gravidity between child loss categories of EW aged 40–44 | | | | | |
| | Semi-urban area | | | Urban area | | |
	0 versus 1	0 versus 2 + 3	1 versus 2 + 3	0 versus 1	0 versus 2 + 3	1 versus 2 + 3
t values	1.3	1.7	0.7	2.1[a]	2.3[a]	0.8
df (degrees of freedom)	305	245	180	375	296	131

[a] $P < 0.05$.

For women in the age group 40–44 years in the urban area the mean numbers of pregnancies were 7.8, 8.6, and 9.1 for those who had experienced no child loss, one child loss, and 2–3 child losses, respectively, among their first 3 live-born children. The corresponding figures for the semi-urban area were 8.2, 8.7, and 9.0 for 0, 1, and 2–3 losses respectively.

The results of t-tests run for the differences in mean gravidity at ages 40–44 showed that in the urban area the differences in the mean number of pregnancies between women who had not lost any children and those who had lost 1 child or those who had lost 2 or 3 children among their first 3 live births were

327

statistically significant at the 0.05 level (for 0 versus 1 child loss, $t = 2.1$ ($df = 375$); for 0 versus 2 + 3 child losses, $t = 2.3$ ($df - 296$)). The difference in mean gravidity between those with no child loss and those with some child loss was significant at the 0.01 level. Although the same trends were observed in the semi-urban area the differences were not statistically significant ($P < 0.10$) (Table 7.C.7(b)).

Child loss among the first three live births and mean parity

A pattern similar to that for child loss and mean gravidity emerged when parity was examined (Table 7.C.8(a)). Looking at the age group 40–44, it was observed that the number of children born increased with increasing child losses. There was an element of over-compensation for almost all groups compared with the ideal family size stated by the same women. In the case of child loss, this compensation is an indicator of replacement. In the case of no child loss, this over-compensation (e.g., having 6 children when they needed

TABLE 7.C.8. MEAN PARITY AND CHILD LOSS AMONG FIRST THREE LIVE BIRTHS*

(a) By age of EW and residence

| Age of EW | Mean parity of EW in each residential area with child loss of: | | | | | | | |
| | Semi-urban area | | | | Urban area | | | |
	0	1	2–3	N[a]	0	1	2–3	N[a]
<20	(3.0)	(3.0)	—	4	(3.0)	—	—	2
20–24	3.5	(3.6)	(3.8)	117	3.4	(3.1)	—	92
25–29	4.5	5.0	(5.6)	412	4.0	4.2	(5.6)	389
30–34	5.8	6.4	7.2	474	5.2	5.7	(8.6)	376
35–39	6.4	7.6	8.1	391	5.9	6.8	(8.0)	327
40–44	7.3	7.9	8.3	368	6.9	7.6	8.1	404
All ages	5.6	6.7	7.5	1766	5.3	6.3	7.7	1590

* Figures in parentheses refer to fewer than 25 eligible women.
[a] N = total number of eligible women in the sample (excludes women with fewer than 3 live births).

(b) Statistical tests for the 40–44 age group

| | Significance of differences in mean parity between child loss categories of EW aged 40–44 | | | | | |
| | Semi-urban area | | | Urban area | | |
	0 versus 1	0 versus 2 + 3	1 versus 2 + 3	0 versus 1	0 versus 2 + 3	1 versus 2 + 3
t values	1.9	2.5[a]	0.9	2.2[a]	2.4[a]	1.0
df (degrees of freedom)	305	245	180	385	296	131

[a] $P < 0.05$.

only 4 to make up their ideal family size) could stem from a desire to ensure that they would ultimately end up with the number of children they wanted.

The results of the t-tests showed that the differences in mean parity between those with no child loss and those who had lost one child or 2 or 3 children were statistically significant for both the urban and semi-urban areas (Table 7.C.8(b)). In both areas the difference in mean parity between those with no child loss and those with some child loss among their first 3 live births was statistically significant at the 0.01 level.

Child loss among the first three live births and family size

In contrast with the trends seen for mean gravidity and mean parity, mean family size was inversely associated with child loss among the first 3 live births in all the age groups in both the semi-urban area and the urban area (Table 7.C.9).

TABLE 7.C.9. MEAN FAMILY SIZE AND CHILD LOSS AMONG THE FIRST THREE LIVE BIRTHS*

(a) By age of EW and residence

Age of EW	Mean family size of EW in each residential area with child loss of:							
	Semi-urban area				Urban area			
	0	1	2–3	N[a]	0	1	2–3	N[a]
<20	(3.0)	(2.0)	—	4	(3.0)	—	—	2
20–24	3.5	(2.6)	(1.2)	117	3	(2.1)	—	92
25–29	4.4	3.8	(2.8)	412	4.0	3.2	(3.4)	389
30–34	5.6	5.0	4.2	474	5.2	4.6	(5.5)	376
35–39	6.1	6.0	4.9	391	5.8	5.3	(5.2)	327
40–44	6.8	5.8	4.1	368	6.6	6.0	5.3	404
All ages	5.4	5.1	4.0	1766	5.2	4.9	4.9	1590

* Figures in parentheses refer to fewer than 25 eligible women
[a] N = total number of eligible women in the sample (excludes women with fewer than 3 live births).

(b) Statistical tests for the 40–44 age group

	Significance of differences in mean family size between child loss categories of EW aged 40–44					
	Semi-urban area			Urban area		
	0 versus 1	0 versus 2 + 3	1 versus 2 + 3	0 versus 1	0 versus 2 + 3	1 versus 2 + 3
t values	3.7[a]	8.3[a]	4.9[a]	2.4[b]	3.3[a]	1.6
df (degrees of freedom)	305	245	180	375	296	131

[a] $P < 0.01$.
[b] $P < 0.05$.

329

Mean family size declined consistently with increases in child loss in both areas. At age 40–44 the mean family sizes for women in the urban area with losses of 0, 1, and 2 or 3 children were 6.6, 6.0, and 5.3, respectively. In the semi-urban area, the corresponding mean family sizes were 6.8, 5.8, and 4.1. The results of t-tests showed that these differences were statistically significant (Table 7.C.9(b)).

Approval and ever-use of birth control in relation to child loss among the first three live births

Birth control methods had actually been used by only about 45% of the women, although more than 85% said they approved of it. There was a marked difference between the semi-urban and urban areas, the ever-use being higher in the urban areas. A negative association between ever-use of birth control and child loss was observed in both the study areas. Among women with no child loss among the first 3 live births, 55.6% had used birth control methods compared with only 34.7% of those who had experienced 2–3 child losses (Table 7.C.10).

TABLE 7.C.10. APPROVAL AND EVER-USE OF BIRTH CONTROL BY RESIDENCE AND CHILD LOSS AMONG FIRST THREE LIVE BIRTHS

Residence	Percentage approval of birth control among EW with child loss of:			Percentage ever-use of birth control among EW with child loss of:			Total no. of EW in sample[a]
	0	1	2 & 3	0	1	2 & 3	
Semi-urban	91.5	94.3	85.6	42.6	37.3	31.3	1766
Urban	91.7	89.5	84.7	67.9	64.2	44.1	1590
Both areas	91.6	92.4	85.4	55.6	48.1	34.7	3356

[a] Excludes women with fewer than 3 live births.

Child Loss and Subsequent Birth Interval

The birth interval that follows a live birth, especially when it occurs early in the reproductive span, is assumed to be longer than that following the death of a child. This difference exists because of a biological mechanism (post partum amenorrhoea, which may be prolonged by lactation) and/or absence of replacement motivation. The present data came from a lactating community and it is possible that biological mechanisms may have been involved, at least partly, in prolonging the interval after a live-born child who was breast fed (Table 7.C.11).

In the present data, the interval between the end of two successive pregnancies was calculated both for a live-born child who had survived the first year and for one who died in infancy (during the first year). The average interval between the birth of a child who survived the first year of life and the end of the subsequent pregnancy was about 26 months in both the semi-urban

TABLE 7.C.11. MEAN SUBSEQUENT BIRTH INTERVAL BY RESIDENCE, CHILD SURVIVAL, AND BIRTH ORDER

Residence and child survival	Mean subsequent birth interval (months) for birth order:							
	1	2	3	4	5	6 and over	All birth orders	Reported no. live births
Semi-urban								
Child alive at age 1	26.5	26.0	25.7	26.1	26.0	25.9	26.1	8558
Child died at age <1	20.5	21.3	22.3	20.9	21.2	18.7	20.6	899
Urban								
Child alive at age 1	25.0	26.1	25.9	27.3	26.9	25.8	26.0	7467
Child died at age <1	20.1	19.8	21.0	18.4	22.9	21.0	20.3	450

and the urban area. When the child died during the first year, the interval was shortened by about 5 months in both areas. This means that improved child survival will tend to prolong spacing between pregnancy and may reduce fertility. These results are only tentative, since the subsequent interval may be affected by the length of the second pregnancy.

D. SYRIAN ARAB REPUBLIC

N. Ghabra, M. Gharib & A. R. Omran

Total Child Loss and Family Formation

Child loss seems to be high in the three areas examined; on the average, 36.8% of the women lost one or more of their children (Table 7.D.1). Rural women had more child losses than women in towns and large cities; the figures for Rural Aleppo, Sweida, and Damascus were 44.6%, 36.4% and 29.1%, respectively.

TABLE 7.D.1. DISTRIBUTION OF ELIGIBLE WOMEN BY RESIDENCE AND CHILD LOSS EXPERIENCE

Residence	Percentage of EW with child loss of:			Total no. of EW interviewed
	0	1–2	3 and over	
Damascus	70.9	25.5	3.6	1975
Sweida	73.6	30.6	5.8	1711
Rural Aleppo	54.9	32.6	12.0	1935
All areas	63.2	29.5	7.3	5621

Total child loss and mean ideal family size

The variations in mean ideal family size among the different residential areas are evident from Table 7.D.2, which shows that, in general, rural women preferred larger families than did women in towns and large cities. Likewise, there was a positive association between achieved family size and ideal family size, which persisted within each residential group and child loss experience category.

TABLE 7.D.2. MEAN IDEAL FAMILY SIZE BY RESIDENCE, ACTUAL FAMILY SIZE, AND TOTAL CHILD LOSS EXPERIENCE*

Residence and actual family size	Mean ideal family size of EW with child loss of:			Total no. of EW interviewed
	0	1–2	3 and over	
Damascus				
0–3	3.3	3.8	(3.9)	615
4–5	3.9	4.0	(4.1)	400
6 and over	4.5	4.3	(4.7)	471
All family sizes	3.8	4.1	4.4	1486
Sweida				
0–3	3.8	4.1	(4.5)	612
4–5	4.5	4.7	5.2	412
6 and over	5.4	5.5	6.4	511
All family sizes	4.4	5.0	5.7	1535
Rural Aleppo				
0–3	6.4	6.0	(5.7)	431
4–5	6.4	6.5	6.1	209
6 and over	6.7	6.9	6.5	329
All family sizes	6.4	6.6	6.3	969

* Figures in parentheses refer to fewer than 25 eligible women.

There was a tendency for the mean ideal family size of Damascus and Sweida women to increase slightly with total child loss experience, but no such tendency was evident for Rural Aleppo. Among Damascus women, the mean ideal family size increased from 3.8 for those with no child loss to 4.1 for those with 1–2 losses and 4.4 for those with 3 or more losses. The corresponding means for the Sweida women were 4.4, 5.0, and 5.7; and for the women of Rural Aleppo they were 6.4, 6.6, and 6.3, respectively.

Total child loss and mean gravidity

In all three areas, fertility was unquestionably high, as judged by the average number of pregnancies a woman experienced before menopause. As expected, mean gravidity increased progressively with age. At age 40–44 years, a woman in these areas had on the average from 7 to 12 pregnancies, depending on child loss experience (Tables 7.D.3). The differences among the three areas were slight. If anything, women in Damascus experienced slightly higher gravidity than in the other two areas, while those in Sweida had the lowest gravidity.

TABLE 7.D.3. MEAN NUMBER OF PREGNANCIES, BY RESIDENCE, TOTAL CHILD LOSS
EXPERIENCE, AND AGE OF ELIGIBLE WOMEN*

Residence and child loss	Mean number of pregnancies of EW aged:						
	15–19	20–24	25–29	30–34	35–39	40–44	All EW
Damascus							
0	0.9	2.5	4.0	5.8	7.0	7.6	4.8
1–2	(2.8)	4.3	6.0	7.8	9.1	10.4	8.1
3 or more	—	—	(8.6)	(10.0)	(10.1)	12.4	11.0
Sweida							
0	0.9	2.2	3.8	5.3	6.3	7.3	4.6
1–2	(2.5)	3.7	5.4	6.9	8.1	9.2	7.5
3 or more	—	—	(9.0)	(9.1)	(10.6)	10.8	(10.4)
Rural Aleppo							
0	0.7	2.1	4.1	6.1	7.9	8.1	4.3
1–2	(1.8)	3.7	5.8	7.9	8.7	10.3	8.1
3 or more	—	(5.6)	(7.2)	9.5	10.7	11.4	10.5

* Figures in parentheses refer to fewer than 25 eligible women.

The mean gravidity was directly related to total child loss. This relationship was maintained within each residential group and each class of eligible women. By age 40–44, which corresponds approximately to completed gravidity, the pattern was well established. At this age, for example, urban women with no child loss had on the average 7.6 pregnancies, compared with 10.4 for those with 1–2 child losses and 12.4 for those with 3 or more losses. Similar relative rises in gravidity with increasing child loss experience were observed for both Sweida and Rural Aleppo, as shown in Table 7.D.3.

Total child loss and mean parity

The pattern of association between total child loss and mean parity specific for age (Table 7.D.4) was quite similar to that described for mean gravidity (Table 7.D.3).

At age 40–44, for example, the mean parity of Rural Aleppo women increased from 6.1 for those with no child loss to 8.4 for those who had lost 1–2 children, and to 10.1 for those who had lost 3 or more children. The corresponding means for Sweida women were 5.6, 8.0 and 9.5, and for Damascus women 5.8, 8.5 and 11.2.

Total child loss and mean family size

There was a positive relationship between family size and child loss within each residential group. Damascus women who had not lost any children had an average family size of 3.8, while those who had lost 1–2 children averaged 5.5 living children, and those with 3 or more losses averaged 6.2 living children.

TABLE 7.D.4. MEAN PARITY BY RESIDENCE, TOTAL CHILD LOSS EXPERIENCE, AND AGE OF ELIGIBLE WOMEN*

Residence and child loss	Mean parity of EW aged:							Total no. of EW interviewed
	15–19	20–24	25–29	30–34	35–39	40–44	All EW	
Damascus								
0	0.7	2.1	3.4	4.8	5.8	5.8	3.8	1401
1–2	(2.5)	3.9	5.2	6.7	7.7	8.5	6.8	503
3 or more	—	—	(6.5)	(8.3)	(9.4)	11.2	9.8	71
Sweida								
0	0.8	1.9	3.3	4.6	5.3	5.6	3.8	1088
1–2	(2.5)	3.3	4.8	6.0	7.0	8.0	6.4	524
3 or more	—	—	(8.3)	(8.2)	(9.6)	9.5	(9.3)	99
Rural Aleppo								
0	0.6	1.8	3.6	5.1	6.3	6.1	3.3	1063
1–2	(1.6)	3.2	5.2	6.9	7.7	8.4	6.7	630
3 or more	—	(5.2)	(6.8)	8.8	9.6	10.1	9.4	242

* Figures in parentheses refer to fewer than 25 eligible women.

The corresponding figures for Sweida women were 3.8, 5.2, and 5.6, and for Rural Aleppo women 3.3, 5.3, and 5.4. Among Damascus women aged 40–44, the same trend was apparent; the mean family size rose from 5.8 for those with no child loss experience, to.7.1 for those with 1–2 losses, and to 7.4 for those with 3 or more losses. However, for women aged 40–44 in Sweida and Rural Aleppo, the pattern was somewhat different; family size was positively related to child loss for those who had lost 1 or 2 children, but it decreased again for

TABLE 7.D.5. MEAN FAMILY SIZE BY RESIDENCE, TOTAL CHILD LOSS EXPERIENCE, AND AGE OF ELIGIBLE WOMEN*

Residence and child loss	Mean family size of EW aged:							Total no. of EW interviewed
	15–19	20–24	25–29	30–34	35–39	40–44	All EW	
Damascus								
0	0.7	2.1	3.4	4.8	5.8	5.8	3.8	1401
1–2	(1.5)	2.8	4.0	5.5	6.4	7.1	5.5	503
3 or more	—	—	(3.5)	(5.0)	(5.7)	7.4	6.2	71
Sweida								
0	0.8	1.9	3.3	4.6	5.3	5.9	3.8	1088
1–2	(1.5)	2.2	3.6	4.8	5.7	6.8	5.2	524
3 or more	—	—	(5.0)	(4.5)	(5.7)	6.0	(5.6)	99
Rural Aleppo								
0	0.6	1.8	3.6	5.0	6.4	6.0	3.3	1063
1–2	(0.6)	2.1	3.9	5.6	6.2	7.0	5.3	630
3 or more	—	(1.8)	(3.3)	5.2	5.6	6.0	5.4	242

* Figures in parentheses refer to fewer than 25 eligible women.

those who had lost 3 or more children. The actual figures for family size were 5.9, 6.8, and 6.0 for Sweida and 6.0, 7.0, and 6.0 for Rural Aleppo. These figures reflect the high child loss in rural areas where health and sanitary conditions are inferior to those in urban areas.

Child Loss among the First Three Live Births

The birth order of children lost is important in examining the relationship of family formation to child loss experience. Family formation is therefore examined here in relation to the loss of children under 5 years of age among the first 3 live-born children only, for each woman who had achieved this parity. Data relating to women who had had fewer than 3 live births are therefore excluded from Tables 7.D.6 to 7.D.10.

Child loss among the first three live births and mean ideal family size

When the data for child loss experience among the first three live births were analysed by residence (Table 7.D.6), little difference was found in the ideal family preferred by women with different child losses. The mean ideal family size preferred by women with no child loss was 4.9, while for women with 1 child loss and 2–3 child losses the figures were 5.1 and 5.2, respectively.

Women in Rural Aleppo chose higher mean ideal family sizes than those in either Sweida or Damascus.

TABLE 7.D.6. MEAN IDEAL FAMILY SIZE BY RESIDENCE AND CHILD LOSS AMONG THE FIRST THREE LIVE BIRTHS

Residence	Mean ideal family size of EW with child loss of:			No. of EW in sample[a]
	0	1	2–3	
Damascus	4.1	4.0	4.1	1096
Sweida	4.8	5.0	5.0	1152
Rural Aleppo	6.6	6.5	6.0	652
All areas	4.9	5.1	5.2	2900

[a] Excludes women with fewer than 3 live births.

Child loss among the first three live births and mean gravidity

The mean number of pregnancies per woman specific for age not only reflected residential differences (with women in Rural Aleppo having larger averages than those in Damascus and Sweida ($P < 0.01$)) but also showed a direct positive association with child loss experiences among the first 3 live births (Table 7.D.7). In Rural Aleppo women aged 40–44 years reported averages of 9.5, 10.7, and 10.6 pregnancies for those with 0, 1, and 2–3 child losses, respectively. The corresponding figures for Sweida women were 8.6, 9.1, and 10.0, and for Damascus women 8.7, 10.3, and 10.8.

335

TABLE 7.D.7. MEAN NUMBER OF PREGNANCIES AND CHILD LOSS AMONG FIRST THREE
LIVE BIRTHS*

(a) By age of EW and residence

| Age of EW | Mean no. of pregnancies of EW in each residential area with child loss of: | | | | | | | | | | | |
| | Damascus | | | | Sweida | | | | Rural Aleppo | | | |
	0	1	2–3	N[a]	0	1	2–3	N[a]	0	1	2–3	N[a]
<20	(3.0)	(4.0)	—	9	(3.0)	(3.0)	—	2	(3.0)	(3.0)	—	6
20–24	4.0	4.5	(4.7)	159	3.8	(4.0)	(3.7)	92	3.9	4.3	(4.8)	128
25–29	5.0	6.0	(5.9)	292	4.7	5.5	(5.1)	286	5.0	5.5	6.0	287
30–34	6.5	8.0	(7.5)	382	6.2	7.0	(7.1)	323	7.0	7.9	8.7	320
35–39	8.0	8.5	(9.5)	328	7.5	8.1	(9.9)	246	8.5	8.9	9.6	315
40–44	8.7	10.3	(10.8)	290	8.6	9.1	10.0	335	9.5	10.7	10.6	320
All ages	6.6	7.9	8.7	1460	6.4	7.4	8.7	1284	6.8	8.3	9.1	1376

* Figures in parentheses refer to fewer than 25 eligible women.
[a] N = total number of eligible women in the sample (excludes women with fewer than 3 live births).

(b) Statistical tests for the 40–44 age group

| | Significance of differences in mean gravidity between child loss categories of EW aged 40–44: | | | | | | | | |
| | Damascus | | | Sweida | | | Rural Aleppo | | |
	0 v. 1	0 v. 2 + 3	1 v. 2 + 3	0 v. 1	0 v. 2 + 3	1 v. 2 + 3	0 v. 1	0 v. 2 + 3	1 v. 2 + 3
t values	4.15[a]	2.82[a]	0.72	1.62	2.56[b]	1.49	3.61[a]	2.56[b]	0.32
df (degrees of freedom)	270	196	108	292	225	147	244	193	197

[a] $P < 0.01$.
[b] $P < 0.05$.

The results of t-tests run for the differences in mean gravidity at ages 40–44 in all three residential areas showed that the differences in mean number of pregnancies for women who had lost one child and for those who had lost none were statistically significant for Damascus and for Rural Aleppo, but not for Sweida (Table 7.D.7(b)). The differences in mean number of pregnancies for other categories of child loss experience were also tested, with the results given in Table 7.D.7(b). The differences in mean gravidity between those with no child loss experience among the first 3 live births and those with 1–3 child losses were statistically significant for all three areas ($P < 0.01$ for Damascus and Rural Aleppo, $P < 0.05$ for Sweida).

Child loss among the first three live births and mean parity

A pattern similar to that for child loss and mean gravidity emerged when child loss was analysed in relation to parity (Table 7.D.8). Rural women aged 40–44 years reported averages of 8.2, 9.2, and 10.0 live births for those with 0, 1, and 2–3 child losses among their first 3 live births. The corresponding figures for Sweida women were 7.6, 8.3, and 8.9, and for Damascus women 7.2, 8.9, and 9.1. It was evident that in all three residential areas the women were trying to compensate for their child losses.

TABLE 7.D.8. MEAN PARITY AND CHILD LOSS AMONG FIRST THREE LIVE BIRTHS*

(a) By age of EW and residence

	Mean parity of EW in each residential area with child loss of:											
Age of EW	Damascus				Sweida				Rural Aleppo			
	0	1	2–3	N[a]	0	1	2–3	N[a]	0	1	2–3	N[a]
<20	(3.0)	(3.3)	—	9	(3.0)	(3.0)	—	2	3.0	3.0	—	6
20–24	3.6	4.1	(4.6)	559	3.6	(3.5)	(3.7)	92	3.5	4.1	(4.5)	128
25–29	4.5	5.3	(5.2)	292	4.3	5.1	(4.8)	286	4.7	5.1	5.6	287
30–34	5.7	6.9	(6.9)	382	5.6	6.3	(6.5)	323	6.2	7.3	8.2	320
35–39	7.0	7.3	(8.4)	328	6.7	7.4	(8.2)	246	7.5	8.0	8.7	315
40–44	7.2	8.9	(9.1)	290	7.6	8.3	8.9	335	8.2	9.2	10.0	320
All ages	5.7	6.9	7.6	1460	5.7	6.7	7.8	1284	6.1	7.4	8.3	1370

* Figures in parentheses refer to fewer than 25 eligible women.
[a] N = total number of eligible women in the sample (excludes women with fewer than 3 live births).

(b) Statistical tests for the 40–44 age group

	Significance of differences in mean parity between child loss categories of EW aged 40–44:								
	Damascus			Sweida			Rural Aleppo		
	0 v. 1	0 v. 2 + 3	1 v. 2 + 3	0 v. 1	0 v. 2 + 3	1 v. 2 + 3	0 v. 1	0 v. 2 + 3	1 v. 2 + 3
t values	5.25[a]	2.97[a]	0.27	2.49[b]	2.94[a]	1.36	2.96[a]	3.37[a]	0.90
df (degrees of freedom)	270	196	108	292	225	147	244	193	197

[a] $P < 0.01$.
[b] $P < 0.05$.

If the data from this table are compared with those for mean ideal family size, it can be seen that women aged 40–44 years had mean parities higher than their mean ideal family sizes, even among those who had had child losses. This may have been due to fear of child loss, compensation for child loss, and lack of birth control resources.

The results of the *t*-tests showed the differences in the mean parity for women who had lost one child and for those women who had lost none to be statistically significant ($P < 0.01$ for Damascus and Rural Aleppo, $P < 0.05$ for Sweida) (Table 7.D.8(*b*)). The differences were also significant ($P < 0.01$) for no child loss versus 2 or 3 children lost and for no child loss versus some child loss.

Child loss among the first three live births and mean family size

Family size seems to have been influenced by child loss in all three areas. Taking all ages together, women in Rural Aleppo reported mean family sizes of 5.7, 5.6, and 4.9 for those with 0, 1, and 2–3 losses, respectively. The corresponding figures for Sweida were 5.5, 5.1, and 4.8, and for Damascus 5.5, 5.5, and 4.8 (Table 7.D.9).

TABLE 7.D.9. MEAN FAMILY SIZE AND CHILD LOSS AMONG FIRST THREE LIVE BIRTHS*

(*a*) By age of EW and residence

| Age of EW | Mean family size in each residential area with child loss of: | | | | | | | | | | | |
| | Damascus | | | | Sweida | | | | Rural Aleppo | | | |
	0	1	2–3	N^a	0	1	2–3	N^a	0	1	2–3	N^a
< 20	(3.0)	(2.3)	—	9	(3.0)	(2.0)	—	2	(3.0)	(2.0)	—	6
20–24	3.6	3.0	(2.6)	159	3.5	2.5	(1.7)	92	3.4	2.9	(1.9)	128
25–29	4.4	4.1	(3.0)	292	4.3	3.8	(2.9)	286	4.5	3.8	2.9	287
30–34	5.5	5.5	(4.3)	382	5.4	4.9	(3.6)	323	5.9	5.7	4.9	320
35–39	6.7	6.0	(5.5)	328	6.4	5.8	(4.6)	246	7.0	6.1	5.4	315
40–44	6.9	7.1	(5.8)	290	7.1	6.3	6.0	335	7.5	6.9	5.6	320
All ages	5.5	5.5	4.8	1460	5.5	5.1	4.8	1284	5.7	5.6	4.9	1376

  * Figures in parentheses refer to fewer than 25 eligible women.
  ^{a} N = total number of eligible women in the sample (excludes women with fewer than 3 live births).

(*b*) Statistical tests for the 40–44 age group

| | Significance of differences in mean family size between child loss categories of EW aged 40–44: | | | | | | | | |
| | Damascus | | | Sweida | | | Rural Aleppo | | |
	0 v. 1	0 v. 2 + 3	1 v. 2 + 3	0 v. 1	0 v. 2 + 3	1 v. 2 + 3	0 v. 1	0 v. 2 + 3	1 v. 2 + 3
t values	0.84	2.11^a	2.48^a	3.02^b	2.73^b	0.90	2.19^a	5.25^b	3.69^b
df (degrees of freedom)	270	196	108	292	225	147	244	193	197

  ^{a} $P < 0.05$.
  ^{b} $P < 0.01$.

338

For rural women aged 40–44 years, the mean family size decreased from 7.5 for those with no child loss, to 6.9 for those with 1 child loss, and 5.6 for those with 2.3 child losses. The corresponding figures for Sweida women were 7.1, 6.3, and 6.0, and for Damascus 6.9, 7.1, and 5.8.

The results of the t-tests confirmed the negative association between family size and child loss (Table 7.D.9(b)).

Approval and ever-use of birth control in relation to child loss among the first three live births

The data summarized in Table 7.D.10 reflect the expected residential differences, with rural women showing the lowest rates of both approval and ever-use of contraception. The mean approval rates were 13.4% of women with no child loss, 19.6% of those who had lost 1 child, and 13.4% of those who had lost 2–3 children among the first 3 live births. The corresponding rates for Sweida women were 68.1%, 59.2%, and 49.4%, and for Damascus women 76.6%, 73.0%, and 62.5%. The mean rates for use of birth control in all three residential areas were decidedly lower than those for approval. In Rural Aleppo, 3.7% of the women with no child loss, 4.6% of those who had lost 1 child, and 3.8% of those who had lost 2–3 children used birth control. The corresponding rates for Sweida women were 38.5%, 28.5%, and 25.3%; and for Damascus women 58.6%, 57.6%, and 42.2%.

TABLE 7.D.10. APPROVAL AND EVER-USE OF BIRTH CONTROL BY RESIDENCE, PARITY AND CHILD LOSS AMONG FIRST THREE LIVE BIRTHS*

Residence and parity	Percentage approval of birth control among EW with child loss of:			Percentage ever-use of birth control among EW with child loss of:			Total EW in sample[a]
	0	1	2–3	0	1	2–3	
Damascus							
<4	74.8	72.7	—	46.3	(43.2)	—	734
4 and over	77.9	73.0	65.6	68.5	59.6	44.3	1237
All parities	76.6	73.0	62.5	58.6	57.6	42.2	1971
Sweida							
<4	71.5	56.1	(33.3)	35.2	(22.7)	(33.3)	594
4 and over	65.7	59.8	50.6	40.8	29.7	(24.7)	1114
All parities	68.1	59.2	49.4	38.5	28.5	(25.3)	1708
Rural Aleppo							
<4	10.8	(19.2)	—	(1.1)	—	—	724
4 and over	16.3	19.7	13.9	6.5	(5.5)	(4.0)	1207
All parities	13.4	19.6	13.4	3.7	(4.6)	(3.8)	1931

* Figures in parentheses refer to fewer than 25 eligible women.
[a] Excludes women with fewer than 3 live births.

Among both Damascus and Sweida women, the rates of both approval and ever-use of birth control decreased as child loss among the first 3 live births increased. For women in Rural Aleppo, these rates decreased only after the second child loss.

It is also noticeable that in all three residential areas, the rates of both approval and ever-use of birth control increased with increasing parity.

Child Loss and Subsequent Birth Interval

It is generally assumed that because of a biological mechanism (post-partum amenorrhoea, which may be prolonged by lactation) and/or absence of replacement motivation, the interval that follows a live birth, especially when it occurs early in the reproductive span, is longer than that following the birth of a child who died in infancy.

It should be emphasized that the data used here came from a lactating community and that biological mechanisms may have been involved, at least partly, in prolonging the birth interval after a live-born child who was breast fed. In the present data the mean interval between the ends of two successive pregnancies was calculated, a distinction being made between live-born children who survived the first year and those who died in infancy (during the first year). The results are given in Table 7.D.11.

TABLE 7.D.11. MEAN SUBSEQUENT BIRTH INTERVAL BY RESIDENCE, CHILD SURVIVAL, AND BIRTH ORDER

Residence and child survival	Mean subsequent birth interval (months) for birth order:							Reported no. live births
	1	2	3	4	5	6 and over	All birth orders	
Damascus								
Child alive at age 1	14.0	15.5	16.0	17.5	17.1	17.8	16.2	7306
Child died at age < 1	10.5	11.1	11.4	13.6	9.6	9.6	12.4	535
Sweida								
Child alive at age 1	15.1	16.7	17.5	18.0	17.5	18.5	17.1	6301
Child died at age < 1	11.2	11.4	12.4	12.1	12.5	13.6	12.2	631
Rural Aleppo								
Child alive at age 1	15.0	15.9	16.0	15.8	16.2	15.9	15.8	7472
Child died at age < 1	10.2	11.8	12.7	13.3	12.1	12.0	11.8	966

There were small differences between the different residential groups in the means of both intervals (when the child survived the first year, and when it did not). The mean intervals between the birth of a child who survived the first year of life and the end of the subsequent pregnancy were 16.2 months for Damascus, 17.1 months for Sweida, and 15.8 months for Rural Aleppo. This interval was shortened by 3.8–4.9 months when the child died during the first year, when the means became 12.4 months for Damascus, 12.2 months for Sweida and 11.8 months for Rural Aleppo.

340

When the birth order of the index live-birth was considered, however, greater differences were observed between the mean interval following a surviving live-born and the mean interval following a live-born child who died in the first year. These differences ranged between 3.5 and 8.2 months for Damascus, 3.9 and 5.9 months for Sweida, and 2.5 and 4.8 months for Rural Aleppo.

Chapter Eight

FAMILY FORMATION AND BIRTH CONTROL: BEHAVIOUR AND ATTITUDES

INTRODUCTION

A. R. Omran

This chapter presents information on opinions and attitudes (examined in relation to age, parity, and family size), on family formation patterns, and on the correlation between these patterns and health. It includes data on the woman's judgement of changing natality and child mortality and whether the latter might affect fertility behaviour. It also comprises information on knowledge and practice of fertility control and attitudes towards it. The eligible women answered questions concerning the health of mothers and children in small versus large families, spacing (birth intervals of 1 versus 3 years), and the ability of a mother to provide child care.

In addition to the usual KAP (Knowledge, Attitudes and Practice) assessment of family planning, an effort was made to determine whether contraception would be used by women to avoid health hazards to themselves or their children. Some questions were general in nature, with the aim of discovering whether the woman would approve of contraception for health reasons, while others were more specific and were designed to investigate her willingness to use birth control if a physician told her that further pregnancies would be dangerous. Discrepancies existed in certain areas between the general approval of and the hypothetical willingness personally to use birth control. Similarly, a gap appeared between acceptance and actual use.

A. COLOMBIA

G. Ochoa, A. Gil & A. R. Omran

This chapter may be considered as an expanded KAP (Knowledge, Attitudes, and Practice) study designed to ascertain the views of the interviewed women regarding family formation and health, family planning behaviour, and related subjects relevant to health. Because of the high literacy rate among the study population in Colombia, this chapter is particularly pertinent to policy considerations.

Opinions on Family Formation and Health

Opinions on ideal family size

The ideal family size that the interviewed women preferred has already been discussed in chapter 2.

Opinions on ideal age at marriage

Women were asked what they considered to be the ideal age at marriage for boys and girls. Women in the NSZ preferred lower ages at marriage for both boys and girls than did women in the OUZ. There was no significant variation by social status in either zone. As might be expected, women in both zones preferred higher ages at marriage for boys (27.7 in the OUZ and 26.4 in the NSZ) than for girls (22.5 in the OUZ, 21.2 in the NSZ), the average age difference being 5 years (Table 8.A.1). For both boys and girls, women who

TABLE 8.A.1. MEAN IDEAL AGE AT MARRIAGE FOR BOYS AND GIRLS, BY RESIDENCE, SOCIAL STATUS, AND AGE AT MARRIAGE OF ELIGIBLE WOMEN*

Sex of child; residence and social status	Mean ideal age at marriage in the opinion of EW who married at age:								Total no. of EW interviewed
	12–14	15–17	18–20	21–23	24–26	27–29	30–34	All EW	
BOYS									
Old urban zone									
Middle	28.7	27.4	27.6	27.8	27.9	28.2	29.1	27.8	2513
Low	(27.1)	27.9	27.3	27.7	(26.9)	(28.4)	28.1	27.6	153
Both categories	28.5	27.5	27.6	27.8	27.8	28.2	29.0	27.7	2666
Newly settled zone									
Middle	25.1	26.3	26.5	26.4	27.0	27.3	29.0	26.5	965
Low	25.9	26.4	26.2	26.2	26.2	27.5	26.8	26.3	1633
Both categories	25.9	26.4	26.3	26.3	26.5	27.4	27.2	26.4	2598
GIRLS									
Old urban zone									
Middle	21.9	21.8	21.8	22.7	23.4	24.0	24.5	22.5	2514
Low	20.8	21.9	21.7	22.9	(23.7)	(26.8)	(23.6)	22.5	153
Both categories	21.8	21.8	21.8	22.7	23.4	24.2	24.4	22.5	2667
Newly settled zone									
Middle	(20.9)	20.9	21.1	21.6	21.8	22.0	(23.9)	21.4	965
Low	21.4	20.8	21.0	21.4	21.3	22.8	23.0	21.1	1633
Both categories	21.2	20.8	21.1	21.4	21.5	22.4	23.4	21.2	2598

* Figures in parentheses refer to fewer than 25 eligible women.

TABLE 8.A.2. VIEWS OF ELIGIBLE WOMEN ON FAMILY FORMATION AND HEALTH, BY RESIDENCE AND SOCIAL STATUS

Percentage of EW giving replies indicated

Statements on which women's views were obtained:	Middle status				Low status				Both categories			
	Yes	No	Same	No opinion	Yes	No	Same	No opinion	Yes	No	Same	No opinion
Newly settled zone[a]												
A child's health is better in a small family	80.2	1.8	15.5	2.5	82.4	3.3	13.7	0.7	80.3	1.9	15.4	2.4
The mother's health is better in a small family	80.6	3.4	13.2	2.8	83.7	5.9	9.8	0.7	80.7	3.6	13.0	2.7
A child's health is better when the birth interval is 3 years rather than 1 year	81.2	6.6	11.2	1.0	86.9	5.9	7.2	0.0	81.5	6.6	10.9	1.0
The mother's health is better when the birth interval is 3 years rather than 1 year	84.1	6.5	8.4	0.9	86.3	6.5	7.2	0.0	84.3	6.5	8.4	0.4
A mother who is sick for a long time should have fewer children	95.4	4.6	—	0.2	95.4	4.6	0.0	0.0	95.3	4.5	—	0.2
A decrease in child mortality would result in fewer children being born	28.4	68.7	0.0	3.0	28.1	66.0	0.0	5.9	28.4	68.3	—	3.3
Old urban zone[b]												
A child's health is better in a small family	88.7	1.2	7.9	2.2	90.2	1.7	5.7	2.4	89.6	1.5	6.5	2.3
The mother's health is better in a small family	86.2	3.7	7.0	3.0	88.1	2.4	6.2	3.3	87.4	2.9	6.5	3.2
A child's health is better when the birth interval is 3 years rather than 1 year	91.5	4.2	3.5	0.6	93.0	3.0	3.3	0.7	92.4	3.5	3.4	0.7
The mother's health is better when the birth interval is 3 years rather than 1 year	90.8	4.7	3.3	1.2	92.0	3.1	3.5	1.3	91.6	3.7	3.5	1.3
A mother who is sick for a long time should have fewer children	91.9	8.0	—	0.1	96.6	3.2	—	0.1	94.8	5.0	0.0	0.1
A decrease in child mortality would result in fewer children being born	32.0	66.5	—	1.6	31.1	66.0	—	2.9	31.4	66.2	0.0	2.4

[a] Numbers of EW responding: middle status, 2516; low status, 153; both categories, 2669.
[b] Numbers of EW responding: middle status, 966; low status, 1635; both categories 2601.

345

themselves married at later ages (over 26) preferred higher ages at marriage than did women who married at younger ages.

Opinions on small families and spacing

Opinions of eligible women on maternal and child health status in small as opposed to large families and on child spacing are shown by social status in Table 8.A.2 and by education in Table 8.A.3. Most of the women felt that there were health advantages in having small families and well-spaced pregnancies. Such an opinion was held more frequently by women in the OUZ than in the NSZ, with no significant social status differences in either zone. Small and sometimes inconsistent variations with educational level are shown in Table 8.A.3.

As examples, 80.3% of the women from the NSZ and 89.6% of the women from the OUZ believed that *child health* would be better in small families; likewise, 80.7% of the women from the NSZ and 87.4% of those from the OUZ believed that *maternal health* would be better in small families. Women in both regions believed that a 3-year spacing between births would result in better maternal and child health than a 1-year spacing. This view was held by over 90% of the eligible women in the OUZ and over 80% in the NSZ.

An overwhelming majority (over 90%) of the women in both zones and of both middle and low social status believed that a mother who was sick for a long time should not have any more children.

Opinions on changes in natality and child mortality

Approximately one-third of the women interviewed believed that a decrease in childhood mortality would result in fewer children being born, and two-thirds believed it would not. There were only small differences by social status and residential area (Table 8.A.2). In the NSZ, the percentage of positive answers decreased with an increase in educational level. In the OUZ, no consistent pattern by education was found.

Opinions on Birth Control

Approval of birth control

An overwhelming majority (over 90%) of women approved of birth control (Table 8.A.4). This was true in both residential areas and for all parities and ages. Nearly all the women approving of birth control claimed to have used contraception at some time. The only exception was that women who had no living children (parity 0) were less likely to have used birth control than women who had living children. Among women with children, no consistent increase in practice was observed when parity increased. The approval rate was also high for both spacing and limiting pregnancies, with no significant variation by education (Table 8.A.5).

346

TABLE 8.A.3. VIEWS OF ELIGIBLE WOMEN ON FAMILY FORMATION, BY RESIDENCE AND EDUCATION

Statements on which women's views were obtained	Percentage of women agreeing with statements in left-hand column					
	Old urban zone[a]			Newly settled zone[b]		
	No school	Primary	Secondary	No school	Primary	Secondary
A child's health is better in a small family	80.7	80.8	79.1	90.3	89.2	89.8
The mother's health is better in a small family	85.1	80.6	80.1	86.9	87.8	85.7
A child's health is better when the birth interval is 3 years rather than 1 year	89.4	82.2	78.0	93.3	92.0	89.8
The mother's health is better when the birth interval is 3 years rather than 1 year	90.7	84.0	83.4	91.6	91.6	90.8
A decrease in child mortality would result in fewer children being born	24.8	29.6	26.1	32.5	28.1	18.4
A mother who is sick for a long time should not have any more children	94.4	96.0	94.3	97.3	96.2	94.9
A woman should use birth control if the additional pregnancies would affect the health of her children	95.0	98.1	98.7	97.1	98.3	98.0
A woman should use birth control if her health would suffer from a further pregnancy	95.7	97.5	98.2	96.9	97.4	96.6

[a] No. of women responding: 2601.
[b] No. of women responding: 2669.

TABLE 8.A.4. APPROVAL AND USE OF BIRTH CONTROL BY ELIGIBLE WOMEN, BY RESIDENCE, AGE, AND PARITY*

Residence, age, and parity of EW	EW approving of birth control		Use of birth control among women who approve (%)			Use of birth control among women who disapprove (%)		
	%	N[a]	Ever used	Never used	Not known	Ever used	Never used	Not known
AGE								
Old urban zone								
<25	97.4	464	88.1	0.2	11.7	(66.7)	(0.0)	(33.3)
25–34	97.4	1256	92.7	0.3	7.0	(62.5)	(4.2)	(33.3)
35–44	94.7	949	86.0	0.7	13.3	40.5	0.0	59.5
All ages	96.4	2669	89.5	0.4	10.0	50.7	1.5	47.8
Newly settled zone								
<25	94.4	522	76.5	1.0	22.5	(43.5)	(4.3)	(52.2)
25–34	95.6	1216	89.9	0.9	9.3	52.6	7.9	39.5
35–44	89.6	183	83.4	2.7	13.8	32.4	5.4	62.2
All ages	93.4	2601	85.1	1.5	13.4	40.0	5.9	54.1
PARITY								
Old urban zone								
0	95.1	287	60.8	1.8	37.4	(33.3)	(11.1)	(55.6)
1–3	97.1	1438	91.8	0.4	7.8	51.7	0.0	48.3
4–5	95.4	500	95.4	0.0	4.6	(50.0)	(0.0)	(50.0)
6 and over	96.4	444	93.9	0.2	5.8	(63.6)	(0.0)	(36.4)
All parities	96.4	2669	89.5	0.4	10.0	50.7	1.5	47.8
Newly settled zone								
0	89.5	181	30.9	2.5	66.7	(18.8)	(0.0)	(81.3)
1–3	93.7	1055	87.4	1.1	11.5	39.1	8.7	52.2
4–5	94.4	535	92.9	1.6	5.5	52.0	0.0	48.0
6 and over	93.1	830	88.5	1.7	9.8	41.7	8.3	50.0
All parities	93.4	2601	85.1	1.5	13.4	40.0	5.9	54.1

* Figures in parentheses refer to fewer than 25 eligible women.
[a] N = total number of eligible women responding.

TABLE 8.A.5. APPROVAL AND EVER USE OF BIRTH CONTROL, BY RESIDENCE AND EDUCATION

Attitude to birth control	Percentage of EW with attitude shown in left-hand column					
	Old urban zone			Newly settled zone		
	No school	Primary	Secondary or higher	No school	Primary	Secondary or higher
Approve birth control to limit pregnancy	77.6	86.4	88.2	75.5	82.3	79.6
Approve birth control to space pregnancy	76.4	87.2	89.1	76.3	82.7	71.4
Ever used birth control	78.3	88.4	89.9	79.0	84.5	83.7
No. of EW responding	161	1803	705	1016	1487	98

TABLE 8.A.6. REASONS FOR APPROVAL OR DISAPPROVAL OF BIRTH CONTROL, BY RESIDENCE AND FAMILY SIZE

Residence and family size	Percentage of EW who approve for reasons stated					Percentage of EW who disapprove for reasons stated					
	Preserve health of mother	Care of child	Improve child health	Reduce costs	N[a]	Religion	Maternal risks	Husband disapproves	Desire more children	Mother-in-law disapproves	N[a]
Old urban zone											
0–3	84.8	98.1	95.0	98.3	1707	50.0	80.0	67.5	40.0	15.0	40
4 and over	85.8	96.9	93.6	99.1	865	66.7	96.3	74.1	44.4	18.5	27
All OUZ	85.1	97.7	94.6	98.6	2572	56.7	86.6	70.1	41.8	16.4	67
Newly settled zone											
0–3	90.5	99.2	98.3	99.5	1206	52.9	92.0	61.2	47.1	20.6	68
4 and over	92.5	98.7	98.7	99.8	1223	59.1	89.4	65.2	49.2	30.8	66
All NSZ	91.5	98.9	98.5	99.6	2429	56.0	91.0	63.2	48.1	25.6	134

[a] N = total number of eligible women responding.

It is worth noting that among women who disapproved in principle of birth control, 51% in the OUZ and 40% in the NSZ had themselves used contraception at some time. However, a high proportion of these women claimed not to know whether they had ever used contraception (Table 8.A.4).

Among women who approved of birth control, the reasons given for approval were related to both health and economic benefits (Table 8.A.6).

The minority of women disapproving of birth control gave as reasons for disapproval: safeguarding maternal health (presumably from risks of contraception), husband's disapproval, religion, and desire for more children (Table 8.A.6). Only 15 (31%) mentioned the mother-in-law's disapproval. There were no marked differences between zones in the percentages of women in favour of birth control and those disapproving.

Willingness to use birth control for health reasons

The women were also asked *specifically* whether they would be willing to use birth control if they were to be told by a physician that more pregnancies would harm either their own health or their child's health (Table 8.A.7). A substantial proportion of women responded that they would use birth control in such cases.

TABLE 8.A.7. ATTITUDE OF ELIGIBLE WOMEN TOWARDS BIRTH CONTROL, BY RESIDENCE AND FAMILY SIZE

Residence and family size	Percentage of EW approving birth control in principle who would use it for stated reason:			Percentage of EW disapproving birth control in principle who would use it for stated reason:		
	to safeguard health of child	to safeguard health of mother	N[a]	to safeguard health of child	to safeguard health of mother	N[a]
Old urban zone						
0–3	98.7	97.9	1709	85.0	87.5	40
4 and over	98.2	98.5	865	85.2	77.8	27
All OUZ	98.5	98.1	2574	85.1	83.6	67
Newly settled zone						
0–3	98.6	98.3	1206	82.4	80.9	68
4 and over	99.1	98.3	1223	76.1	79.1	67
All NSZ	98.8	98.3	2429	79.3	80.0	135

[a] N = total number of eligible women responding.

Almost all the women in the study (98%) who approved of birth control were willing to use birth control for health reasons. What is more interesting is that a great majority (over 80%) of the women who opposed the principle of birth control said they would approve of its use for the sake of the child's and/or the mother's health. As is shown in Table 8.A.7 there was very little difference in opinion by family size or by residence.

Knowledge and Practice of Specific Methods of Birth Control

Knowledge of specific methods of birth control

The women were asked whether they had heard of and whether they had previously used or were currently using specific methods of birth control (Table 8.A.8). Knowledge of methods of birth control was generally better in the OUZ than in the NSZ. Almost all the women had heard of the "pill", the IUD, and the rhythm method. The diaphragm was the least known method. More than half (50%) in the OUZ and three-quarters (75%) of the women in the NSZ had never heard of the diaphragm. Other methods of birth control not well known included vasectomy, tubectomy, and abortion. The percentage of women who had never heard of these methods was higher in the low than in the middle social status groups.

Use of specific methods of birth control

The 5 methods most commonly being used by the women in the OUZ, in descending order of frequency, were: oral contraceptives (33.8%), rhythm method (19.1%), withdrawal (10.8%), douche (9.5%), and IUD (6.9%). In the NSZ, the corresponding figures were: oral contraception (27.4%), rhythm method (12.5%), IUD (11.7%), withdrawal (10.0%), and douche (4.5%) (Table 8.A.8).

Opinions on breast feeding as a birth control method

Some 17% of women in the OUZ and 24% of those in the NSZ believed that breast feeding could prevent pregnancy (Table 8.A.9): 63.79% of the women in the OUZ and 67.1% of the women in the NSZ did not believe that breast feeding was an effective method of birth control; the remainder of the women were not certain about its effectiveness.

While there were no differences by social status, there was a positive association between the size of the family and the belief that breast feeding could prevent pregnancy.

Opinions on Induced Abortion

As might be expected in a predominantly Catholic country, the expressed approval of induced abortion was low. However, when certain health indications were mentioned, approval rates increased (Table 8.A.10). The use of induced abortion because of the failure of another birth control method was approved by the smallest proportion of the women (approximately 4% in the OUZ, and 3.2% in the NSZ). A slightly higher proportion of the women approved of induced abortion if the child was unwanted and the family could not afford more children. However, a larger proportion (about one-third of the women in the OUZ and one-fifth of the women in the NSZ) said they would approve of terminating pregnancy if it would endanger the woman's health or if there was a possibility that it would result in a deformed child.

351

TABLE 8.A.8. KNOWLEDGE AND USE OF FERTILITY CONTROL METHODS AMONG ELIGIBLE WOMEN, BY RESIDENCE, SOCIAL STATUS, USE, AND METHOD

Knowledge and use of fertility control methods among EW (%)

Social status and method	Old urban zone				Newly settled zone			
	Never heard of	Heard of and used	Heard of and using[a]	Heard of but never used	Never heard of	Heard of and used	Heard of and using	Heard of but never used
Middle	N = 2516				N = 966			
Condom	9.3	14.8	4.3	71.7	11.3	12.1	3.0	73.6
Withdrawal	10.8	19.4	10.5	59.3	14.7	22.5	8.9	53.9
Rhythm	1.5	29.4	19.1	50.0	4.0	22.4	15.1	58.5
Diaphragm	49.7	1.0	0.1	49.2	70.1	0.2	0.0	29.7
Douche, etc.	7.1	14.9	9.3	68.2	17.2	9.6	5.6	67.6
Coil or IUD	0.8	4.1	7.0	88.1	1.3	4.8	9.8	84.1
Orals	0.0	30.2	34.0	35.8	0.1	23.8	28.0	48.1
Tubectomy	13.9	0.0	1.1	84.9	29.6	0.0	0.6	69.8
Vasectomy	15.7	0.0	0.2	84.0	35.2	0.0	0.1	64.7
Abortion	13.1	0.2	0.0	86.4	23.4	0.0	0.0	76.4
Low	N = 153				N = 1635			
Condom	13.1	15.0	4.6	67.3	14.3	12.8	2.6	70.4
Withdrawal	16.3	19.0	15.7	49.0	19.8	22.6	10.6	46.9
Rhythm	7.8	21.6	19.6	51.0	6.4	20.9	10.9	61.6
Diaphragm	69.9	0.7	0.0	29.4	77.5	0.2	0.1	22.1
Douche, etc.	19.0	10.5	4.6	66.0	23.9	9.1	3.9	63.2
Coil or IUD	3.9	4.6	5.9	85.6	1.5	5.1	12.8	80.6
Orals	0.0	22.2	29.4	48.4	0.2	25.7	27.1	47.0
Tubectomy	25.5	0.0	0.0	74.5	36.7	0.0	0.9	62.4
Vasectomy	34.6	0.0	0.0	65.4	41.3	0.0	0.2	58.5
Abortion	19.0	0.7	0.0	80.4	26.9	0.4	0.1	72.3

[a] N = total number of eligible women responding.

TABLE 8.A.8 (continued)

Knowledge and use of fertility control methods among EW (%)

Social status and method	Old urban zone				Newly settled zone			
	Never heard of	Heard of and used	Heard of and using	Heard of but never used	Never heard of	Heard of and used	Heard of and using	Heard of but never used
	N = 2669				N = 2601			
Both categories								
Condom	9.5	11.8	4.3	71.4	13.1	12.5	2.7	71.6
Withdrawal	11.1	13.4	10.8	58.7	17.9	22.6	10.0	49.5
Rhythm	1.9	23.9	19.1	50.0	5.5	21.5	12.5	60.6
Diaphragm	50.8	1.0	0.1	48.1	74.7	0.2	0.1	25.0
Douche, etc.	7.8	14.6	9.5	68.1	21.4	9.3	4.5	64.8
Coil or IUD	1.0	4.1	6.9	88.0	1.5	5.0	11.7	81.9
Orals	0.0	29.7	33.8	36.5	0.2	25.0	27.4	47.4
Tubectomy	14.6	0.0	1.0	84.3	34.1	0.0	0.8	65.2
Vasectomy	16.8	0.0	0.2	83.0	39.1	0.0	0.2	60.8
Abortion	13.5	0.2	0.0	86.1	25.6	0.3	0.1	73.8

[a] N = total number of eligible women responding.

Opinions on Sterilization

Approval rates for sterilization were higher than those for induced abortion. A higher proportion of women in the NSZ than in the OUZ were in favour of sterilization (Table 8.A.11). The figures were 57.3% and 45.7%, respectively. While the differences by social status were slight, approval rates for sterilization generally increased with parity.

When the women were asked whether they thought the husband or the wife should be the one to be sterilized, those favouring the wife outnumbered those favouring the husband by 3:1. A small number of women (4.2% in the OUZ and 3.2% in the NSZ) considered it acceptable to sterilize either the husband or the wife. However, 50.1% of women in the OUZ and 40.1% in the NSZ felt that neither should be sterilized.

TABLE 8.A.9. VIEWS OF ELIGIBLE WOMEN ON WHETHER BREAST FEEDING PREVENTS PREGNANCY, BY RESIDENCE, SOCIAL STATUS, AND FAMILY SIZE

(a) By residence and social status

Residence and social status	Percentage of EW believing breast feeding does or does not prevent pregnancy			Total no. of EW responding
	Yes	No	No opinion	
Old urban zone				
Middle	17.2	67.2	15.7	2516
Low	17.6	69.3	13.1	153
All OUZ	17.2	63.7	15.5	2669
Newly settled zone				
Middle	23.0	67.4	9.6	966
Low	24.6	67.0	8.4	1635
All NSZ	24.0	67.1	8.8	2601

(b) By residence and family size

Residence and family size	Percentage of EW believing breast feeding does or does not prevent pregnancy			Total no. of EW responding
	Yes	No	No opinion	
Old urban zone				
0–3	15.4	66.4	18.2	1767
4–5	17.9	71.1	11.0	492
6 and over	24.1	66.6	9.3	410
All OUZ	17.2	67.3	15.5	2669
Newly settled zone				
0–3	20.7	67.7	11.6	1298
4–5	26.7	66.0	7.3	550
6 and over	27.8	66.9	5.3	752
All NSZ	24.0	67.1	8.8	2601

Of the women who preferred that the wife rather than the husband should be sterilized 67.9% in the OUZ and 58.6% in the NSZ gave as a reason that the husband would refuse (Table 8.A.12). The next most common reason was that the wife should be the one to be sterilized as she was the child bearer (18.4% in the OUZ and 19.8% in the NSZ).

Of the women who preferred that the husband rather than the wife should be sterilized, 40.4% of the women in the OUZ and 31.8% of the women in the NSZ believed that the husband should be sterilized because he should be sharing in limiting the pregnancies. The reason next in order of frequency was that the wife would refuse to have it done. A third reason was that it would be healthier for the husband rather than the wife to be sterilized, a view expressed by 16.7% of the women in the OUZ and 14.1% in the NSZ (Table 8.A.12).

Timing Failure of Last Pregnancy

In an attempt to provide some indication of the adequacy of pregnancy planning, women were asked if they felt that their last pregnancy came sooner than they had wanted. We will call such an occurrence timing failure. The frequency of timing failure was surprisingly high among the study population

TABLE 8.A.10. PERCENTAGE OF ELIGIBLE WOMEN APPROVING ABORTION FOR VARIOUS REASONS, BY RESIDENCE, PARITY, AND FAMILY SIZE

| Residence and reasons for approving abortion | Percentage of EW approving abortion[a] | | | |
| | Parity | | Family size | |
	0–3	4 and over	0–3	4 and over
Old urban zone	N = 1725[b]	N = 944	N = 1767	N = 902
Failure of birth control	3.7	4.1	3.6	4.3
Reluctance to have more children	4.5	4.2	4.4	4.4
Pregnancy endangers woman's health	33.0	32.6	32.9	32.7
Possibility of deformed child	31.7	29.8	31.7	29.7
Inability to afford more children	8.9	8.5	8.8	8.8
Newly settled zone	N = 1236	N = 1365	N = 1298	N = 1303
Failure of birth control	2.2	3.9	2.2	4.0
Reluctance to have more children	2.6	4.5	2.5	4.6
Pregnancy endangers woman's health	22.9	23.7	22.9	23.7
Possibility of deformed children	18.1	18.0	17.9	18.3
Inability to afford more children	6.0	5.9	5.8	6.1

[a] The majority of the women not shown as approving abortion expressed disapproval of it; less than 4% of the women gave no opinion. The 5 categories in which the reasons for approval have been placed are not mutually exclusive.
[b] N = total number of eligible women responding.

TABLE 8.A.11. VIEWS OF ELIGIBLE WOMEN AS TO WHETHER HUSBAND OR WIFE SHOULD
BE STERILIZED, BY RESIDENCE, SOCIAL STATUS, AND PARITY

Residence, social status, and parity	Percentage of EW with views on who should be sterilized					No. of EW responding
	Husband	Wife	Either	Neither	No opinion	
OLD URBAN ZONE						
Middle						
0–3	11.0	27.4	4.6	53.0	4.1	1647
4–5	8.5	36.5	3.8	46.5	4.7	469
6 and over	12.0	37.3	3.8	43.5	3.5	400
All parities	10.7	30.6	4.3	50.3	4.1	2516
Low						
0–3	7.7	33.3	1.3	53.8	3.8	78
4–5	3.2	32.3	0.0	54.8	9.7	31
6 and over	13.6	40.9	6.8	31.8	6.8	44
All parities	8.5	35.3	2.6	47.7	5.9	153
Both categories						
0–3	10.8	27.7	4.4	53.0	4.1	1725
4–5	8.2	36.2	3.6	47.0	5.0	500
6 and over	12.2	37.6	4.1	42.3	3.8	444
All parities	10.6	30.9	4.2	50.1	4.2	2669
NEWLY SETTLED ZONE						
Middle						
0–3	11.6	37.7	2.6	46.3	1.8	613
4–5	11.9	40.5	5.4	38.7	3.6	168
6 and over	13.5	45.9	2.2	38.4	0.0	185
All parities	12.0	39.8	3.0	43.5	1.8	966
Low						
0–3	15.4	34.2	2.9	43.5	4.0	623
4–5	10.4	47.1	4.1	34.6	3.8	367
6 and over	11.5	48.4	3.4	34.7	2.0	645
All parities	12.7	42.7	3.4	38.0	3.2	1635
Both categories						
0–3	13.5	35.9	2.8	44.9	2.9	1236
4–5	10.8	45.0	4.5	35.9	3.7	535
6 and over	11.9	47.8	3.1	35.5	1.6	830
All parities	12.5	41.6	3.2	40.1	2.7	2601

(Table 8.A.13). The frequency was higher in both social classes of the NSZ (middle, 48%; low, 61%) than in the OUZ (middle, 43%; low, 51.4%); and in each zone it was more frequent among women of low social status than among those of middle social status. In both zones and among both social classes timing failure was positively associated with parity while no consistent pattern was discernible by age. Likewise, timing failure was positively associated with gravidity and family size (tables not given).

356

TABLE 8.A.12. REASONS WHY WIFE OR HUSBAND SHOULD BE STERILIZED, BY RESIDENCE AND PARITY

(a) Reasons wife should be sterilized

Residence and parity	Percentage of EW giving indicated reason:						No. of EW approving sterilization
	Husband would refuse	Reduce husband's sexual activity	Make husband physically weak	Woman is child-bearer	Man's operation ineffective	Man is wage-earner	
Old urban zone							
0–3	68.0	7.8	4.6	17.2	0.7	1.7	460
4–5	68.0	7.5	2.8	20.2	0.6	1.1	178
6 and over	67.5	7.2	3.6	19.9	0.6	1.2	166
All parities	67.9	7.6	4.0	18.4	0.6	1.5	804
Newly settled zone							
0–3	55.2	10.8	5.6	22.1	3.3	3.1	426
4–5	59.5	11.2	4.3	20.3	2.6	2.2	232
6 and over	62.0	10.4	3.6	16.9	3.1	3.9	384
All parities	58.6	10.7	4.6	19.8	3.1	3.2	1042

(b) Reasons husband should be sterilized

Residence and parity	Percentage of EW giving indicated reason:						No. of EW approving sterilization
	Healthier	Easier	No hospitilization necessary	Wife would refuse	Health of wife bad	Sharing in limiting pregnancies	Wife's operation might have complications	
Old urban zone							
0–3	17.4	13.6	0.5	22.3	3.3	38.6	3.8	184
4–5	10.0	12.5	0.0	12.5	10.0	50.0	2.5	40
6 and over	19.6	11.8	0.0	17.6	5.9	39.2	5.9	51
All parities	16.7	13.1	0.4	20.0	4.7	40.4	4.0	225
Newly settled zone							
0–3	15.1	14.5	0.6	25.8	6.9	28.3	8.2	159
4–5	17.2	13.8	3.4	15.5	1.7	32.8	15.5	58
6 and over	10.6	14.9	2.1	12.8	9.6	37.2	10.6	94
All parities	14.1	14.5	1.6	19.9	6.8	31.8	10.3	311

357

TABLE 8.A.13. TIMING FAILURE OF LAST PREGNANCY, BY RESIDENCE, SOCIAL STATUS, AGE OF ELIGIBLE WOMAN, AND PARITY*

Percentage of EW who felt last pregnancy came too soon, at indicated parities

Social status and age of EW	Old urban zone				Newly settled zone			
	1–3	4–5	6 and over	All parities	1–3	4–5	6 and over	All parities
Middle								
<20	(41.7)	—	—	38.5	42.3	—	—	40.7
20–24	36.8	(75.0)	—	32.3	50.4	(75.0)	—	50.7
25–29	34.0	47.4	(100.0)	35.5	42.9	76.1	87.5	50.4
30–34	35.0	64.7	74.0	47.2	37.7	55.0	61.9	47.1
35–39	33.7	52.6	66.0	50.1	30.3	48.5	58.6	48.2
40–44	22.4	49.0	58.5	47.9	31.0	44.0	52.3	45.4
All ages	33.5	55.4	63.8	43.0	42.2	58.3	58.4	48.3
Low								
<20	(0.0)	—	—	(50.0)	48.5	—	—	47.2
20–24	(57.9)	—	—	(57.9)	59.6	(68.4)	—	60.4
25–29	(21.1)	(50.0)	(50.0)	31.0	57.5	70.0	77.8	64.3
30–34	(68.8)	(37.5)	(60.0)	58.8	44.3	57.1	73.2	61.1
35–39	(20.0)	(60.0)	(72.7)	60.5	50.0	50.0	68.4	62.5
40–44	(37.5)	(40.0)	(60.0)	(45.8)	(40.0)	56.7	64.9	61.8
All ages	44.1	48.4	65.9	51.4	54.5	60.5	69.1	61.8

* Figures in parentheses refer to fewer than 25 eligible women.
Dashes indicate no eligible women with given parameters.

The frequency of timing failure declined with increasing educational level in both regions, although some inconsistency was noted when parity was held constant (Table 8.A.14).

Timing failure was also more frequent among those disapproving of birth control than among those favourable towards it, suggesting that the regularity of contraceptive use (coupled with the educational level analysed above) had something to do with the ability and desire of women to plan their pregnancy.

Ideal Pregnancy Interval

Because of the health benefits of spacing, women were asked how many months there should be between the termination of one pregnancy and the beginning of another. The responses indicated that in both zones the general preference was for a reasonable interval of 2–4 years. The mean interval preferred by women was 32.6 months in the OUZ and 34.1 months in the NSZ. In the OUZ, only 14% of the women preferred an interval of less than 2 years and some 15.5% preferred an interval of 4 or more years; the majority (70.6%) preferred an interval of 2–4 years. The corresponding figures in the NSZ were generally comparable: 11.9%, 22.3%, and 65.8% (Table 8.A.15). There were small differences in the mean interval by age and social status (except in the NSZ where women of middle social status preferred an interval

358

TABLE 8.A.14. TIMING FAILURE OF LAST PREGNANCY, BY RESIDENCE, EDUCATION OF
ELIGIBLE WOMAN, AND PARITY*

Residence and parity	Percentage of EW at indicated educational level who experienced timing failure of last pregnancy				
	No school	Primary	Secondary	College+	All educational levels
Old urban zone					
0–3	44.4	35.6	26.8	30.4	33.4
4–5	53.1	56.3	49.4	(50.0)	55.0
6 and over	58.9	66.6	52.1	(60.0)	64.0
All parities	51.7	46.6	32.7	32.7	43.5
Newly settled zone					
0–3	47.8	49.0	36.7	(100.0)	48.1
4–5	60.9	59.1	(63.6)	(0.0)	59.8
6 and over	67.4	65.7	(80.0)	(100.0)	66.7
All parities	59.1	56.1	45.7	(80.0)	57.0
Both zones					
0–3	47.3	41.2	28.2	32.6	39.6
4–5	59.9	57.6	51.1	(40.0)	57.5
6 and over	66.4	66.1	56.9	(66.7)	65.8
All parities	58.1	50.9	34.5	34.9	50.3

* Figures in parentheses refer to fewer than 25 eligible women.

TABLE 8.A.15. PERCENTAGE DISTRIBUTION OF ELIGIBLE WOMEN BY RESIDENCE,
SOCIAL STATUS, AND IDEAL PREGNANCY INTERVAL

Residence/social status	Percentage of EW specifying an ideal pregnancy interval (months) of:					
	12	12–23	24–35	36–47	48+	No. of EW responding
Old urban zone[a]	1.6	12.4	37.1	33.5	15.5	2669
Newly settled zone[b]	0.6	11.3	33.6	32.2	22.3	2601
Middle social status	1.4	12.5	36.6	32.8	16.6	3402
Low social status	0.5	10.6	32.8	32.9	23.2	1788

[a] Mean ideal pregnancy interval in OUZ: 32.6 months.
[b] Mean ideal pregnancy interval in NSZ: 34.1 months.

of 31 months compared with 35 months for those of low social status) (Table
8.A.16). However, women with secondary or college education preferred
shorter intervals than women of lower education. This was more evident in the
NSZ than in the OUZ (table not given). Taking both areas combined, there
was little difference in the mean interval by child loss (Table 8.A.16). Neither
was there any noticeable difference by family size (data not given).

TABLE 8.A.16. MEAN IDEAL PREGNANCY INTERVAL BY VARIOUS CHARACTERISTICS

Characteristic	Mean ideal pregnancy interval (months)	No. of EW responding
Husband's education		
No school	33.9	1059
Primary	33.0	2587
Secondary	31.4	922
College or higher	29.1	702
EW's education		
No school	33.1	1177
Primary	32.9	3290
Secondary	29.7	668
College or higher	27.5	135
Age of EW		
<20	30.2	164
20–24	32.1	822
25–29	32.2	1280
30–34	33.6	1192
35–39	31.8	1012
40–44	32.2	800
Residence and social status		
Old urban zone		
Middle	32.7	966
Low	33.8	1635
All OUZ	33.4	2601
Newly settled zone		
Middle	31.2	2516
Low	35.0	153
All NSZ	34.1	2669
Child loss		
0	33.5	
1	33.1	
2–3	33.1	

Additional Children Wanted

Women were asked about how many additional children they wanted and their preference by sex (i.e., how many boys and how many girls). The desired numbers of children were analysed according to the parity of the respondents, their social status, their expressed opinions on ideal family size, and the sex of children they already had. The results are summarized in Tables 8.A.17, 18 and 19.

The mean number of the additional children wanted was slightly higher for women in the OUZ than for women in the NSZ, the means being 0.81 and 0.69, respectively. The parity-specific means, however, showed some variation, those in the NSZ being generally higher than those in the OUZ. The relationship between the number of additional children desired and parity was

360

somewhat peculiar. At first, as parity increased from 1–3 to 4–5, the mean desired number decreased from 0.9 to 0.15 in the OUZ and from 1.03 to 0.3 in the NSZ; it then increased again to 0.54 and 0.84 as parity increased to 6 or more in the respective zones. The initial decline was expected in view of the small family size norm in the study population (about 3–4 children). The higher mean number of additional children wanted by women of higher parity (6 and over) may be a generation effect. With a constant mean ideal family size (Table 8.A.17), there was a general tendency for the number of additional children desired to decline with parity (with a few exceptions at parities of 6 and over in both the OUZ and the NSZ). In both zones, the number of additional children desired generally increased with an increase in the ideal family size preferred by the women, although there were a few exceptions.

TABLE 8.A.17. MEAN NUMBER OF ADDITIONAL CHILDREN WANTED, BY RESIDENCE, IDEAL FAMILY SIZE, PARITY, AND SOCIAL STATUS*

(a) By parity

	Mean no. of additional children wanted by EW of indicated parities							
Ideal family size	Old urban zone				Newly settled zone			
	1–3	4–5	6 and over	All parities	1–3	4–5	6 and over	All parities
0	(0.64)	(0.17)	(0.0)	0.32	(0.25)	(0.67)	(0.35)	0.42
1	(0.63)	(0.0)	(0.0)	(0.83)	(0.38)	(0.0)	(0.0)	0.27
2	0.48	0.11	0.0	0.58	0.62	0.24	0.44	0.51
3	0.90	0.83	0.29	0.91	0.95	0.23	0.54 -	0.71
4	1.17	0.12	0.31	0.88	1.32	0.21	0.95	0.77
5	1.63	0.30	(0.48)	0.99	1.98	0.42	0.17	0.92
6 and over	(20.0)	0.41	0.28	0.88	2.23	1.05	0.12	1.07
All family sizes	0.90	0.15	0.54	0.81	1.03	0.30	0.84	0.69

(b) By social status

	Mean no. of additional children wanted by EW of indicated social status					
Ideal family size	Old urban zone			Newly settled zone		
	Middle	Low	All OUZ	Middle	Low	All NSZ
0	(0.25)	(2.00)	0.32	(0.0)	0.56	0.42
1	(0.09)	(0.0)	(0.83)	(0.37)	(0.17)	0.27
2	0.59	0.44	0.58	0.72	0.40	0.51
3	0.92	0.79	0.91	0.93	0.55	0.71
4	0.91	0.43	0.88	1.09	0.58	0.77
5	1.02	(0.67)	0.99	1.51	0.57	0.92
6 and over	0.87	(1.00)	0.88	1.56	0.81	1.07
All family sizes	0.82	0.57	0.81	0.97	0.53	0.69

* Figures in parentheses refer to fewer than 25 eligible women.

361

TABLE 8.A.18. MEAN NUMBER OF ADDITIONAL BOYS WANTED, BY RESIDENCE AND BY NUMBER OF GIRLS AND NUMBER OF BOYS ALREADY PRESENT IN THE FAMILY*

Residence and number of boys present in family	Mean no. of additional boys wanted by EW with indicated no. of girls in family							
	0	1	2	3	4	5	6 and over	All EW
Old urban zone								
0	1.29	0.96	0.77	0.59	(0.45)	(0.00)	(0.00)	0.94
1	0.47	0.42	0.43	0.26	0.22	(0.14)	(0.00)	0.39
2	0.03	0.14	0.14	0.16	0.08	(0.14)	0.06	0.12
3	0.11	0.09	0.06	0.04	0.05	(0.00)	(0.04)	0.07
4	(0.00)	0.06	0.00	0.08	0.00	(0.00)	(0.03)	0.03
5	(0.00)	(0.00)	(0.00)	(0.08)	(0.04)	(0.00)	(0.00)	0.03
6 and over	(0.00)	(0.07)	(0.00)	(0.00)	(0.16)	(0.00)	(0.00)	0.03
All OUZ	0.60	0.40	0.29	0.18	0.13	0.05	0.03	0.36
Newly settled zone								
0	1.30	0.91	0.52	0.29	(0.08)	(0.00)	(0.00)	0.92
1	0.58	0.29	0.22	0.10	0.08	(0.00)	(0.00)	0.34
2	0.11	0.06	0.07	0.03	0.00	0.00	0.00	0.06
3	0.00	0.00	0.02	0.02	0.04	(0.00)	(0.00)	0.01
4	(0.00)	0.00	0.09	0.00	0.00	0.00	0.00	0.02
5	(0.00)	(0.07)	0.29	0.06	(0.00)	(0.00)	(0.00)	0.08
6 and over	(0.00)	(0.00)	0.00	0.00	(0.00)	(0.00)	0.00	0.00
All NSZ	0.70	0.37	0.22	0.08	0.03	0.00	0.00	0.36

* Figures in parentheses refer to fewer than 25 eligible women.

TABLE 8.A.19. MEAN NUMBER OF ADDITIONAL GIRLS WANTED, BY RESIDENCE AND BY NUMBER OF GIRLS AND NUMBER OF BOYS ALREADY PRESENT IN THE FAMILY*

Residence and number of boys present in family	Mean no. of additional girls wanted by EW with indicated no. of girls in family							
	0	1	2	3	4	5	6 and over	All EW
Old urban zone								
0	1.42	0.64	0.19	0.17	(0.00)	(0.00)	(0.00)	0.80
1	1.03	0.33	0.11	0.07	0.00	(0.00)	(0.00)	0.46
2	0.72	0.29	0.14	0.08	0.00	(0.00)	(0.00)	0.30
3	0.34	0.11	0.15	0.02	0.00	(0.00)	(0.00)	0.13
4	(0.08)	0.07	0.06	0.03	0.04	(0.00)	(0.00)	0.05
5	(0.00)	0.07	0.29	(0.00)	(0.17)	(0.00)	(0.00)	0.09
6 and over	(0.00)	(0.00)	(0.00)	(0.11)	(0.00)	(0.00)	(0.00)	0.02
All OUZ	1.04	0.37	0.14	0.07	0.02	0.00	(0.00)	0.43
Newly settled zone								
0	1.33	0.62	0.15	0.07	(0.05)	(0.00)	(0.00)	0.66
1	0.92	0.58	0.24	0.03	0.03	(0.00)	(0.00)	0.48
2	0.81	0.38	0.15	0.10	0.03	0.00	0.00	0.27
3	0.70	0.27	0.13	0.04	0.08	(0.00)	0.11	0.20
4	(0.38)	0.34	0.15	0.02	0.00	0.03	0.10	0.12
5	(0.33)	(0.20)	0.12	0.05	(0.04)	(0.00)	(0.00)	0.07
6 and over	(0.00)	(0.13)	0.05	0.09	0.07	(0.17)	(0.22)	0.06
All NSZ	0.98	0.47	0.16	0.05	0.04	0.01	0.07	0.04

* Figures in parentheses refer to fewer than 25 eligible women.

In both zones, women of middle social status desired more children than women of low social status. The respective means were 0.82 and 0.57 in the OUZ, 0.97 and 0.53 in the NSZ. This differential persisted when the mean ideal family size was held constant. In other words, the ideal-family-size-specific means of additional children desired were higher for the middle than for the low social status women, with only a few exceptions.

The sex of the additional children desired in relation to the sex of the living children is examined in Tables 8.A.18 and 19. When women had not yet had any children, the mean number of girls wanted was somewhat higher than that of boys, especially in the OUZ. In the OUZ, these women wanted 1.42 girls compared with 1.29 boys, and in the NSZ the corresponding figures were 1.33 boys and 1.30 girls. However, women who had had one or more girls but no boys wanted more additional boys than girls, although the means declined with increases in the number of girls already present in the family. Likewise, women who had had one or more boys but no girls wanted on the average more girls than boys. When women already had both boys and girls, the pattern of sex preference was not clear (Tables 8.A.18 and 19).

B. EGYPT

A. F. Moustafa, H. M. Hammam, M. E. Abdel Fattah,
L. M. Hassanein, E. Abdel Kader, A. F. El-Sherbini
& A. R. Omran

Opinions on Family Formation and Health

Opinions on ideal age at marriage

Women were asked what they considered to be the ideal age at marriage for boys and girls. Table 8.B.1 shows that the ideal age at marriage for boys was given by women in the rural, urban, and industrial areas, as 22.5, 24.9, and 26.3 years, respectively. The corresponding ages for girls were 17.7, 20.3, and 21·3 years. Thus, in all 3 areas boys were expected to marry at a higher age than girls. The lowest ideal ages for marriage were given by rural women: 22.5 years for boys and 17.7 years for girls. The highest ideal ages for marriage were given by women in the industrial area: 26.3 years for boys and 21.3 years for girls. The difference between ideal age at marriage for boys and that for girls was about 4.5 years. Women of middle social status gave a higher mean ideal age at marriage for both sexes than those of low social status.

With very few exceptions there was a direct relationship between the age at marriage of the eligible women themselves and mean ideal age at marriage for both boys and girls. The pattern was more pronounced and regular for marriage of girls than for marriage of boys.

TABLE 8.B.1. MEAN IDEAL AGE AT MARRIAGE FOR BOYS AND GIRLS, BY RESIDENCE, SOCIAL STATUS AND AGE AT MARRIAGE OF ELIGIBLE WOMEN*

Sex of child; residence and social status	Mean ideal age at marriage in opinion of EW who married at age:							
	<15	15–17	18–20	21–23	24–26	27–29	30–44	All EW
BOYS								
Rural								
Middle	25.3	24.8	25.0	25.6	(25.8)	(26.0)	(25.0)	24.8
Low	20.9	21.2	21.6	22.1	22.4	(23.8)	(28.0)	21.3
Both categories	22.5	22.4	22.6	23.6	23.4	(24.6)	(26.6)	22.5
Urban								
Middle	26.3	26.5	26.5	26.6	(26.6)	(27.6)	(26.3)	26.5
Low	22.6	22.5	22.7	22.9	(22.9)	(22.0)	(28.4)	22.7
Both categories	24.7	24.9	24.9	25.3	25.2	(26.5)	(27.3)	24.9
Industrial								
Middle	(26.4)	26.8	26.8	28.0	(27.4)	(28.0)	—	26.8
Low	(24.7)	25.9	26.1	(26.3)	(26.7)	—	—	25.9
Both categories	25.3	26.3	26.5	(27.1)	(27.0)	(28.0)	—	26.3
GIRLS								
Rural								
Middle	19.4	19.7	20.3	21.3	(17.9)	(22.7)	(20.3)	19.9
Low	15.9	16.4	16.9	17.1	17.4	(16.6)	(23.7)	16.5
Both categories	17.2	17.5	18.0	18.9	17.6	(19.3)	(22.0)	17.7
Urban								
Middle	21.0	21.5	22.0	22.9	23.6	(23.6)	(19.9)	21.7
Low	17.9	18.0	18.1	18.9	(19.2)	(19.0)	(22.0)	18.1
Both categories	19.7	20.2	20.6	21.7	22.3	(23.0)	(20.9)	20.3
Industrial								
Middle	(20.9)	22.3	22.5	(15.1)	(22.5)	(27.0)	(28.0)	22.5
Low	(19.4)	19.4	19.4	(20.7)	(22.0)	—	(31.0)	19.6
Both categories	20.1	21.1	21.2	16.7	(22.2)	27.0	(29.5)	21.3

* Figures in parentheses refer to fewer than 25 eligible women.

Opinions on family size and spacing

Table 8.B.2 shows that the majority of women in all 3 areas expressed the view that both maternal and child health were better in a small family. As Table 8.B.3 shows, over 89% of the mothers with no schooling believed that maternal and child health were better in a small family. The percentage was even higher for women who had been to school.

Women in all 3 areas believed that a 3-year spacing between births would be preferable to a 1-year spacing and would result in better maternal and child health.

364

TABLE 8.B.2. VIEWS OF ELIGIBLE WOMEN ON FAMILY FORMATION AND HEALTH, BY RESIDENCE

Statements on which women's views were obtained	Percentage of EW giving replies indicated											
	Rural				Urban				Industrial			
	Yes	No	Same	No opinion	Yes	No	Same	No opinion	Yes	No	Same	No opinion
A child's health is better in a small family	91.7	0.5	3.9	3.9	93.4	0.4	2.2	4.0	82.2	1.1	0.3	16.4
The mother's health is better in a small family	91.3	1.0	3.5	4.2	93.2	0.5	1.8	4.5	82.2	1.6	0.6	15.6
A child's health is better when the birth interval is 3 years rather than 1 year	95.2	1.4	0.8	2.6	94.7	1.1	0.3	3.9	79.6	3.4	2.6	14.4
The mother's health is better when the birth interval is 3 years rather than 1 year	94.8	1.3	1.3	2.6	94.6	0.9	0.5	4.0	78.4	6.0	1.0	14.6

TABLE 8.B.3. VIEWS OF ELIGIBLE WOMEN ON FAMILY FORMATION AND HEALTH, BY RESIDENCE AND EDUCATION*

Percentage of EW agreeing with statements in left-hand column

Statements on which women's views were obtained	Rural				Urban				Industrial			
	No school	Primary	Secondary	College	No school	Primary	Secondary	College	No school	Primary	Secondary	College
A child's health is better in a small family	89.6	98.0	(100.0)	—	95.0	97.2	97.1	(50.0)	91.6	89.0	(100.0)	—
The mother's health is better in a small family	89.3	99.0	(100.0)	—	94.7	96.8	95.6	(50.0)	92.0	90.7	(100.0)	—
A child's health is better when the birth interval is 3 years rather than 1 year	98.5	97.1	—	—	99.2	99.2	98.5	—	91.6	90.2	—	—
The mother's health is better when the birth interval is 3 years rather than 1 year	98.7	93.4	—	—	98.9	99.6	97.1	—	91.6	90.8	—	—
A decrease in child mortality would result in fewer children being born	52.8	77.7	83.3	—	73.7	80.9	92.6	(50.0)	36.4	38.7	(50.0)	—

* Figures in parentheses refer to fewer than 25 eligible women.

Opinions on Birth Control

Approval of birth control

Table 8.B.4 shows that, in order of importance, the following 4 reasons for favouring birth control were given by women in both the rural and the urban areas and with both small and larger families: (1) preservation of the mother's health (81.1% rural and 90.9% urban), (2) improvement of child care (48.9% rural and 71.1% urban), (3) improvement of the child's health (42.8% rural and 66.7% urban), and (4) the expense of raising large families (40.6% rural and 63.2% urban). In the industrial area no one reason for approval of birth control predominated. The proportion giving each of the 4 reasons listed was 98%.

Urban women gave much greater importance to birth control than rural women. The smallest difference between residential areas was observed in the percentage of women giving the reason "preservation of mother's health". However, rural women attached less importance to improvement of child care and child health than did urban women. The expense of raising a large family was of much greater concern to the urban group than the rural group.

Family size affected the opinions of rural and urban women differently. In the rural area, all 4 reasons were advanced more frequently by women with large families. Preservation of the mother's health was given as a reason for approval of birth control more often by women with large families in the urban area while improvement of child health and the expense of raising large families were reasons advanced less frequently by these women. In the industrial area almost equal percentages of women advanced each of the 4 reasons, whether they had small or large families (Table 8.B.3).

Table 8.B.4 also shows the reasons for disapproval of birth control by residence and family size. Among women who disapproved of birth control, desire for more children was the reason most often given (59.4% rural and 48.3% urban), followed by preservation of maternal health (20.3% rural and 49.8% urban), husband's disapproval (31.3% rural and 37.7% urban), mother-in-law's opposition (9.1% rural and 12.7% urban), and finally religious objections (4.8% rural and 10.6% urban). In the industrial area, almost equal percentages of women advanced each of the reasons for disapproval, with a slightly higher percentage giving religious reasons.

Family size affected the mother's disapproval of birth control in both the rural and urban groups, but to varying degrees. The relationship between family size and religious objections and between family size and maternal health was a direct one. The percentage of women who wanted more children, as well as the percentage who claimed that the mother-in-law would object, decreased with increase in family size. In the industrial area, all 4 reasons were advanced more frequently by women with large families.

Knowledge and use of birth control

Women were asked whether they had heard of and whether they had previously used or were currently using any of several fertility control methods. Table 8.B.5 shows that in all 3 areas, the most commonly known methods of

TABLE 8.B.4. REASONS FOR APPROVAL OR DISAPPROVAL OF BIRTH CONTROL BY RESIDENCE AND FAMILY SIZE

Residence and family size	Percentage of EW who approve for reasons stated					Percentage of EW who disapprove for reasons stated					
	Preserve health of mother	Care of child	Improve child health	Reduce costs	Total no. of EW in sample	Religion	Maternal health	Husband disapproved	Desire more children	Mother-in-law disapproved	N[a]
Rural											
0–3	76.8	46.9	40.9	35.4	542	3.9	14.6	31.2	65.9	10.6	689
4 and over	84.7	50.4	44.4	45.6	566	6.6	31.5	31.5	46.5	6.1	348
All family sizes	81.1	48.9	42.8	40.6	1108	4.8	20.3	31.3	59.4	9.1	1037
Urban											
0–3	88.5	74.0	68.5	63.9	649	9.3	39.9	39.9	58.7	13.4	442
4 and over	92.5	68.5	64.3	62.8	744	13.0	69.0	34.0	28.1	10.9	230
All family sizes	90.9	71.1	66.7	63.2	1393	10.6	49.8	37.7	48.3	12.7	672
Industrial											
0–3	97.9	98.0	97.9	98.0	245	36.4	28.6	31.0	28.6	28.6	29
4 and over	97.3	97.4	97.7	97.7	304	79.5	76.9	76.9	76.9	76.9	39
All family sizes	97.6	97.6	97.8	97.8	549	61.0	56.7	57.3	56.7	56.7	68

[a] N = total number of eligible women responding.

TABLE 8.B.5. KNOWLEDGE AND USE OF FERTILITY CONTROL METHODS AMONG ELIGIBLE WOMEN, BY RESIDENCE, USE, AND METHOD

Knowledge and use of fertility control methods among EW (%)

Method	Rural (N = 1156[a])				Urban (N = 1044[a])				Industrial (N = 260[a])			
	Never heard of	Heard of and used	Heard of and using	Heard of but never used	Never heard of	Heard of and used	Heard of and using	Heard of but never used	Never heard of	Heard of and used	Heard of and using	Heard of but never used
Condom	78.5	0.1	0.0	9.3	67.5	1.1	1.1	29.6	41.1	0.5	1.1	40.0
Withdrawal	81.7	0.0	0.0	3.0	94.0	0.2	0.4	4.5	58.8	5.0	2.7	20.0
Rhythm	82.0	3.8	2.0	4.0	91.6	0.4	0.5	6.4	69.6	3.5	1.5	11.9
Diaphragm	77.0	0.3	0.6	14.5	66.8	0.5	0.3	31.3	61.2	0.0	0.0	25.4
Douche, etc	70.8	0.3	0.0	14.1	71.0	0.5	0.7	25.4	68.5	0.4	0.8	17.7
Coil or IUD	23.5	2.9	0.4	67.3	6.2	3.7	3.3	85.3	3.1	8.1	7.7	69.6
Orals	5.0	3.3	4.2	77.3	7.2	12.1	11.0	68.3	5.4	16.1	33.8	37.3
Tubectomy	72.7	2.8	0.2	14.6	69.4	0.5	1.0	27.3	70.0	0.4	2.0	14.7
Vasectomy	75.5	0.2	0.0	6.9	84.3	0.1	0.0	12.4	72.7	0.0	0.0	13.1
Abortion	61.7	0.3	0.1	10.5	62.8	0.3	0.2	20.9	19.2	2.7	0.0	57.3
Others	41.9	0.3	0.3	5.4	40.5	0.6	1.2	4.6	11.9	0.0	0.0	5.4

[a] N = total number of eligible women responding

369

fertility control were oral contraceptives ("pills") and the coil (IUD). These contraceptive methods had been used in the past or were currently being used by fewer women in the rural area (7.5% pills and 3.3% IUD) than in the urban area (23.1% pills and 7.0% IUD), while in the industrial area usage was much higher (49.9% pills and 15.8% IUD).

About 60% of both rural and urban women had never heard of abortion as a means of fertility control and very few reported its use (0.4% among rural women and 0.5% among urban women). In the industrial area, 19.2% of women had never heard of abortion, but 2.7% reported its use.

Other methods, such as withdrawal, vasectomy, and tubectomy were largely unknown in all 3 areas. Thus withdrawal was unknown to 81.7% of women in the rural area, 94% in the urban area, and 58.8% in the industrial area, while around 70–80% of women in the 3 areas had never heard of vasectomy or tubectomy.

Opinions on breast feeding as a birth control method

Table 8.B.6(*a*) shows that 35.6% of rural and 36.9% of urban women thought that breast feeding could prevent pregnancy, as compared with only 12.1% among industrial area women. In all 3 residential areas, more women of low than of middle social status believed that breast feeding was capable of preventing pregnancy. The figures for low and middle social status, respectively, were 38.4% and 30.6% in the rural area, 40.8% and 34.7% in the urban area, and 18.7% and 8.6% in the industrial area.

The proportions of women who did not believe that breast feeding could be used to prevent pregnancy were 45.9% in the rural and 47.1% in the urban area, as compared with 78.9% in the industrial area.

The highest percentages of women who were uncertain that breast feeding could be used as a method of birth control were found among those with small families of 0–3 children in the rural and urban areas (Table 8.B.6(*b*)). A higher percentage of women who believed that breast feeding could prevent pregnancy were found among those with families of 4–5 children in both the rural and urban areas (38.6% and 41.5%, respectively).

Opinions on Induced Abortion

Table 8.B.7 shows that few women approved of abortion for socioeconomic or health reasons, especially in the rural and urban areas. The reported figures for those who favoured abortion for any reason ranged from 0.4% to 1.5% in the rural area and from 0.2% to 2.2% in the urban area; the corresponding figures for the industrial area were considerably higher (4.7% to 18.4%). It is also evident that in the rural area the percentage of women who approved of abortion increased with an increase in parity while it remained at the same level for different family sizes. On the other hand, it increased consistently with both parity and family size in the urban and industrial areas.

370

TABLE 8.B.6. VIEWS OF ELIGIBLE WOMEN ON WHETHER BREAST FEEDING PREVENTS PREGNANCY, BY RESIDENCE, SOCIAL STATUS, AND FAMILY SIZE

(a) By residence and social status

Residence and social status	Percentage of EW believing breast feeding does or does not prevent pregnancy			Total no. of EW responding
	Yes	No	No opinion	
Rural				
Middle	30.6	51.3	17.3	353
Low	38.4	42.9	18.1	656
Both categories	35.6	45.9	17.9	1009
Urban				
Middle	34.7	49.3	15.0	608
Low	40.8	43.2	15.5	336
Both categories	36.9	47.1	15.1	944
Industrial				
Middle	8.6	82.2	6.6	152
Low	18.7	72.5	1.3	80
Both categories	12.1	78.9	4.7	232

(b) By residence and family size

Residence and family size	Percentage of EW believing breast feeding does or does not prevent pregnancy			Total no. of EW responding
	Yes	No	No opinion	
Rural				
0–3	34.5	43.7	21.7	586
4–5	38.6	48.4	12.2	254
6 and over	35.5	49.7	13.6	169
All family sizes	35.8	45.9	17.9	1009
Urban				
0–3	34.9	41.9	21.9	484
4–5	41.5	50.0	8.1	258
6 and over	35.6	55.9	7.9	202
All family sizes	36.9	47.1	15.1	944
Industrial				
0–3	13.0	77.2	6.5	92
4–5	11.5	76.9	7.7	52
6 and over	11.3	81.8	1.2	88
All family sizes	12.1	78.9	4.7	232

Failure of other methods of birth control headed the list of reasons for approval of abortion. This reason was given by 0.7–6.3% of women of low parity (0–3) in the 3 residential areas, and by 1.5–18.4% of women of high parity (4 or more). Industrial area women showed the highest percentages for both low and high parity, the figures being 6.3% and 18.4%, respectively.

TABLE 8.B.7. PERCENTAGE OF ELIGIBLE WOMEN APPROVING ABORTION FOR VARIOUS REASONS, BY RESIDENCE, PARITY, AND FAMILY SIZE

Residence and reasons for approving abortion	Percentage of EW approving abortion				Total no. of EW responding
	Parity		Family size		
	0–3	4 and over	0–3	4 and over	
Rural					
Failure of birth control	0.7	1.5	0.9	1.3	2145
Reluctance to have more children	0.5	0.8	0.6	0.6	2145
Pregnancy endangers woman's health	0.5	0.8	0.6	0.6	2145
Possibility of deformed child	0.4	0.9	0.7	0.7	2145
Inability to afford more children	0.0	0.0	0.0	0.0	0
Urban					
Failure of birth control	0.8	2.1	1.2	1.6	2097
Reluctance to have more children	0.7	1.9	1.2	1.6	2097
Pregnancy endangers woman's health	0.9	2.2	1.1	1.6	2097
Possibility of deformed child	0.8	1.9	1.1	1.6	2097
Inability to afford more children	0.0	0.0	0.0	0.0	0
Industrial					
Failure of birth control	6.3	18.4	5.3	12.8	619
Reluctance to have more children	6.3	18.4	5.3	12.8	619
Pregnancy endangers woman's health	4.7	13.4	5.3	12.8	619
Possibility of deformed child	4.7	13.4	5.3	12.8	619
Inability to afford more children	0.0	0.0	0.0	0.0	0

TABLE 8.B.8. VIEWS OF ELIGIBLE WOMEN AS TO WHETHER THE HUSBAND OR THE WIFE SHOULD BE STERILIZED, BY RESIDENCE, SOCIAL STATUS, AND PARITY

Residence, social status, and parity	Percentage of EW with views on who should be sterilized					Total No. of EW responding
	Husband	Wife	Either	Neither	No opinion	
RURAL						
Middle						
0–3	0.7	10.2	0.7	85.7	2.7	147
4–5	3.3	8.3	1.6	86.8	0.0	60
6 and over	2.7	12.3	0.0	82.9	0.7	144
All parities	1.9	10.8	0.6	84.7	1.4	351
Low						
0–3	0.8	3.8	2.6	89.8	2.6	234
4–5	0.7	5.2	0.0	92.2	1.3	152
6 and over	3.4	8.2	0.7	85.5	2.2	268
All parities	1.8	5.9	1.2	89.0	2.1	654
Both categories						
0–3	0.8	6.3	1.8	88.2	2.6	381
4–5	1.4	6.1	0.5	90.6	0.9	212
6 and over	3.1	9.7	0.5	84.5	1.7	412
All parities	1.9	7.6	1.0	87.2	1.9	1005

TABLE 8.B.8 (continued)

Residence, social status, and parity	Percentage of EW with views on who should be sterilized					Total no. of EW responding
	Husband	Wife	Either	Neither	No opinion	
URBAN						
Middle						
0–3	1.2	11.2	2.8	82.4	2.4	250
4–5	3.8	16.9	0.8	76.2	2.3	130
6 and over	2.2	19.3	3.1	72.8	2.6	228
All parities	2.1	15.5	2.5	77.5	2.4	608
Low						
0–3	0.9	8.6	0.0	87.9	1.7	115
4–5	1.9	13.2	1.9	81.1	1.9	53
6 and over	1.8	10.2	0.6	85.0	1.8	166
All parities	1.5	10.1	0.6	85.9	1.9	334
Both categories						
0–3	1.1	10.4	1.9	84.2	2.2	365
4–5	3.3	15.8	1.1	77.6	2.2	183
6 and over	2.0	15.4	2.0	78.0	2.2	394
All parities	1.9	13.5	1.8	80.4	2.2	942
INDUSTRIAL						
Middle						
0–3	16.9	61.1	1.7	18.6	1.7	59
4–5	5.7	77.1	2.9	14.3	0.0	35
6 and over	15.5	55.2	5.2	20.7	3.4	58
All parities	13.8	62.5	3.3	18.4	2.0	152
Low						
0–3	5.3	63.2	0.0	31.6	0.0	19
4–5	0.0	76.9	0.0	23.1	0.0	13
6 and over	12.5	54.2	2.1	27.1	4.1	48
All parities	8.8	60.0	1.2	27.5	2.5	80
Both categories						
0–3	14.1	61.5	1.3	21.8	1.3	78
4–5	4.2	77.0	2.1	16.7	0.0	48
6 and over	14.1	54.7	3.8	23.6	3.8	106
All parities	12.1	61.6	2.6	21.6	2.1	232

Reluctance to have more children was indicated as a reason for termination of pregnancy by a higher proportion of women in the industrial area than in the other two areas. For women of low and high parity, respectively, the figures were: industrial area, 6.3% and 18.4%; urban area, 0.7% and 1.9%; rural area, 0.5% and 0.8%.

The two health reasons suggested for termination of pregnancy—danger to the mother's health and possibility of a deformed child—were accorded almost equal importance by women of both low and high parity and in both family size categories, as can be seen from the percentages in the table. Not a single woman approved of abortion for the socioeconomic reason that the family was unable to afford more children.

Opinions on Sterilization

Although more than 3 women in 4 in the rural and urban areas (80.4–87.2%) did not approve of sterilization, yet the rate of approval was higher than that for abortion (Table 8.B.8). More urban than rural women were in favour of sterilization. Women in the idustrial area had the lowest rate of disapproval of sterilization (21.6%). The cultural and traditional differences between Upper Egypt (comprising both rural and urban areas) and Lower Egypt near Alexandria (industrial area) probably explain the big difference in attitudes towards abortion and sterilization.

Table 8.B.8 also shows that the majority of women who approved of sterilization felt that it was the wife, and not the husband, who should be sterilized (7.6% in the rural area, 13.5% in the urban area, and 61.6% in the industrial area thought the wife should be sterilized, whereas only 1.9% of rural and urban women and 12.1% of industrial area women thought the husband should be sterilized). Sterilization of either spouse was approved of by a low percentage (1.0%, 1.8%, and 2.6% in the rural, urban and industrial areas, respectively).

Women who approved of sterilization were usually of middle rather than low social status in all 3 three residential areas. No consistent relationship existed between parity and sterilization.

Table 8.B.9(a) shows the 6 reasons given by the women for preferring that the wife rather than the husband should be sterilized. The reason advanced most frequently was that the wife is the child-bearing partner (52.9% of rural women, 37.7% of urban women, and 34.5% of industrial area women). Many women thought that the husband would refuse sterilization, especially in the rural and urban areas (31.4% and 36.9%, respectively), although this reason was given much less often by women in the industrial area (9.9%). However, 52.8% of women in the industrial area thought that the wife should be the one

TABLE 8.B.9. REASONS WHY WIFE OR HUSBAND SHOULD BE STERILIZED, BY RESIDENCE, SOCIAL STATUS, AND PARITY

(a) Reasons wife should be sterilized

Residence, social status, and parity	Percentage of EW giving indicated reason:						
	Husband would refuse	Reduce husband's sexual activity	Make husband physically weak	Woman is child bearer	Man's operation ineffective	Man is wage-earner	No. of EW approving of sterilization
RURAL							
Middle							
0–3	50.0	8.3	0.0	41.7	0.0	0.0	12
4–5	40.0	0.0	0.0	60.0	0.0	0.0	5
6 and over	25.0	6.3	6.2	62.5	0.0	0.0	16
All parities	36.4	6.1	3.0	54.5	0.0	0.0	33

TABLE 8.B.9 (continued)

Residence, social status, and parity	Percentage of EW giving indicated reason:						
	Husband would refuse	Reduce husband's sexual activity	Make husband physically weak	Woman is child-bearer	Man's operation ineffective	Man is wage-earner	No. of EW approving of sterilization
Low							
0–3	20.0	0.0	10.0	70.0	0.0	0.0	10
4–5	0.0	12.5	0.0	62.5	12.5	12.5	8
6 and over	42.1	5.3	10.5	36.8	0.0	5.3	19
All parities	27.0	5.4	8.1	51.4	2.7	5.4	37
Both categories							
0–3	36.4	4.5	4.5	54.5	0.0	0.0	22
4–5	15.4	7.7	0.0	61.5	7.7	7.7	13
6 and over	34.3	5.7	8.6	48.6	0.0	2.8	35
All parities	31.4	5.7	5.7	52.9	1.4	2.9	70
URBAN							
Middle							
0–3	28.6	10.7	7.1	46.4	7.2	0.0	28
4–5	33.3	9.5	14.3	33.4	0.0	9.5	21
6 and over	38.5	5.1	7.7	43.6	0.0	5.1	39
All parities	34.1	7.9	9.1	42.0	2.3	4.6	88
Low							
0–3	50.0	20.0	0.0	20.0	0.0	10.0	10
4–5	57.1	14.3	14.3	14.3	0.0	0.0	7
6 and over	35.3	0.0	23.5	35.3	0.0	5.9	17
All parities	44.2	8.8	14.9	26.4	0.0	5.9	34
Both categories							
0–3	34.2	13.2	5.3	39.5	5.3	2.6	38
4–5	39.2	10.7	14.3	28.6	0.0	7.2	28
6 and over	37.5	3.6	12.5	41.1	0.0	5.4	56
All parities	36.9	8.2	10.2	37.7	1.6	4.9	122
INDUSTRIAL							
Middle							
0–3	11.4	2.9	0.0	37.1	0.0	48.6	35
4–5	3.8	3.8	0.0	65.5	3.8	23.1	26
6 and over	12.1	3.0	0.0	39.4	0.0	45.5	33
All parities	9.6	3.2	0.0	45.7	1.1	40.4	94
Low							
0–3	0.0	0.0	0.0	8.3	0.0	91.7	12
4–5	10.0	0.0	0.0	0.0	0.0	90.0	10
6 and over	15.4	0.0	0.0	19.2	0.0	65.4	26
All parities	10.4	0.0	0.0	12.5	0.0	77.1	48
Both categories							
0–3	8.5	2.1	0.0	29.8	0.0	59.6	47
4–5	5.6	2.8	0.0	47.2	2.8	41.6	36
6 and over	13.6	1.7	0.0	30.5	0.0	54.2	59
All parities	9.9	2.1	0.0	34.5	0.7	52.8	142

TABLE 8.B.9 (continued)

(b) Reasons husband should be sterilized

Residence and parity	Percentage of EW giving indicated reason:							No. of EW approving of sterilization
	Healthier	Easier	No hospitilization necessary	Wife would refuse	Health of wife bad	Sharing in limiting pregnancies	Wife's operation might have complications	
Rural								
0–3	100.0	0.0	0.0	0.0	0.0	0.0	0.0	3
4–5	80.0	0.0	0.0	20.0	0.0	0.0	0.0	5
6 and over	35.3	11.8	0.0	29.4	11.8	5.8	5.9	17
All parities	52.0	8.0	0.0	24.0	8.0	4.0	4.0	25
Urban								
0–3	35.3	33.3	16.7	16.7	0.0	0.0	0.0	6
4–5	0.0	14.3	14.3	57.1	0.0	14.3	0.0	7
6 and over	44.5	0.0	11.1	33.3	0.0	11.1	0.0	9
All parities	27.3	13.6	13.6	36.4	0.0	9.1	0.0	22
Industrial								
0–3	72.7	0.0	0.0	9.1	9.1	0.0	9.1	11
4–5	100.0	0.0	0.0	0.0	0.0	0.0	0.0	2
6 and over	33.3	6.7	0.0	26.7	33.3	0.0	0.0	15
All parities	53.6	3.6	0.0	17.8	21.4	0.0	3.6	28

to be sterilized because the husband is the wage earner; the corresponding proportions in the rural and urban areas were only 2.9% and 4.9%. Rather higher percentages of women in the latter areas thought that sterilization would make the husband weak or reduce his sexual activity, but in the industrial area these reasons received little or no support. In all 3 areas, very few, if any, women thought that sterilization was an ineffective method of birth control.

Table 8.B.9(b) shows that in the rural and urban areas, the two most important reasons for preferring sterilization of the husband were that he was healthier and that the wife would refuse (52.0% and 24.0%, respectively, in the rural area and 27.3% and 36.4%, respectively, in the urban area). In the industrial area, the 3 reasons most often advanced were that the husband was healthier (53.6%), that the health of the wife would suffer (21.4%), and that the wife would refuse (17.8%). The reasons given for preferring sterilization of the husband showed no consistent relationship with parity.

Timing Failure of Last Pregnancy

Table 8.B.10 shows that in the rural and urban areas, women who felt that their last pregnancy had come sooner than they had wanted ("timing failure"), desired more children than women who had not failed. The mean ideal family size among women who had experienced timing failure was 4.3 in the rural area and 3.8 in the urban area, compared with 3.7 and 3.6, respectively, among women who had not experienced timing failure of their last pregnancy. In the industrial area, the mean ideal family size was 3.5 for both women who had and who had not experienced timing failure of their last pregnancy. The higher mean ideal family size among women who had experienced timing failure may be an indication that women who want a large family tend to be more lax in the use of birth control.

TABLE 8.B.10. MEAN IDEAL FAMILY SIZE BY RESIDENCE AND TIMING FAILURE OF LAST PREGNANCY

Residence	Mean ideal family size among women with and without timing failure of last pregnancy				No. of EW responding
	With	Without	Unknown	All EW responding	
Rural	4.3	3.7	4.2	3.8	562
Urban	3.8	3.6	3.6	3.6	827
Industrial	3.5	3.5	3.4	3.5	574

Ideal Pregnancy Interval

Table 8.B.11 shows that more rural than urban women believed in pregnancy intervals of less than 24 months (37.8% rural and 32.1% urban). A similar difference was noted for an ideal pregnancy interval of less than 36 months (66.6% rural and 63.9% urban). However, a pregnancy interval of

377

TABLE 8.B.11. PERCENTAGE DISTRIBUTION OF ELIGIBLE WOMEN, BY RESIDENCE, SOCIAL STATUS, IDEAL PREGNANCY INTERVAL, AND FAMILY SIZE

Residence, social status, and ideal pregnancy interval (months)	Percentage of EW with following family sizes who specified ideal pregnancy intervals indicated in left-hand column:							
	0	1	2	3	4	5	6 and over	All family sizes
RURAL								
Middle								
<12	4.4	—	1.3	1.6	—	—	1.5	1.4
12–23	37.8	40.0	44.4	42.2	44.4	41.4	40.3	40.9
24–35	15.5	31.3	26.4	28.1	27.0	34.5	23.9	25.4
36–47	6.7	8.8	8.3	9.4	1.6	12.1	9.1	8.3
48 and over	12.2	6.3	8.3	6.3	8.0	8.6	10.5	9.5
No opinion	23.4	13.6	11.3	12.4	19.0	3.4	14.3	14.5
Low								
<12	2.3	2.6	2.6	0.8	2.8	1.9	0.5	1.4
12–23	27.3	41.6	40.0	32.8	33.8	40.8	30.7	33.7
24–25	23.9	21.2	36.5	31.2	37.3	24.2	32.0	30.6
36–47	1.1	1.8	4.3	4.7	4.2	5.7	5.5	4.7
48 and over	12.5	6.2	2.6	8.6	9.1	7.0	7.2	7.3
No opinion	32.9	26.2	14.0	21.9	12.8	20.4	24.1	22.3
Both categories								
<12	3.4	1.6	2.1	1.0	1.9	1.4	0.9	1.4
12–23	32.6	40.9	41.7	35.9	37.1	40.9	33.9	36.4
24–35	19.7	25.4	32.6	30.2	34.1	27.0	29.3	28.8
36–47	3.9	4.7	5.9	6.3	3.4	7.4	6.7	6.0
48 and over	12.3	6.2	4.8	7.8	8.8	7.4	8.5	8.1
No opinion	28.1	21.2	12.9	18.8	14.7	15.9	20.7	19.3
URBAN								
Middle								
<12	6.8	2.5	3.5	3.2	—	—	2.4	2.5
12–23	24.5	29.7	39.5	23.4	22.8	30.3	29.2	28.5
24–35	25.4	33.0	27.1	34.6	36.8	29.5	31.7	31.3
36–47	12.7	11.9	9.0	11.3	12.5	13.9	10.9	11.4
48 and over	18.6	15.2	15.3	22.6	19.8	20.5	18.2	18.6
No opinion	12.0	7.7	5.5	4.9	8.1	5.8	7.6	7.3
Low								
<12	2.7	1.4	6.1	2.4	3.0	2.6	1.4	2.2
12–23	22.2	28.1	26.5	30.9	27.7	29.3	33.4	31.0
24–35	25.0	37.7	28.5	30.9	29.2	38.7	32.7	32.6
36–47	2.7	7.2	16.3	7.4	10.7	6.7	8.4	8.5
48 and over	5.6	8.7	8.2	11.1	21.5	13.3	12.3	12.1
No opinion	41.8	16.9	14.3	17.3	7.9	9.4	11.8	13.6
Both categories								
<12	5.8	2.1	4.1	2.9	1.0	1.0	2.0	2.4
12–23	24.0	29.4	36.3	26.3	24.4	29.9	31.0	29.7
24–35	25.3	34.7	27.5	33.2	34.3	33.0	32.1	31.8
36–47	10.4	10.2	10.9	9.7	11.9	11.2	9.9	10.3
48 and over	15.6	12.8	13.5	18.0	20.4	17.8	15.7	16.1
No opinion	18.9	10.8	7.7	9.9	8.0	7.1	9.3	9.7

TABLE 8.B.11 (continued)

Residence, social status, and ideal pregnancy interval (months)	Percentage of EW with following family sizes who specified ideal pregnancy intervals indicated in left-hand column:							
	0	1	2	3	4	5	6 and over	All family sizes
INDUSTRIAL[a]								
Middle								
<12	—	—	—	—	—	5.7	1.5	1.1
12–23	8.9	—	—	3.0	3.0	5.7	5.9	4.6
24–35	42.8	45.9	35.0	39.4	24.2	34.3	29.9	34.8
36–47	32.1	40.5	42.5	48.5	60.6	34.3	37.2	40.2
48 and over	12.5	8.1	22.5	9.1	3.0	20.0	22.6	16.4
No opinion	11.7	5.5	0.0	0.0	9.2	0.0	2.9	2.9
Low								
<12	—	(7.1)	—	—	—	—	—	0.4
12–23	3.4	—	—	—	—	—	2.3	1.6
24–35	41.4	(42.8)	(35.0)	(27.8)	(43.5)	(17.6)	37.5	36.5
36–47	41.4	(28.6)	(50.0)	(61.1)	(43.5)	(64.8)	37.5	42.6
48 and over	6.9	(14.3)	(5.0)	(11.1)	(13.0)	(17.6)	19.0	15.3
No opinion	6.9	(7.2)	(10.0)	(0.0)	(0.0)	(0.0)	3.2	3.6
Both categories								
<12	—	2.0	—	—	—	3.8	0.7	0.8
12–23	7.1	—	—	2.0	1.8	3.8	4.1	3.4
24–35	12.4	16.1	35.0	35.3	32.1	28.8	33.8	35.5
36–47	35.3	37.2	45.0	52.9	53.6	44.2	37.3	41.2
48 and over	10.6	9.8	16.7	9.8	7.1	19.2	21.1	16.0
No opinion	4.6	5.9	3.3	0.0	5.4	0.2	3.2	3.1

[a] Figures in parentheses refer to fewer than 25 eligible women.

24–35 months was preferred by more urban than rural women (31.8% and 28.8%, respectively). Industrial area women preferred a longer ideal pregnancy interval (41.2% preferred 36–47 months). It was interesting to find that the percentage of women who favoured an interval of over 48 months was 16.0% in both the urban and the industrial area. However, the percentage was lower among rural women (8.1%).

Preference for a pregnancy interval of 36 months or more was more prevalent among women of middle than of low social status in both the rural and the urban areas (17.8% middle and 12.0% low social status in the rural area) compared with 30.0% middle and 20.6% low social status in the urban area). In the industrial area, the percentage of women preferring a long pregnancy interval was high in both social status categories (56.6% middle and 57.9% low social status). No clear relationship between actual family size and ideal pregnancy interval was observed.

Mean ideal pregnancy interval by various characteristics

Table 8.B.12 shows the mean ideal pregnancy interval by education of the husband and the wife, by age of the wife, and by social status. Education of the husband showed no relationship to ideal pregnancy interval, except in the industrial area where the mean ideal pregnancy interval decreased with increasing education of the husband.

In the rural area, women with no education preferred a shorter pregnancy interval than women with primary or secondary education. However, in the urban and industrial areas, the preferred pregnancy interval became shorter with an increase in the educational level of the woman.

TABLE 8.B.12. MEAN IDEAL PREGNANCY INTERVAL BY VARIOUS CHARACTERISTICS*

Characteristic	Rural		Urban		Industrial	
	Mean ideal pregnancy interval (months)	No. of EW in sample	Mean ideal pregnancy interval (months)	No. of EW in sample	Mean ideal pregnancy interval (months)	No. of EW in sample
Husband's education						
No school	20.1	1376	23.3	505	35.4	57
Primary	21.6	316	23.7	929	34.4	360
Secondary	21.3	62	22.8	281	26.9	60
College +	(37.0)	6	23.1	61	—	—
Unknown	—	384	—	314	—	142
EW's education						
No school	20.4	1668	23.7	1317	35.7	350
Primary	22.1	84	22.4	408	28.6	123
Secondary	(22.0)	6	22.8	51	(15.8)	4
College +	—	—	(17.5)	6	—	—
Unknown	—	384	—	314	—	—
Age of EW						
<20	13.0	102	12.0	77	(12.6)	16
20–24	15.1	328	14.3	335	16.2	93
25–29	16.9	412	18.8	381	25.2	87
30–34	19.1	351	22.3	351	31.8	62
35–39	24.1	338	27.6	362	37.4	109
40–44	34.9	230	40.3	277	55.9	110
Unknown	—	384	—	314	—	142
Social status						
Middle	21.8	586	24.8	1078	34.4	288
Low	19.9	1175	21.5	705	32.2	189
Unknown	—	384	—	314	—	142
Parity of EW's mother						
1	21.9	57	27.2	66	(39.6)	19
2–3	21.5	297	24.4	333	37.6	74
4–5	19.5	541	24.9	556	35.6	137
6–7	25.8	359	21.5	405	31.9	138
8–9	17.9	249	21.4	187	31.1	74
10–11	21.3	60	23.6	52	(21.4)	14
12–13	(19.7)	9	(20.3)	17	(55.0)	3
14–15	(21.6)	5	(19.0)	3	(9.0)	1
16 and over	(21.5)	11	(24.6)	15	(16.5)	4
Unknown	—	384	—	314	—	142

* Figures in parentheses refer to fewer than 25 eligible women.

380

There was an increase in mean ideal pregnancy interval with an increase in the mother's age in all 3 areas of residence. Women of middle social status preferred a longer pregnancy interval than those of low social status.

There was an inverse relationship between the ideal pregnancy interval and parity by residence, except at parities 6 and 7 in the rural area. For the most part, the mean ideal pregnancy interval became shorter with increasing parity. After parity 10, this relationship was reversed; however, the small sample with such high parities did not allow for further follow-up (table not shown).

C. PAKISTAN

Afroze Qazi & A. R. Omran

Opinions on Family Formation and Health

Opinions on ideal family size

The ideal family size that the interviewed women preferred has already been discussed in detail in Table 2.C.6 of chapter 2. It was found that, on the average, the women preferred an ideal family size of about 4 children.

TABLE 8.C.1. MEAN IDEAL AGE AT MARRIAGE FOR BOYS AND GIRLS, BY RESIDENCE, SOCIAL STATUS, AND AGE AT MARRIAGE OF ELIGIBLE WOMAN*

Sex of child, residence, and social status	Mean ideal age at marriage in the opinion of EW who married at age:								
	<12	12–14	15–17	18–20	21–23	24–26	27–29	30 and over	All EW
BOYS									
Semi-urban									
Middle	(22.5)	25.8	26.1	26.4	26.4	(27.4)	(26.6)	—	26.1
Low	23.9	25.5	25.2	25.1	25.7	(25.2)	(27.5)	—	25.3
Both categories	23.6	25.6	25.7	25.9	26.2	26.7	(26.8)	—	25.7
Urban									
Middle	(25.9)	26.6	26.6	26.9	27.7	27.8	28.0	(27.4)	26.9
Low	(25.8)	25.3	25.9	26.2	(24.5)	(28.0)	(22.0)	—	25.7
Both categories	(25.8)	26.4	26.6	26.8	27.7	27.8	27.8	(27.4)	26.8
GIRLS									
Semi-urban									
Middle	(18.0)	19.0	19.4	20.0	20.2	(20.0)	(20.8)	—	19.5
Low	17.8	18.6	18.8	18.9	19.4	(20.2)	(20.0)	—	18.8
Both categories	17.8	18.8	19.1	19.5	20.0	20.1	(20.7)	—	19.1
Urban									
Middle	(19.3)	19.1	19.3	19.6	20.2	21.0	21.3	(21.1)	19.6
Low	(17.9)	17.3	18.0	18.9	(18.5)	(21.5)	(20.0)	—	18.0
Both categories	18.4	18.9	19.2	19.5	20.2	21.0	21.2	(21.1)	19.5

* Figures in parentheses refer to fewer than 25 eligible women.

TABLE 8.C.2. VIEWS OF ELIGIBLE WOMEN ON FAMILY FORMATION AND HEALTH, BY RESIDENCE AND SOCIAL STATUS

(a) Urban

Statements or questions on which women's views obtained	Percentage of EW giving replies indicated											
	Middle status				Low status				Both categories			
	Yes	No	Same	No opinion	Yes	No	Same	No opinion	Yes	No	Same	No opinion
A child's health is better in a small family	94.4	0.3	4.3	1.0	89.3	0.0	3.4	7.3	94.0	0.3	4.3	1.4
The mother's health is better in a small family	94.6	0.4	4.0	1.0	89.9	0.0	3.4	6.7	94.1	0.4	4.0	1.5
A child's health is better when the birth interval is 3 years rather than 1 year	96.1	1.6	1.8	0.5	91.6	0.0	2.8	5.6	95.8	1.4	1.9	0.9
The mother's health is better when the birth interval is 3 years rather than 1 year	96.3	1.4	1.7	0.6	92.2	0.0	2.2	5.6	96.0	1.3	1.8	0.9
A decrease in childhood mortality would result in fewer children being born	65.2	20.7	0.0	14.1	57.6	15.6	0.0	26.8	64.6	20.3	0.0	15.1
A mother who is sick for a long time should not have any more children	3,4	95.8	0.0	0.8	1.7	93.3	0.0	5.0	3.3	95.6	0.0	1.1
Would you use birth control if the health of your children would suffer from an additional pregnancy?	89.7	6.7	—	3.6	75.4	17.9	—	6.7	88.6	7.5	0.0	3.9
Would you use birth control if your health would suffer from becoming pregnant?	89.8	6.5	—	3.7	75.4	17.9	—	6.7	88.7	7.4	0.0	3.9

(b) Semi-urban

TABLE 8.C.2 (continued)

Statements or questions on which women's views obtained	Percentage of EW giving replies indicated											
	Middle status				Low status				Both categories			
	Yes	No	Same	No opinion	Yes	No	Same	No opinion	Yes	No	Same	No opinion
A child's health is better in a small family	98.6	0.0	0.6	0.8	99.2	0.2	0.3	0.3	98.9	0.1	0.5	0.5
The mother's health is better in a small family	98.7	0.1	0.5	0.7	99.2	0.2	0.3	0.3	99.0	0.1	0.4	0.5
A child's health is better when the birth interval is 3 years rather than 1 year	98.4	0.3	0.6	0.7	98.7	0.3	0.3	0.8	98.5	0.3	0.5	0.7
The mother's health is better when the birth interval is 3 years rather than 1 year	98.3	0.3	0.7	0.7	98.7	0.2	0.3	0.8	98.5	0.3	0.5	0.7
A decrease in childhood mortality would result in fewer children being born	65.8	19.3	—	14.9	61.5	19.5	—	19.0	63.4	19.4	0.2	17.0
A mother who is sick for a long time should not have any more children	2.9	95.5	0.0	1.6	3.3	95.5	0.0	1.3	3.1	95.5	—	1.4
Would you use birth control if the health of your children would suffer from an additional pregnancy?	89.7	5.0	—	5.3	88.7	5.7	—	5.6	89.2	5.4	—	5.4
Would you use birth control if your health would suffer from becoming pregnant?	90.4	4.4	—	5.2	89.1	5.4	—	5.5	89.8	4.9	—	5.3

383

Opinions on ideal age at marriage

The women selected for this study were asked what they considered to be the ideal age at marriage for boys and girls. The ideal ages at marriage stated by women of the semi-urban and urban areas for boys was 25.7 and 26.8 years, respectively, and for girls 19.1 and 19.5 years, respectively. Women of middle social status in both areas preferred the age at marriage a little higher than those of low social status (Table 8.C.1). On the average, a difference of 7 years between the ideal ages at marriage for boys and girls was found. In all cases, there was a tendency for women married at a young age (less than 12) to give a low ideal age of marriage.

Opinions on family formation

Almost all the women, whatever their social status, educational standard, or place of residence, expressed the view that maternal and child health were better in a small family than in a larger one. Women of both middle and low social status believed that the health of both mother and child was better with a birth interval of 3 years than with an interval of 1 year (Table 8.C.2). About 65% of the women believed that a decrease in child mortality would result in fewer children being born.

It was suggested by 95.6% of the respondents that if a woman had been sick for a long time she should not have any more children, while more than 80% thought that if additional pregnancies would affect the health of the children, then birth control methods should be used by the mothers. A majority of women (about 89%) also believed that if their health were to suffer as a result of becoming pregnant they would use some method of birth control (Table 8.C.3).

Opinions on Birth Control

Approval of birth control

An overwhelming majority of women interviewed approved of birth control irrespective of their age, parity, or residence (Table 8.C.4). In the semi-urban area, 90.8% of the women expressed approval of birth control; in the urban area, the figure was 91.3%.

The proportion who expressed approval increased only slightly with education, the increase being greater in the urban area (Table 8.C.5). In both areas, birth control was approved of more often as a method of spacing pregnancies than for limiting their number.

The reasons given for approval of birth control were preservation of the mother's health, better care of the child, improved child health, and economic considerations. All of these reasons were supported by almost all the women (99%), irrespective of family size or residence.

Among the women who disapproved of birth control, the main reasons given were religious objections, harm to maternal health, and husband's disapproval. Less frequently stated reasons were a desire for more children and mother-in-law's disapproval (Table 8.C.6).

TABLE 8.C.3. VIEWS OF ELIGIBLE WOMEN ON FAMILY FORMATION, BY RESIDENCE AND EDUCATION

Statements or questions on which women's views obtained	Percentage of women giving affirmative answer					
	Semi-urban			Urban		
	No school	Primary	Secondary	No school	Primary	Secondary
A child's health is better in a small family	98.7	99.2	99.5	91.1	95.6	95.4
The mother's health is better in a small family	98.7	99.2	100.0	91.5	95.5	95.6
A child's health is better when the birth interval is 3 years rather than 1 year	98.2	99.4	99.5	94.6	97.0	96.1
The mother's health is better when the birth interval is 3 years rather than 1 year	98.2	99.4	99.5	94.7	97.5	96.2
A decrease in childhood mortality would result in fewer children being born	62.3	64.9	71.8	63.7	65.4	64.8
A mother who is sick for a long time should not have any more children	60.3	23.3	16.4	34.6	25.9	39.5
Would you use birth control if the health of your children would suffer from an additional pregnancy?	31.6	28.7	39.7	69.7	21.7	8.6
Would you use birth control if your health would suffer from becoming pregnant?	69.6	21.7	8.7	31.5	28.7	39.8

385

TABLE 8.C.4. APPROVAL AND USE OF BIRTH CONTROL BY ELIGIBLE WOMEN, BY RESIDENCE, AGE, AND PARITY

Residence, age and parity of EW	EW approving of birth control		Use of birth control among women who approve (%)			Use of birth control among women who disapprove (%)		
	%	N[a]	Ever used	Never used	Not known	Ever used	Never used	Not known
AGE								
Semi-urban								
<25	89.7	513	18.9	78.5	2.6	—	100.0	—
25–34	91.3	1051	44.2	54.6	1.2	7.1	92.9	0.0
35–44	90.8	825	36.0	63.0	0.9	—	98.3	1.7
All ages	90.8	2389	36.0	62.6	1.4	2.8	96.5	0.7
Urban								
<25	91.3	519	41.8	55.9	2.3	—	91.7	8.3
25–34	92.8	1128	67.6	31.6	0.8	6.1	90.9	3.0
35–44	89.1	826	61.8	37.4	0.8	0.4	87.0	2.6
All ages	91.3	2473	60.3	38.6	1.1	6.7	89.4	3.9
PARITY								
Semi-urban								
0	84.3	197	1.2	94.6	4.2	0.0	100.0	0.0
1–3	90.4	668	24.3	74.3	1.3	4.9	95.1	0.0
4–5	92.5	563	42.4	55.7	1.9	3.3	96.7	0.0
6 and over	91.4	961	46.8	52.5	0.7	1.5	96.9	1.5
All parities	90.8	2389	36.0	62.6	1.4	2.8	96.5	0.7
Urban								
0	90.2	256	3.9	90.5	5.6	0.0	100.0	0.0
1–3	92.8	971	59.9	39.2	0.9	3.4	87.9	8.6
4–5	92.5	533	74.2	25.4	0.4	2.9	97.1	0.0
6 and over	88.6	713	70.6	29.1	0.3	13.0	84.1	2.9
All parities	91.3	2473	60.3	38.6	1.1	6.7	89.4	3.9

[a] N = total number of eligible women responding.

TABLE 8.C.5. APPROVAL AND EVER USE OF BIRTH CONTROL, BY RESIDENCE AND EDUCATION

Attitude to birth control	Percentage of EW with attitude shown in left-hand column					
	Semi-urban			Urban		
	No school	Primary	Secondary or higher	No school	Primary	Secondary or higher
Approve use	90.2	91.6	93.8	85.7	92.6	95.1
Approve use to limit pregnancy	31.3	38.2	32.3	47.0	61.3	58.8
Approve use to space pregnancy	91.0	92.3	95.3	86.0	91.9	94.0
Ever used birth control[a]	31.4	38.2	32.3	47.0	61.3	58.8
No. of EW responding	1680	513	195	827	706	940

[a] Among EW approving of contraception.

Residence and family size	Percentage of EW who approve for reasons stated					Percentage of EW who disapprove for reasons stated					
	Preserve health of mother	Care of child	Improve child health	Reduce costs	N[a]	Religion	Maternal health	Husband disapproves	Desire more children	Mother-in-law disapproves	N[a]
Semi-urban											
0–3	99.8	100.0	100.0	99.8	895	90.4	84.0	72.0	32.0	33.3	52
4 and over	99.4	99.9	99.8	99.8	1274	90.0	83.1	66.3	34.8	34.1	90
All family sizes	99.5	100.0	99.9	99.8	2169	90.1	83.5	68.3	33.8	33.8	142
Urban											
0–3	98.0	100.0	99.4	99.6	1195	81.0	65.8	29.5	20.5	29.1	79
4 and over	98.3	99.9	99.4	99.6	1061	91.9	82.0	59.0	36.0	32.3	100
All family sizes	98.1	100.0	99.4	99.6	2256	86.6	74.9	59.2	29.2	30.9	179

[a] N = total number of eligible women responding.

Willingness to use birth control for health reasons

The women were asked whether they would want to use birth control if additional pregnancies would constitute a definite threat to their own health or to the health of their children. About 95% of the women in both the urban and semi-urban areas who approved of birth control in principle said they would be willing to use contraception for the sake of their children's health, while approximately the same percentage expressed a willingness to use birth control to safeguard their own health.

Among the women who disapproved of birth control in principle, 22.5% in the semi-urban area and 19.6% in the urban area said that they would be willing to use contraceptives if the health of their children were threatened. In both areas, about 20% of the women who disapproved of birth control expressed a willingness to use it to safeguard their own health (Table 8.C.7).

TABLE 8.C.7. ATTITUDE OF ELIGIBLE WOMEN TOWARDS BIRTH CONTROL, BY RESIDENCE AND FAMILY SIZE

Residence and family size	Percentage of EW approving birth control in principle who would use it for stated reason:		Percentage of EW disapproving birth control in principle who would use it for stated reason:	
	to safeguard health of child	to safeguard health of mother	to safeguard health of child	to safeguard health of mother
Semi-urban				
0–3	92.5	93.4	15.4	13.5
4 and over	96.8	97.4	26.7	25.6
All family sizes	95.0	95.8	22.5	21.1
Urban				
0–3	94.5	94.6	20.3	19.0
4 and over	95.5	95.7	19.0	19.0
All family sizes	94.9	95.1	19.6	19.0

Knowledge of birth control

A substantial proportion (68.8%) had some knowledge or a general awareness of contraceptive methods. This was probably due to the fact that the areas selected for the study were well covered by family planning programmes. In both the semi-urban and urban areas there were a number of family planning clinics to which field workers were attached. These field workers or motivators visit the homes and diffuse information about family planning.

Although the knowledge had become widespread as a result of the mass media campaign that formed part of the national programme, not all the methods were equally well known. The overwhelming majority of women interviewed in the semi-urban area had heard of the condom (91.0%), the IUD (94.7%), oral contraceptives (96.9%), and abortion (95.7%). The corresponding proportions in the urban area were 90.6%, 89.8%, 95.9%, and 92.2%. The women were also well informed about tubectomy and vesectomy but only about half of them were familiar with the withdrawal, rhythm, and diaphragm methods (Table 8.C.8).

No substantial differences in knowledge were noted between women of middle and low social status or between women of urban and semi-urban areas, except in the case of the withdrawal method, which was known to 55.3% of semi-urban women but to only 37.2% of urban women.

TABLE 8.C.8. KNOWLEDGE AND USE OF FERTILITY CONTROL METHODS AMONG ELIGIBLE WOMEN, BY RESIDENCE, SOCIAL STATUS, USE, AND METHOD

Social status and method	Knowledge and use of fertility control methods among EW (%)							
	Semi-urban				Urban			
	Never heard of	Heard of and used	Heard of and using	Heard of but never used	Never heard of	Heard of and used	Heard of and using	Heard of but never used
Middle								
Condom	0.4	5.4	11.7	74.2	8.5	14.4	23.1	53.3
Withdrawal	43.9	0.4	0.8	44.2	62.0	2.2	6.4	29.1
Rhythm	54.5	0.7	0.9	43.6	50.3	3.0	4.3	42.1
Diaphragm	44.1	0.7	0.3	53.8	52.6	2.0	0.5	44.1
Douche, etc.	27.3	1.8	1.6	69.1	39.4	3.1	2.0	55.1
Coil or IUD	4.8	5.0	1.8	87.8	10.2	5.7	1.3	82.2
Orals	3.0	7.9	4.3	84.6	3.9	13.0	5.3	77.4
Tubectomy	7.1	0.0	1.7	91.0	7.4	—	3.5	88.9
Vasectomy	11.0	0.0	0.5	88.3	12.6	—	1.1	86.0
Abortion	2.9	0.8	0.0	95.0	7.3	3.7	—	87.5
Others	5.3	0.2	0.3	0.8	7.1	0.1	0.2	0.6
Low								
Condom	9.5	4.6	7.1	78.6	21.2	10.1	10.1	56.4
Withdrawal	45.5	0.3	0.4	53.3	72.1	1.1	4.5	20.7
Rhythm	61.1	0.5	0.8	37.3	66.5	1.1	3.9	27.4
Diaphragm	48.5	0.6	0.1	50.1	60.9	—	1.1	36.3
Douche, etc.	30.9	1.8	0.8	66.6	46.4	0.6	1.1	49.7
Coil or IUD	5.3	5.5	2.8	85.9	10.1	5.0	1.1	82.1
Orals	3.1	8.8	7.0	81.1	6.7	9.4	3.0	70.0
Tubectomy	7.4	0.0	1.7	90.9	13.4	0.0	2.2	83.2
Vasectomy	13.4	—	0.4	86.1	20.1	—	—	78.2
Abortion	3.2	0.5	0.0	95.1	15.1	0.6	—	81.0
Others	5.9	0.9	0.7	1.6	10.1	—	—	0.6
Both categories								
Condom	9.0	5.0	9.4	76.4	9.4	14.1	22.2	53.9
Withdrawal	44.7	0.4	0.6	53.7	62.8	2.1	6.3	28.5
Rhythm	57.8	0.6	0.9	40.4	51.5	2.8	4.2	41.0
Diaphragm	46.7	0.6	0.2	51.9	53.2	1.8	0.6	43.6
Douche, etc.	29.1	1.8	1.2	67.8	39.9	3.0	1.9	54.8
Coil or IUD	5.1	5.3	2.3	86.9	10.2	5.7	1.3	82.2
Orals	3.1	8.3	5.7	82.5	4.1	12.7	5.2	77.6
Tubectomy	7.2	0.0	1.7	91.0	7.8	—	3.4	88.5
Vasectomy	12.2	0.0	0.5	87.2	13.1	—	1.0	85.5
Abortion	3.1	0.6	0.0	95.1	7.8	3.5	—	87.1
Others	5.6	0.6	0.5	1.2	7.3	0.1	0.2	0.6

NOTE: Percentages do not add up to 100 as ''no response' cases were not included.

Use of birth control

Although the number of women who approved of birth control was large, only one third to one half of them had ever practised or were practising contraception. Among the semi-urban women who approved the use of birth control, only 36% had ever used a contraceptive, while the remaining 62.6% had never used any method. Of the urban women, 60.3% had used contraception at some time; thus more urban than semi-urban women had at some time been users of contraceptives. The lowest proportion who had ever been users was found among women under 25. More users were found among women having four or more children (Table 8.C.4). It was further observed that 2.8% of semi-urban women and 6.7% of urban women who disapproved of birth control had at some time used birth control methods.

The most popular methods in the urban area were condoms (14.4%), followed by oral contraceptives (12.7%), while in the semi-urban area the most widely used methods were oral contraceptives (18.3%) followed by IUDs (5.3%) (Table 8.C.8).

In Muslim culture, withdrawal is a traditionally accepted method of contraception. It is therefore surprising that only 62.8% of the urban women had heard about it and only 6.3% said their husbands practised it. In the urban area, the condom was again the most popular method and was being used by 22.2% of the couples currently using contraception. In the semi-urban area, the condom was likewise the most widely used method (9.4%), followed by oral contraceptives (5.7%). The diaphragm was the least used method in both areas. The number of women who had had tubectomy performed was greater in the urban area (3.4%) than in the semi-urban area (1.7%). Similarly, vasectomy had been performed more often on men in the urban area (1.0%) than in the semi-urban area (0.5%).

From the above data, it can be safely concluded that in the population under study there was a wide gap between knowledge of contraception and its actual use. The percentage of users was higher among women in the urban area than among their counterparts in the semi-urban area.

Opinions on breast feeding as a birth control method

The women were asked whether they believed that breast feeding prevented pregnancies. About two-fifths (40.5%) of the women in the semi-urban area believed breast feeding to be a method of birth control, while in the urban area the corresponding proportion was only about a quarter (25.6%). The proportion who replied that breast feeding was not a method of birth control was 48.6% in the semi-urban area and 58.4% in the urban area. The proportion of women who were uncertain whether breast feeding prevented pregnancies was higher among women with small families (0–3) than among women with 4 or more children (Table 8.C.9).

TABLE 8.C.9. VIEWS OF ELIGIBLE WOMEN ON WHETHER BREAST FEEDING PREVENTS PREGNANCY, BY RESIDENCE, SOCIAL STATUS, AND FAMILY SIZE

(a) By residence and social status

Residence and social status	Percentage of EW believing breast feeding does or does not prevent pregnancy			Total no. of EW responding
	Yes	No	No opinion	
Semi-urban				
Middle	40.2	47.3	12.5	1189
Low	40.7	50.0	9.3	1199
Both categories	40.5	48.6	10.9	2388
Urban				
Middle	25.4	58.3	16.3	2294
Low	29.1	59.2	11.7	179
Both categories	25.6	58.4	16.0	2473

(b) By residence and family size

Residence and family size	Percentage of EW believing breast feeding does or does not prevent pregnancy			Total no. of EW responding
	Yes	No	No opinion	
Semi-urban				
0–3	35.6	44.6	19.8	997
4–5	43.9	51.2	4.8	660
6 and over	43.9	51.7	4.4	731
All family sizes	40.5	48.6	10.9	2388
Urban				
0–3	23.2	52.0	24.8	1298
4–5	28.0	63.7	8.3	578
6 and over	28.6	67.2	4.2	597
All family sizes	25.6	58.4	16.0	2473

Opinions on Induced Abortion

It was noted that women of high parity and those having large families favoured abortions slightly more than women of low parity.

The women who approved of abortions were asked their reasons for doing so. The majority replied that if pregnancy endangered the health of the woman, it was justified to resort to abortion. In the semi-urban area, 65% of the women with a family size of 4 or more children approved of abortion for this reason, while in the urban area the corresponding proportion was 46.5%. Another important reason given for approval of abortion was the possibility of a deformed child. Smaller numbers approved of termination of pregnancy in cases of failure of birth control (33.2%) or for economic reasons (39.3%) (Table 8.C.10).

TABLE 8.C.10. PERCENTAGE OF ELIGIBLE WOMEN APPROVING ABORTION FOR VARIOUS
REASONS, BY RESIDENCE, PARITY, AND FAMILY SIZE

Residence and reasons for approving abortion	Percentage of EW approving of abortion[a]			
	Parity		Family size	
	0–3	4 and over	0–3	4 and over
Semi-urban	N = 865[b]	N = 1524	N = 998	N = 1391
Failure of birth control	17.5	20.3	17.9	20.2
Reluctance to have more children	19.9	22.6	20.2	22.6
Pregnancy endangers woman's health	62.3	64.5	61.9	65.0
Possibility of deformed child	37.1	41.6	38.0	41.4
Inability to afford more children	22.1	25.1	22.4	25.2
Urban	N = 1227	N = 1246	N = 1298	N = 1175
Failure of birth control	13.8	14.8	13.3	15.3
Reluctance to have more children	14.8	15.7	14.5	16.1
Pregnancy endangers woman's health	46.5	46.1	46.1	46.5
Possibility of deformed child	32.2	33.9	32.0	34.1
Inability to afford more children	15.0	16.4	14.7	16.8

[a] The majority of the women not shown as approving abortion expressed disapproval of it; only 3% of the women or fewer gave no opinion. The 5 categories in which the reasons for approval have been placed are not mutually exclusive.

[b] N = total number of eligible women responding.

Opinions on Sterilization

The inclusion of sterilization in the national family planning programme and the advent of minilaparotomy and laparoscopy have aroused interest in this permanent method of family limitation. An overwhelming majority of women knew about the operations of tubectomy and vasectomy. These women were asked their opinions about which partner should be sterilized. In both the semi-urban and the urban area, the majority of women were of the opinion that neither partner should accept sterilization. Among those women who approved of the method, the proportion who considered that the wife should undergo the operation was much higher than the proportion who favoured the husband as the partner to be sterilized. In the semi-urban area, 4.3% of the women said that the husband should undergo vasectomy, while 7.7% believed that the wife should be sterilized. In the urban area, the corresponding proportions were 6.6% and 16.4% (Table 8.C.11). The number of women wanting their husbands to be sterilized was greater among those of middle social status than among those of low social status. In both populations, low status women considered that neither the husband nor the wife should be sterilized.

The main reason given for preferring that the wife should be the one to be sterilized was that she was the child bearer. Many women also thought that the husband would refuse. A smaller proportion thought that the husband should not be sterilized because he was the wage earner or because it would reduce his sexual activity or make him physically weak (Table 8.C.12(a)).

392

TABLE 8.C.11. VIEWS OF ELIGIBLE WOMEN AS TO WHETHER THE HUSBAND OR THE WIFE
SHOULD BE STERILIZED, BY RESIDENCE, SOCIAL STATUS, AND PARITY

Residence, social status, and parity	Percentage of EW with views on who should be sterilized					No. of EW responding
	Husband	Wife	Either	Neither	No opinion	
SEMI-URBAN						
Middle						
0–3	3.9	6.3	11.9	55.9	22.1	512
4–5	6.7	10.6	12.7	59.0	10.1	283
6 and over	6.6	9.1	13.7	59.8	10.9	395
All parities	5.5	8.2	12.7	57.9	15.7	1190
Low						
0–3	1.7	4.0	7.1	62.3	24.9	353
4–5	2.5	7.5	6.1	67.5	16.4	280
6 and over	4.4	9.2	10.6	62.7	13.1	565
All parities	3.2	7.3	8.5	63.7	17.3	1198
Both categories						
0–3	3.0	5.3	9.9	58.5	23.2	865
4–5	4.6	9.1	9.4	63.2	13.7	563
6 and over	5.3	9.2	11.9	61.5	12.2	960
All parities	4.3	7.7	10.6	60.8	16.5	2388
URBAN						
Middle						
0–3	5.9	14.6	5.7	63.4	10.4	1168
4–5	6.8	19.5	6.8	63.1	3.8	502
6 and over	9.1	18.6	6.7	60.9	4.6	624
All parities	7.0	16.8	6.2	62.6	7.4	2294
Low						
0–3	0.0	6.8	1.7	81.4	10.2	59
4–5	3.2	22.6	3.2	67.7	3.2	31
6 and over	1.1	10.1	7.9	73.0	7.9	89
All parities	1.1	11.2	5.0	74.9	7.8	179
Both categories						
0–3	5.6	14.3	5.5	64.2	10.4	1227
4–5	6.6	19.7	6.6	63.4	3.8	533
6 and over	8.1	17.5	6.9	62.4	5.0	713
All parities	6.6	16.4	6.1	63.5	7.4	2473

Those women who considered that the husband should be the one to be sterilized gave as their main reason that vasectomy was an easier operation and some also thought that the husband was healthier. A very small number (2%) thought that the wife would refuse (Table 8.C.12(b)).

Timing Failure of Last Pregnancy

The women were asked whether they felt that their last pregnancy had come sooner than they had wanted ("timing failure"). Such timing failure was found to be quite prevalent in the study area, more than 42% of the women indicating that it had occurred at some time or another. The incidence was found to be slightly higher in the urban than in the semi-urban area. Timing failure tended to be less frequent among younger women than among older women. The frequency also increased with increasing parity (Table 8.C.13(a)). Likewise, timing failure was positively associated with gravidity and family size in both residential areas and in both social status groups (tables not given).

TABLE 8.C.12. REASONS WHY WIFE OR HUSBAND SHOULD BE STERILIZED, BY RESIDENCE, SOCIAL STATUS, AND PARITY

(a) Reasons wife should be sterilized

Residence, social status, and parity	Percentage of EW giving indicated reason:						
	Husband would refuse	Reduce husband's sexual activity	Make husband physically weak	Woman is child bearer	Man's operation in-effective	Man is wage-earner	No. of EW approving steriliza-tion
SEMI-URBAN							
Middle							
0–3	25.0	9.3	6.2	50.0	3.2	6.3	32
4–5	26.6	6.7	—	56.7	6.7	3.3	30
6 and over	31.4	2.9	—	54.3	—	11.4	35
All parities	27.8	6.2	2.1	53.6	3.1	7.2	97
Low							
0–3	7.7	—	—	69.2	—	23.1	13
4–5	14.3	9.5	—	52.4	—	23.8	21
6 and over	20.8	4.2	10.4	52.0	6.3	6.3	48
All parities	17.1	4.9	6.1	54.9	3.7	13.4	82
Both categories							
0–3	20.0	6.7	4.4	55.6	2.2	11.1	45
4–5	21.6	7.8	—	54.9	3.9	11.8	51
6 and over	25.3	3.6	6.0	53.1	3.6	8.4	83
All parities	22.9	5.6	3.9	54.2	3.4	10.0	179
URBAN							
Middle							
0–3	37.5	3.6	6.5	38.7	1.8	11.9	168
4–5	33.7	4.3	10.6	37.9	4.3	9.5	95
6 and over	43.9	3.5	7.0	37.7	2.6	5.3	114
All parities	38.5	3.7	7.7	38.2	2.7	9.2	377
Low							
0–3	25.0	—	—	75.0	—	—	4
4–5	28.6	—	14.3	57.1	—	—	7
6 and over	33.3	11.1	11.1	33.3	—	11.1	9
All parities	30.0	5.6	10.0	50.0	—	5.0	20
Both categories							
0–3	37.3	3.5	6.4	39.5	1.7	11.6	172
4–5	33.3	3.9	10.8	39.3	3.9	8.8	102
6 and over	43.1	4.1	7.8	37.4	2.4	5.7	123
All parities	38.0	3.8	7.8	38.8	2.5	9.1	397

TABLE 8.C.12 (*continued*)

(b) Reasons husband should be sterilized

Residence and parity	Percentage of EW giving indicated reason:						
	Healthier	Easier	No hos- pitalization necessary	Wife would refuse	Health of wife bad	Sharing in limiting pregnancies	Wife's operation might have complications
Semi-urban[a]							
0–3	24.0	36.0	8.0	—	12.0	8.0	8.0
4–5	21.7	56.5	—	4.3	4.3	4.3	8.7
6 and over	14.3	61.2	2.0	2.0	2.0	4.1	10.2
All parities	18.6	53.6	3.1	2.1	5.2	5.2	9.3
Urban[b]							
0–3	19.4	38.8	7.5	4.5	3.0	14.9	11.9
4–5	5.9	41.2	2.9	—	8.8	14.7	17.6
6 and over	23.2	46.4	—	—	7.1	14.3	7.1
All parities	17.8	42.0	3.8	1.9	5.7	14.6	11.5

[a] No. of eligible women responding = 103.
[b] No. of eligible women responding = 163.

TABLE 8.C.13. TIMING FAILURE OF LAST PREGNANCY, BY RESIDENCE, SOCIAL STATUS, AGE OF ELIGIBLE WOMAN, AND PARITY*

Social status and age of EW	Percentage of EW who felt last pregnancy came too soon, at indicated parities:							
	Semi-urban				Urban			
	1–3	4–5	6 and over	All parities	1–3	4–5	6 and over	All parities
Middle								
<20	10.3	—	—	13.6	26.2	—	—	23.5
20–24	18.6	(36.4)	(50.0)	22.0	38.2	48.2	(0.0)	38.2
25–29	32.0	44.4	48.4	38.8	34.1	51.5	47.9	40.0
30–34	8.1	45.3	57.0	44.5	37.4	48.5	61.8	48.9
35–39	29.6	54.4	57.2	51.8	32.0	48.4	57.8	49.6
40–44	(23.8)	35.9	53.4	46.2	19.0	35.8	51.9	46.4
All ages	17.8	44.8	54.5	39.4	34.6	46.7	55.3	43.8
Low								
<20	(8.7)	—	—	12.0	(0.0)	—	—	(0.0)
20–24	20.2	(50.0)	—	24.6	(31.8)	(50.0)	(0.0)	32.0
25–29	32.9	38.8	65.0	43.3	(31.6)	(40.0)	(33.3)	34.9
30–34	22.3	37.2	54.1	45.8	(66.6)	(37.5)	66.6	61.0
35–39	21.7	38.7	52.8	46.9	(33.3)	(0.0)	(45.8)	40.0
40–44	(14.6)	(40.0)	54.7	50.0	(33.3)	(66.6)	56.0	54.8
All ages	22.7	39.2	35.5	42.9	33.3	—	53.9	45.0

* Figures in parentheses refer to fewer than 25 eligible women.
  Dashes indicate no eligible women with given parameters.

It was observed that timing failure of the last pregnancy increased with increasing parity. However, a slight decrease in timing failure was observed with improved education. Timing failure was less frequent in women with college education than in women who had had no schooling or primary and secondary education only. In each of the education categories, timing failure was slightly more frequent in the urban than in the semi-urban area. The difference was quite pronounced for women with college education; in the semi-urban area, 31.6% of such women reported timing failure, compared with 42.3% in the urban area (Table 8.C.14).

TABLE 8.C.14. TIMING FAILURE OF LAST PREGNANCY, BY RESIDENCE, EDUCATION OF ELIGIBLE WOMAN, AND PARITY*

Residence and parity	Percentage of EW at indicated educational level who experienced timing failure of last pregnancy				
	No school	Primary	Secondary	College +	All educational levels
Semi-urban					
0–3	20.3	20.9	26.8	31.3	21.6
4–5	39.7	50.0	44.4	(20.0)	42.0
6 and over	52.5	63.1	(78.6)	(100.0)	54.8
All parities	40.9	43.7	38.0	31.6	41.2
Urban					
0–3	34.9	32.4	32.5	37.9	33.8
4–5	43.6	48.9	51.2	52.4	48.1
6 and over	52.2	57.5	61.1	(80.0)	55.1
All parities	45.2	45.4	41.0	42.3	43.9

* Figures in parentheses refer to fewer than 25 eligible women.

Ideal Pregnancy Interval

The majority of women (51.5%), irrespective of their residence or social status, preferred a pregnancy interval of 48 months or more, while about 40.5% preferred an interval of 36–47 months. In the semi-urban area, 58% of the women preferred a pregnancy interval of 48 months or more, while in the urban area the corresponding proportion was 45%. When the effect of social status was examined, it was found that 57% of the women of low social status preferred an interval of 48 months or more, compared with 49% of the women of middle social status. It was also found that the proportion of women desiring a pregnancy interval of 48 months or more increased with increasing family size (Table 8.C.15).

The mean ideal pregnancy interval advocated by the respondents was about 43 months. Women whose husbands had had primary or secondary level

TABLE 8.C.15. PERCENTAGE DISTRIBUTION OF ELIGIBLE WOMEN BY RESIDENCE, IDEAL PREGNANCY INTERVAL, SOCIAL STATUS, AND FAMILY SIZE

Residence/social status and ideal pregnancy interval (months)	Percentage of EW who specified the indicated pregnancy interval and who had a family size of:							
	0	1	2	3	4	5	6 and over	All family sizes
Semi-urban								
Less than 12	—	—	0.7	0.7	—	—	0.1	0.2
12–23	—	—	—	—	—	—	0.1	0.0
24–35	13.9	9.7	2.9	1.8	3.2	4.8	4.0	5.0
36–47	35.2	38.8	38.7	44.7	32.5	34.7	36.0	36.8
48 and over	50.9	51.5	57.7	52.8	64.3	60.5	59.8	57.9
Number of EW	216	206	274	275	345	314	731	2361
Urban								
Less than 12	1.1	0.4	—	0.3	—	—	0.3	0.3
12–23	1.5	1.1	0.8	—	0.6	1.1	0.2	0.7
24–35	14.9	10.8	9.3	9.9	8.4	7.7	9.5	9.9
36–47	43.1	49.6	47.8	41.4	44.1	42.5	42.2	44.2
48 and over	39.4	38.1	42.1	48.4	46.9	48.7	47.8	44.9
Number of EW	269	268	387	355	311	261	590	2441
Middle status								
Less than 12	0.7	0.3	0.4	0.7	—	—	0.2	0.3
12–23	1.0	0.8	0.6	—	0.4	0.8	0.1	0.6
24–35	14.4	10.1	7.5	7.5	7.2	6.4	7.7	8.4
36–47	38.8	46.5	45.5	42.8	40.5	39.8	39.6	41.7
48 and over	45.1	42.3	46.0	49.0	51.9	53.0	52.4	49.0
Number of EW	397	385	532	453	464	394	820	3445
Low status								
Less than 12	—	—	—	—	—	—	0.2	0.1
12–23	—	—	—	—	—	—	0.2	0.1
24–35	14.8	11.2	3.1	3.4	2.1	5.5	4.4	5.1
36–47	43.2	38.2	38.0	42.9	31.8	34.8	37.5	37.5
48 and over	42.0	50.6	58.9	53.7	66.1	59.7	57.7	57.2
Number of EW	88	89	129	177	192	181	501	1357
All categories								
Less than 12	0.6	0.2	0.3	0.5	—	—	0.2	0.2
12–23	0.8	0.6	0.4	—	0.3	0.5	0.1	0.3
24–35	14.5	10.4	6.7	6.3	5.6	6.1	6.4	7.5
36–47	39.6	44.9	44.0	42.9	38.0	38.3	38.9	40.5
48 and over	44.5	43.9	48.6	50.3	56.1	55.1	54.4	51.5
Number of EW	485	474	661	630	656	575	1321	4802

education preferred slightly longer pregnancy intervals than those whose husbands had not had any schooling or had had college level education. When the education of the eligible women was considered, it was interesting to note that the preferred pregnancy interval declined as their educational level increased. The women with no education preferred an interval of 44.1 months, while those with college education preferred an interval of 40.6 months. The age of the women had little influence on their opinions as to the ideal pregnancy interval (Table 8.C.16).

TABLE 8.C.16. MEAN IDEAL PREGNANCY INTERVAL BY VARIOUS CHARACTERISTICS

Characteristic	Mean ideal pregnancy interval (months)	No. of EW responding
Husband's education		
No school	44.7	1028
Primary	44.4	844
Secondary	43.9	1277
College +	42.7	1653
EW's education		
No school	44.1	2465
Primary	44.2	1206
Secondary	43.5	654
College +	40.6	476
Age of EW		
<20	42.2	208
20–24	43.5	805
25–29	43.9	1173
30–34	44.3	981
35–39	43.5	803
40–44	43.6	832
Residence and social status		
Semi-urban		
Middle	44.2	1175
Low	45.1	1186
Urban		
Middle	42.8	2370
Low	43.4	171
Child loss		
0	43.7	3755
1	43.8	821
2–3	43.9	224
Family size		
0–3	42.9	2249
4–5	44.5	1231
6 and over	44.4	1320

In both the semi-urban and urban areas, women of low social status advocated a slightly higher ideal pregnancy interval than women of middle status. Women with family sizes of 0–3 preferred slightly shorter pregnancy intervals than women with larger family sizes. No significant differences were noted between women of different child loss experience.

Additional Children Wanted

Generally, for a given ideal family size the mean number of additional children wanted decreased with parity in both residential areas and for both social status groups. However, when parity was held constant, the number of additional children wanted did not show any well-defined pattern as the ideal family size increased (it was expected that it would increase with an increase in ideal family size) (Table 8.C.17).

Women having no male issue wanted to have a least one boy even if they had 5 or more girls. But if they already had even 1 boy the desire to produce more sons decreased. Hence, there was an inverse relation between the desire to produce more sons and the number of boys already present in the family (Table 8.C.18).

Women with no children desired one or more girls, and those with one or two children, especially if they were boys, wanted another girl. Among the others, however, there was little or no wish for another daughter (Table 8.C.19).

TABLE 8.C.17. MEAN NUMBER OF ADDITIONAL CHILDREN WANTED, BY RESIDENCE, IDEAL FAMILY SIZE, SOCIAL STATUS, AND PARITY*

Residence/social status and parity	Mean no. of additional children wanted by EW who specified an ideal family size of:						
	1	2	3	4	5	6 and over	All family sizes
Semi-urban							
1–3	—	0.7	1.1	1.8	2.1	(3.6)	1.5
4–5	(1.0)	0.9	0.2	0.3	0.4	1.2	0.3
6 and over	0.0	0.6	0.2	0.1	0.4	0.3	0.1
All parities	(1.0)	0.6	0.8	1.0	0.7	1.0	0.9
Urban							
1–3	(0.5)	(0.7)	0.8	1.7	(2.6)	(3.1)	1.3
4–5	(0.3)	0.3	0.5	0.2	0.2	(0.8)	0.1
6 and over	—	0.5	0.2	0.5	—	—	0.5
All parities	(0.0)	0.8	0.9	1.0	—	0.7	0.9
Middle status							
1–3	(0.5)	0.7	0.9	1.8	2.2	3.0	1.4
4–5	(0.3)	—	—	0.1	0.2	0.8	0.2
6 and over	—	0.3	0.3	0.1	—	0.1	0.1
All parities	(0.5)	0.7	0.9	1.0	0.7	0.7	0.9
Low status							
1–3	—	0.7	0.9	1.6	2.6	(3.8)	1.5
4–5	(1.0)	0.1	0.3	0.4	0.3	(1.7)	0.4
6 and over	—	—	—	0.1	—	0.2	0.1
All parities	(1.0)	0.5	0.5	0.8	0.5	1.1	0.7
All categories							
1–3	0.5	0.7	0.9	1.7	2.3	3.3	1.4
4–5	(0.5)	0.6	0.1	0.2	0.3	1.1	0.2
6 and over	—	0.2	0.2	0.7	0.2	0.2	0.1
All parities	(0.6)	0.7	0.8	1.0	0.7	0.9	0.9

* Figures in parentheses refer to fewer than 25 eligible women.

TABLE 8.C.18. MEAN NUMBER OF ADDITIONAL BOYS WANTED, BY RESIDENCE AND BY THE NUMBER OF GIRLS AND NUMBER OF BOYS ALREADY PRESENT IN THE FAMILY*

Residence and no. of boys present in family	Mean no. of additional boys wanted by EW with indicated no. of girls in family							
	0	1	2	3	4	5	6 and over	All EW
Semi-urban								
0	1.6	1.6	1.6	(1.3)	(0.7)	(0.7)	(1.2)	1.5
1	1.2	0.9	0.9	0.5	0.4	(0.4)	(0.1)	0.8
2	0.5	0.3	0.2	0.2	0.2	0.1	(0.3)	0.3
3	0.1	0.1	0.2	0.2	0.1	0.2	0.1	0.1
4	(0.1)	0.0	0.1	0.1	0.1	0.0	(0.1)	0.1
5	(0.0)	0.0	0.1	0.0	(0.0)	(0.0)	(0.2)	0.1
6 and over	(0.0)	(0.0)	0.0	0.1	(0.0)	(0.1)	(0.0)	0.0
All semi-urban	1.1	0.5	0.4	0.3	0.2	0.2	0.2	0.5
Urban								
0	1.6	1.4	1.4	1.1	(0.6)	(1.0)	(0.4)	1.5
1	0.9	0.7	0.6	0.2	0.2	(0.2)	(0.0)	0.6
2	0.4	0.2	0.1	0.1	0.1	(0.4)	(0.0)	0.2
3	(0.0)	0.2	0.0	0.2	0.0	(0.0)	(0.0)	0.1
4	(0.0)	0.0	0.0	0.0	0.0	(0.0)	(0.0)	0.0
5	(0.0)	(0.0)	0.0	0.1	(0.1)	(0.0)	(0.0)	0.0
6 and over	(0.0)	(0.0)	0.0	0.0	(0.0)	(0.0)	(0.0)	0.0
All urban	1.0	0.4	0.4	0.2	0.1	0.5	0.0	0.5

* Figures in parentheses refer to fewer than 25 eligible women.

TABLE 8.C.19. MEAN NUMBER OF ADDITONAL GIRLS WANTED, BY RESIDENCE AND BY THE NUMBER OF BOYS AND NUMBER OF GIRLS ALREADY PRESENT IN THE FAMILY*

Residence and no. boys present in family	Mean no. of additional girls wanted by EW with indicated no. of girls in family:					
	0	1	2	3	4 and over	All EW
Semi-urban						
0	1.6	0.8	0.2	(0.2)	(0.1)	1.0
1	1.3	0.6	0.1	0.0	0.0	0.5
2	1.0	0.2	0.1	0.1	0.0	0.2
3	0.5	0.1	0.1	0.1	0.0	0.1
4	(0.3)	0.1	0.0	0.1	0.0	0.1
5	(0.4)	0.0	0.0	0.0	0.1	0.0
6 and over	(0.3)	(0.0)	0.0	0.0	0.0	0.0
All semi-urban	1.2	0.3	0.1	0.1	0.0	0.3
Urban						
0	1.3	0.7	0.2	0.0	0.0	0.8
1	1.5	0.4	0.1	0.0	0.1	0.5
2	0.9	0.2	0.1	0.1	0.0	0.2
3	0.5	0.2	0.0	0.2	0.0	0.1
4	(0.1)	0.0	0.0	0.0	0.0	0.0
5	(0.3)	(0.0)	0.0	0.1	0.0	0.0
6 and over	(0.1)	(0.0)	0.0	0.0	0.0	0.0
All urban	1.1	0.3	0.1	0.1	0.2	0.3

* Figures in parentheses refer to fewer than 25 eligible women.

D. SYRIAN ARAB REPUBLIC

N. Hanbali & A. R. Omran

Opinions on Family Formation and Health

Opinions on ideal age at marriage

All eligible women thought that girls should marry at a younger age than boys. From Table 8.D.1, it can be seen that in Damascus the mean ideal age at marriage was considered to be 26.3 for boys and 18.6 for girls; in Sweida, the corresponding figures were 25.7 for boys and 19.4 for girls and in Rural Aleppo they were 22.0 for boys and 16.5 for girls. Thus, rural women gave younger ages for both boys and girls compared with those in more urban areas (Table 8.D.1). Small differences in opinions were observed by social status.

TABLE 8.D.1. MEAN IDEAL AGE AT MARRIAGE FOR BOYS AND GIRLS, BY RESIDENCE, SOCIAL STATUS, AND AGE AT MARRIAGE OF ELIGIBLE WOMEN*

Sex of child; residence, and social status	Mean ideal age at marriage in the opinion of EW who married at age:							
	12–14	15–17	18–20	21–23	24–26	27–29	30–44	All EW
BOYS								
Damascus								
Middle	26.6	26.2	26.3	26.9	27.9	27.5	28.1	26.5
Low	25.2	25.4	24.8	25.0	(24.0)	(24.3)	(24.5)	25.0
Both categories	26.3	26.1	26.1	26.5	27.3	26.9	27.3	26.3
Sweida								
Middle	25.6	25.6	26.1	.26.7	26.3	27.3	(27.0)	26.0
Low	24.7	25.0	25.3	25.7	(23.5)	(23.9)	(21.7)	24.9
Both categories	25.4	25.4	25.9	26.5	25.7	26.4	24.7	25.7
Rural Aleppo								
Middle	22.4	22.0	22.4	22.1	(23.5)	(25.0)	(21.7)	22.2
Low	21.6	21.6	22.2	22.3	22.5	(21.8)	(21.4)	21.9
Both categories	21.9	21.8	22.2	22.2	22.7	(22.2)	(21.4)	22.0
GIRLS								
Damascus								
Middle	18.2	18.5	18.7	19.5	20.5	20.2	20.5	18.8
Low	17.2	17.9	17.6	18.0	(18.0)	(17.4)	(19.0)	17.7
Both categories	18.0	18.3	18.5	19.2	20.0	19.7	20.0	18.6
Sweida								
Middle	19.1	19.2	19.5	20.1	21.0	20.5	(20.2)	19.5
Low	18.1	19.0	19.0	19.3	(17.4)	(17.6)	(17.8)	18.8
Both categories	18.9	19.2	19.4	19.9	19.9	19.7	19.2	19.4
Rural Aleppo								
Middle	16.4	16.4	16.8	16.5	(17.9)	(22.5)	(17.3)	16.6
Low	16.0	16.1	17.0	17.0	17.8	(17.3)	(16.0)	16.5
Both categories	16.2	16.2	16.9	16.8	17.8	(18.0)	(16.3)	16.5

* Figures in parentheses refer to fewer than 25 eligible women.

TABLE 8.D.2. VIEWS OF ELIGIBLE WOMEN ON FAMILY FORMATION AND HEALTH, BY RESIDENCE AND SOCIAL STATUS

Damascus

Percentage of EW giving replies indicated

Statements or questions on which women's views were obtained	Middle status				Low status				Both categories			
	Yes	No	Same	No opinion	Yes	No	Same	No opinion	Yes	No	Same	No opinion
A child's health is better in a small family	91.2	1.2	5.2	2.4	84.2	2.3	9.6	3.9	89.8	1.4	6.1	2.7
The mother's health is better in a small family	91.6	1.3	4.9	2.2	84.7	2.6	9.1	3.6	90.2	1.6	5.7	7.5
A child's health is better when the birth interval is 3 years rather than 1 year	94.1	2.7	2.3	0.9	89.1	4.4	4.9	1.6	93.1	3.0	2.8	1.1
The mother's health is better when the birth interval is 3 years rather than 1 year	94.8	2.6	2.0	0.6	89.4	4.2	4.9	1.6	93.8	2.9	2.5	0.8
A decrease in childhood mortality would result in fewer children being born	79.3	14.2	0.0	6.5	74.5	14.3	0.0	11.2	78.4	14.2	0.0	7.4
Would you use birth control if your children's health would suffer from additional pregnancies?	85.5	13.1	—	1.4	80.0	17.9	—	2.1	84.4	14.0	—	1.6
Would you use birth control if your health would suffer at the next pregnancy?	86.1	12.4	—	1.5	80.8	17.1	—	2.1	85.1	13.3	—	1.6

TABLE 8.D.2 (continued)

Statements or questions on which women's views were obtained	Percentage of EIV giving replies indicated											
	Middle status				Low status				Both categories			
	Yes	No	Same	No opinion	Yes	No	Same	No opinion	Yes	No	Same	No opinion
					Sweida							
A child's health is better in a small family	97.0	0.5	2.0	0.5	96.7	1.0	1.8	0.5	97.0	0.6	1.9	0.5
The mother's health is better in a small family	96.8	0.6	2.1	0.5	97.2	0.5	1.5	0.8	96.9	0.6	2.0	0.5
A child's health is better when the birth interval is 3 years rather than 1 year	98.2	0.7	0.9	0.2	96.2	0.8	2.0	1.0	97.8	0.7	1.2	0.4
The mother's health is better when the birth interval is 3 years rather than 1 year	98.2	0.6	1.0	0.2	96.5	0.5	0.8	1.3	97.8	0.6	1.2	0.5
A decrease in childhood mortality would result in fewer children being born	76.6	18.5	0.0	4.9	70.3	22.7	0.0	7.1	75.1	19.5	0.0	5.4
Would you use birth control if your children's health would suffer from additional pregnancies?	76.3	22.6	1.1	65.0	31.5	—	—	3.5	73.6	24.7	—	1.7
Would you use birth control if your health would suffer at the next pregnancy?	76.2	22.7	—	1.1	67.0	29.5	—	3.5	74.1	24.3	—	1.7

TABLE 8.D.2. (continued)

Percentage of EW giving replies indicated

Statements or questions on which women's views were obtained	Middle status				Low status				Both categories			
	Yes	No	Same	No opinion	Yes	No	Same	No opinion	Yes	No	Same	No opinion
Rural Aleppo												
A child's health is better in a small family	96.1	0.7	1.9	1.2	93.8	0.7	2.7	2.8	94.6	0.7	2.4	2.2
The mother's health is better in a small family	96.3	0.6	1.9	1.2	94.2	0.8	0.3	2.8	24.9	0.7	2.2	2.2
A child's health is better when the birth interval is 3 years rather than 1 year	95.7	2.4	1.3	0.6	94.4	3.7	1.1	0.8	94.8	3.3	1.2	0.7
The mother's health is better when the birth interval is 3 years rather than 1 year	96.0	2.2	1.2	0.6	94.3	3.6	1.3	0.9	94.9	3.1	1.2	0.8
A decrease in childhood mortality would result in fewer children being born	46.2	36.7	0.0	17.1	43.6	31.6	0.0	24.9	44.5	33.4	0.0	22.2
Would you use birth control if your children's health would suffer from additional pregnancies?	24.9	70.4	—	4.8	14.9	77.6	—	7.5	18.4	75.1	—	6.6
Would you use birth control if your health would suffer at the next pregnancy?	25.0	70.5	—	4.5	15.9	76.5	—	7.6	19.0	74.5	—	6.5

TABLE 8.D.3. VIEWS OF ELIGIBLE WOMEN ON FAMILY FORMATION, BY RESIDENCE AND EDUCATION

Percentage of EW agreeing with statements in left-hand column

Statements on which women's views were obtained	Damascus			Sweida			Rural Aleppo		
	No school	Primary	Secondary	No school	Primary	Secondary	No school	Primary	Secondary
A child's health is better in a small family	87.0	95.1	99.4	96.6	98.0	100.0	94.6	100.0	—
The mother's health is better in a small family	87.4	96.0	99.4	96.5	98.0	100.0	94.8	100.0	—
A child's health is better when the birth interval is 3 years rather than 1 year	92.2	94.7	97.1	97.6	98.8	97.4	94.8	94.7	
The mother's health is better when the birth interval is 3 years rather than 1 year	92.9	95.1	97.7	97.6	98.8	98.7	94.9	94.7	—

In general, women who themselves had married at later ages suggested higher ages at marriage, for both sexes, than those who had married at younger ages.

Opinions on small families and spacing

Tables 8.D.2 and 8.D.3 show that over 90% of the women believed that the health of both the child and the mother was better in small families. Less than 2% did not agree. Also, more than 93% of eligible women believed that 3 years' spacing of children would yield better maternal and child health.

Variations in opinions by social status, residence, and education were generally small.

Acceptance of the use of birth control

From Table 8.D.2 it can be seen that a high proportion of eligible women in Damascus and Sweida accepted the use of birth control if their own health or the health of their children would suffer from additional pregnancies, but in Rural Aleppo only 19% of eligible women accepted the use of birth control for these reasons. When women were asked whether a reduction in infant mortality would increase the acceptance of family planning, 3 out of every 4 women in the urban areas and about 2 out of every 4 women in the rural areas responded positively.

Opinions on Birth Control

Approval of birth control

While the majority of women in the towns and cities expressed approval of birth control, very few of them actually practised it. From Table 8.D.4 it can be seen that the proportions of eligible women who approved of birth control were 75.5% in Damascus, 65.2% in Sweida, and 15% in Rural Aleppo. But of those eligible women who expressed approval, only a small proportion reported using birth control, especially in the rural area (Table 8.D.5).

In all areas, the approval rate increased with increasing levels of education. There was no consistent pattern of approval by age in any of the three areas; when the data were analysed by parity, the highest rates of approval for Damascus and Sweida (the urban areas) were found for women who had had 1–3 births (Tables 8.D.4 and 8.D.5).

Among the reasons given for approval of family planning, benefit to the health of the mother or child received particularly frequent mention. Economic reasons were also important, especially in urban areas (Table 8.D.6). Among women in these areas who disapproved of birth control, the main reasons given were the desire for more children and husband's disapproval. In the rural area, however, religious objections were most often cited as the reason for disapproval. It appears that these women, most of whom are Muslim, were under a misconception, since the Islamic religion approves of family planning.

406

Willingness to use birth control for health reasons

The women were also asked specifically whether they would be willing to use birth control if they were told by a physician that more pregnancies would

TABLE 8.D.4. APPROVAL AND USE OF BIRTH CONTROL BY ELIGIBLE WOMEN, BY RESIDENCE, AGE, AND PARITY

Residence, age, and parity of EW	EW approving of birth control		Use of birth control among women who approve (%)			Use of birth control among women who disapprove (%)		
	%	N[a]	Ever used	Never used	Not known	Ever used	Never used	Not known
AGE								
Damascus								
<25	69.5	485	52.5	47.2	0.3	7.3	92.7	0.0
25–34	76.5	818	81.6	18.2	0.2	7.3	92.7	0.0
35–44	78.6	672	78.6	21.4	0.0	10.3	89.7	0.0
All ages	75.5	1975	74.0	25.9	0.1	8.2	91.8	0.0
Sweida								
<25	75.0	316	43.9	55.7	0.4	5.5	93.2	1.4
25–34	69.0	751	53.5	45.8	0.8	7.7	90.9	1.4
35–44	56.1	644	51.5	47.9	0.6	5.0	92.4	0.5
All ages	65.2	1711	50.8	48.6	0.6	—	—	—
Rural Aleppo								
<25	12.5	554	7.2	91.3	1.4	0.5	99.3	0.2
25–34	15.1	702	23.6	75.5	0.9	2.3	97.1	0.6
35–44	17.0	678	19.1	80.9	0.2	1.5	97.8	0.7
All ages	15.0	1934	17.9	81.4	0.7	1.5	98.0	0.5
PARITY								
Damascus								
0	62.1	145	10.0	90.0	0.0	2.0	98.0	0.0
1–3	77.4	589	69.7	30.0	0.2	7.4	92.6	0.0
4–5	74.4	461	81.9	18.1	0.0	10.8	89.2	0.0
6 and over	77.2	780	82.2	17.6	0.2	8.9	91.1	0.0
All parities	75.5	1975	74.0	25.9	0.1	8.2	91.8	0.0
Sweida								
0	65.5	116	14.5	82.9	2.6	0.0	100.0	0.0
1–3	70.3	478	51.5	48.2	0.3	9.4	89.0	1.6
4–5	63.4	418	50.6	48.7	0.8	5.0	91.4	3.6
6 and over	62.8	699	56.7	42.8	0.5	5.9	92.8	1.4
All parities	65.2	1711	50.8	48.6	0.6	6.2	91.9	1.9
Rural Aleppo								
0	8.5	189	0.0	100.0	0.0	0.0	100.0	0.0
1–3	12.7	535	5.9	92.6	1.5	0.5	98.8	0.7
4–5	17.1	298	19.6	80.4	0.0	1.5	98.0	0.5
6 and over	17.0	912	24.5	74.8	0.6	2.4	97.1	0.5
All parities	15.0	1934	17.9	81.4	0.7	1.5	98.0	0.5

[a] N = total number of eligible women responding.

TABLE 8.D.5. APPROVAL AND EVER USE OF BIRTH CONTROL, BY RESIDENCE AND EDUCATION

Percentage of EW with attitude shown in left-hand column

Attitude to birth control	Damascus			Sweida			Rural Aleppo		
	No school	Primary	Secondary	No school	Primary	Secondary	No school	Primary	Secondary
Approve use to limit pregnancy	69.8	86.7	95.4	60.7	83.3	89.7	14.9	21.1	—
Approve use to space pregnancy	70.7	87.7	97.7	59.1	87.6	88.5	14.8	26.3	—
Ever used	50.9	72.2	82.8	30.3	55.1	70.5	3.9	10.5	—
No. of EW responding	1402	399	174	1388	245	78	1915	90	—

TABLE 8.D.6. REASONS FOR APPROVAL OR DISAPPROVAL OF BIRTH CONTROL, BY RESIDENCE AND FAMILY SIZE

Residence and family size	Percentage of EW who approve for reasons stated					Percentage of EW who disapprove for reasons stated					
	Preserve health of mother	Care of child	Improve child health	Reduce costs	N [a]	Religion	Maternal health	Husband disapproves	Desire more children	Mother-in-law disapproves	N [a]
Damascus											
0–3	99.3	100.0	100.0	97.8	590	73.9	89.4	87.4	89.9	63.3	199
4 and over	99.1	99.3	98.8	97.6	899	70.5	90.0	82.6	75.5	56.0	241
All family sizes	99.2	99.6	99.3	97.6	1489	72.0	89.8	84.8	82.0	59.3	440
Sweida											
0–3	96.3	98.2	98.0	92.6	457	61.9	84.5	74.2	73.7	47.9	194
4 and over	97.7	99.4	99.8	95.9	656	62.4	89.7	78.7	62.7	42.5	319
All family sizes	97.1	98.9	99.1	94.5	1113	62.2	87.7	77.0	66.9	44.5	513
Rural Aleppo											
0–3	99.0	95.9	94.9	83.7	98	94.0	89.3	92.4	88.9	60.3	605
4 and over	97.4	93.3	94.8	82.9	193	92.0	90.6	92.5	88.2	58.0	735
All family sizes	97.9	94.2	94.8	83.2	291	92.9	90.0	92.5	88.5	59.0	1340

[a] N = total number of eligible women responding.

TABLE 8.D.7. ATTITUDE OF ELIGIBLE WOMEN TO BIRTH CONTROL, BY RESIDENCE AND FAMILY SIZE

Residence and family size	Percentage of EW approving birth control in principle who would use it for stated reason:		N^a	Percentage of EW disapproving birth control in principle who would use it for stated reason:		N^a
	to safeguard health of child	to safeguard health of mother		to safeguard health of child	to safeguard health of mother	
Damascus						
0–3	96.8	97.5	591	47.2	48.2	199
4 and over	97.7	98.4	900	38.4	38.4	242
All family sizes	97.3	98.1	1491	42.4	42.9	441
Sweida						
0–3	90.2	90.0	459	31.5	31.5	197
4 and over	95.1	96.0	657	36.0	36.6	322
All family sizes	93.1	93.5	1116	34.3	34.7	519
Rural Aleppo						
0–3	73.5	74.5	98	6.9	7.8	606
4 and over	82.8	84.9	192	7.3	7.3	738
All family sizes	79.7	81.4	290	7.1	7.5	1344

[a] N = total number eligible women responding.

harm either their own health or the health of the child (Table 8.D.7). Almost all of the women in the urban areas and 80% of the rural women who approved of birth control in principle said that they would be willing to use contraception for health reasons. Even among women who disapproved of birth control in principle, 42.4% in Damascus and 34.3% in Swedia, but only 7.1% in Rural Aleppo expressed willingness to use contraception to safeguard their own health or that of the child. These opinions were not appreciably influenced by family size.

TABLE 8.D.8. KNOWLEDGE AND USE OF FERTILITY CONTROL METHODS AMONG ELIGIBLE WOMEN, BY RESIDENCE, SOCIAL STATUS, USE, AND METHOD

(a) Damascus

Social status and method	Knowledge and use of fertility control methods among EW (%)			
	Never heard of	Heard of and used	Heard of and using	Heard of but never used
Middle	N = 1590[a]			
Condom	47.4	7.4	1.8	43.4
Withdrawal	33.5	12.6	7.3	46.6
Rhythm	24.3	13.1	7.2	55.3
Diaphragm	61.3	1.0	0.2	37.5
Douche, etc.	21.5	12.9	5.0	60.6
Coil or IUD	41.5	0.7	0.4	57.4
Oral pills	2.1	21.9	23.9	52.1
Tubectomy	49.1	0.0	0.8	50.2
Vasectomy	71.7	0.0	0.0	28.3
Abortion	0.9	6.8	0.3	92.0
Low	N = 385			
Condom	53.5	3.6	0.3	42.6
Withdrawal	44.2	8.3	4.2	43.4
Rhythm	38.7	7.0	2.6	51.7
Diaphragm	71.7	0.0	0.0	28.3
Douche, etc.	25.5	11.7	3.6	59.2
Coil or IUD	57.1	0.8	0.8	41.3
Oral pills	3.9	15.6	16.6	63.9
Tubectomy	63.1	0.0	0.8	36.1
Vasectomy	80.0	0.0	0.0	20.0
Abortion	3.6	6.0	0.3	90.1
Both categories	N = 1975			
Condom	48.6	6.7	1.3	43.2
Withdrawal	35.5	11.7	6.7	46.0
Rhythm	27.1	11.9	6.3	54.6
Diaphragm	63.3	0.8	0.2	35.7
Douche, etc.	22.3	12.7	4.8	60.3
Coil or IUD	44.4	0.7	0.5	54.4
Oral pills	2.4	20.7	22.5	54.4
Tubectomy	51.8	0.0	0.8	47.4
Vasectomy	73.3	0.0	0.0	26.7
Abortion	1.5	6.5	0.3	91.6

[a] N = total number of eligible women responding.

TABLE 8.D.8 *(continued)*

(b) Sweida

Social status and method	Knowledge and use of fertility control methods among EW (%)			
	Never heard of	Heard of and used	Heard of and using	Heard of but never used
Middle	N = 1314[a]			
Condom	70.5	1.8	0.9	26.8
Withdrawal	62.9	5.4	5.3	26.4
Rhythm	44.1	1.9	7.6	41.3
Diaphragm	89.0	0.1	0.1	10.7
Douche, etc.	59.5	2.0	1.7	36.8
Coil or IUD	87.9	0.1	0.1	11.9
Oral pills	7.2	12.0	14.6	66.1
Tubectomy	76.4	0.0	0.2	23.4
Vasectomy	91.3	0.2	0.0	8.4
Abortion	46.3	1.7	1.8	50.2
Low	N = 397			
Condom	88.6	1.0	0.0	10.3
Withdrawal	78.8	3.0	2.5	15.6
Rhythm	67.6	2.1	2.3	27.9
Diaphragm	95.9	0.0	0.0	3.9
Douche, etc.	71.9	0.8	0.5	26.7
Coil or IUD	94.9	0.1	0.0	5.0
Oral pills	11.5	6.6	4.5	77.3
Tubectomy	85.9	0.0	0.0	14.1
Vasectomy	97.5	0.0	0.0	2.5
Abortion	59.2	1.5	0.0	39.0
Both categories	N = 1711			
Condom	74.6	1.6	0.9	22.8
Withdrawal	66.8	4.9	4.4	23.9
Rhythm	49.6	5.8	6.3	38.2
Diaphragm	90.6	0.1	0.1	9.1
Douche, etc.	62.4	1.7	1.4	34.5
Coil or IUD	89.5	0.1	0.1	10.3
Oral pills	8.2	10.7	12.2	68.9
Tubectomy	78.5	0.0	0.2	21.2
Vasectomy	92.9	0.0	0.0	6.9
Abortion	49.9	1.9	0.5	47.6

[a] N = total number of eligible women responding.

Knowledge and use of birth control methods

The women were asked whether they had heard of, and whether they had previously used or were currently using, any specific fertility control methods (Table 8.D.8). In Sweida, the majority of the eligible women had heard of abortion, douches, and oral contraception, while over half had never heard of the diaphragm or vasectomy. In Damascus the methods known to over 50% of the women included oral contraception, abortion, and rhythm or withdrawal. The level of contraceptive knowledge in rural areas was relatively low. Only pills and abortion were known to over 50% of the women. These trends were found in both social status groups.

TABLE 8.D.8 (*continued*)

(c) Rural Aleppo

Social status and method	Knowledge and use of fertility control methods among EW (%)			
	Never heard of	Heard of and used	Heard of and using	Heard of but never used
Middle	N = 668[a]			
Condom	96.3	0.1	0.3	3.3
Withdrawal	93.1	0.7	0.0	6.2
Rhythm	85.9	0.6	0.1	13.3
Diaphragm	97.9	0.5	0.0	1.6
Douche, etc.	80.8	0.6	0.1	18.4
Coil or IUD	92.9	0.1	0.0	7.0
Oral pills	19.2	3.4	1.3	76.0
Tubectomy	91.3	0.0	0.0	8.7
Vasectomy	96.9	0.0	0.6	2.4
Abortion	40.2	0.3	0.0	59.4
Low	N = 1267			
Condom	99.0	0.0	0.0	0.9
Withdrawal	96.8	0.1	0.1	3.0
Rhythm	93.8	0.2	0.1	6.0
Diaphragm	99.5	0.0	0.0	0.5
Douche, etc.	86.9	0.2	0.2	12.8
Coil or IUD	96.9	0.0	0.0	2.9
Oral pills	35.8	1.8	0.6	61.8
Tubectomy	96.5	0.0	0.0	3.3
Vasectomy	98.9	0.0	0.0	0.9
Abortion	47.8	0.1	0.0	51.5
Both categories	N = 1935			
Condom	98.0	0.1	0.0	1.8
Withdrawal	95.5	0.3	0.1	4.0
Rhythm	91.0	0.3	0.1	8.5
Diaphragm	99.0	0.0	0.0	0.9
Douche, etc.	84.8	0.3	0.2	14.7
Coil or IUD	95.2	0.1	0.0	4.5
Oral pills	30.1	2.4	0.8	66.7
Tubectomy	95.2	0.0	0.0	4.9
Vasectomy	97.8	0.0	0.0	1.9
Abortion	44.9	0.2	0.0	54.8

[a] N = total number of eligible women responding.

The level of current use of birth control was extremely low, the highest proportions being for oral contraception: 22.5% in Damascus, 12.2% in Sweida and 0.08% in Rural Aleppo. The level of use of other methods was much lower.

Opinions on breast feeding as a birth control method

The eligible women were asked whether they believed that breast feeding could prevent pregnancy or not. From Table 8.D.9. it is apparent that 19.6%

of eligible women in Damascus believed that breast feeding prevents pregnancy, compared with 36.3% in Sweida and 52.3% in Rural Aleppo. Only small differences were noticed by social status, but women with large family sizes were more inclined to believe in breast feeding as a contraceptive method than those with smaller families.

TABLE 8.D.9. VIEWS OF ELIGIBLE WOMEN ON WHETHER BREAST FEEDING PREVENTS PREGNANCY, BY RESIDENCE, SOCIAL STATUS, AND FAMILY SIZE

(a) By residence and social status

Residence and social status	Percentage of EW believing breast feeding does or does not prevent pregnancy			
	Yes	No	No opinion	Total no. of EW responding
Damascus				
Middle	19.3	73.5	7.2	1590
Low	21.0	75.8	3.1	385
Both categories	19.6	74.0	6.4	1975
Sweida				
Middle	35.1	57.7	7.2	1313
Low	40.1	54.4	5.5	397
Both categories	36.3	56.9	6.8	1710
Rural Aleppo				
Middle	49.3	40.4	10.3	668
Low	53.9	35.1	11.0	1267
Both categories	52.3	37.0	10.7	1935

(b) By residence and family size

Residence and family size	Percentage of EW believing breast feeding does or does not prevent pregnancy			
	Yes	No	No opinion	Total no. of EW responding
Damascus				
0–3	17.3	69.8	13.0	810
4–5	20.7	77.5	1.8	507
6 and over	21.7	76.4	1.8	658
All family sizes	19.6	74.0	6.4	1975
Sweida				
0–3	28.9	56.9	14.2	682
4–5	43.0	55.0	2.0	460
6 and over	39.6	58.5	1.9	568
All family sizes	36.3	56.9	6.8	1710
Rural Aleppo				
0–3	46.9	31.5	21.6	828
4–5	57.7	38.6	3.7	433
6 and over	55.5	42.6	1.9	647
All family sizes	52.3	37.0	10.7	1935

Opinions on Induced Abortion

In general, abortion was approved of more often by urban than by rural women, regardless of reason. In each area, however, the approval rate differed with different indications for abortion. The most acceptable reason for abortion was the possibility of a deformed child or danger to the woman's health. Over two-thirds of the women in Damascus and one half of the women in Sweida approved of abortion performed for these reasons. Abortion for other reasons was approved of by about 30–38% in the two areas (Table 8.D.10). In the rural areas, less than 6% of the women approved of abortion for most of the reasons indicated, although about 9% of those of high parity or with large families approved if there was danger to the woman's health.

TABLE 8.D.10. PERCENTAGE OF ELIGIBLE WOMEN APPROVING ABORTION FOR VARIOUS REASONS, BY RESIDENCE, PARITY, AND FAMILY SIZE

Residence and reasons for approving abortion	Percentage of EW approving abortion[a]			
	Parity		Family size	
	0–3	4 and over	0–3	4 and over
Damascus	N = 734[b]	N = 1241	N = 810	N = 1165
Failure of birth control	37.6	35.6	36.4	36.3
Reluctance to have more children	38.6	39.1	37.5	39.8
Pregnancy endangers woman's health	67.6	64.3	66.3	65.0
Possibility of deformed child	76.7	72.9	75.8	73.3
Inability to afford more children	73.2	38.4	35.9	39.3
Sweida	N = 594	N = 1117	N = 682	N = 1029
Failure of birth control	29.1	28.5	29.5	28.2
Reluctance to have more children	31.6	28.7	32.4	28.0
Pregnancy endangers woman's health	45.6	41.1	45.6	40.7
Possibility of deformed child	50.0	43.1	49.6	42.8
Inability to afford more children	32.5	27.3	32.7	26.7
Rural Aleppo	N = 724	N = 1211	N = 828	N = 1107
Failure of birth control	1.5	2.8	1.6	2.9
Reluctance to have more children	3.9	5.1	3.7	5.3
Pregnancy endangers woman's health	6.2	9.0	6.4	9.1
Possibility of deformed child	3.7	7.4	4.0	7.6
Inability to afford more children	2.9	4.0	2.8	4.2

[a] The majority of the women not shown as approving abortion expressed disapproval of it; only a very small percentage gave no opinion. The 5 categories in which the reasons for approval have been placed are not mutually exclusive.

[b] N = total number of eligible women responding.

Opinions on Sterilization

Sterilization did not seem to be a popular method of contraception in the areas surveyed. As Table 8.D.11 shows, the proportions of eligible women

TABLE 8.D.11. VIEWS OF ELIGIBLE WOMEN AS TO WHETHER HUSBAND OR WIFE SHOULD BE STERILIZED, BY RESIDENCE, SOCIAL STATUS, AND PARITY

Residence, social status, and parity	Percentage of EW with views on who should be sterilized					No. of EW responding
	Husband	Wife	Either	Neither	No opinion	
DAMASCUS						
Middle						
0–3	12.3	26.9	6.6	49.0	5.2	610
4–5	14.8	29.6	3.9	47.2	4.6	392
6 and over	14.3	29.0	5.1	46.7	4.9	587
All parities	14.7	28.3	5.3	47.7	5.0	1589
Low						
0–3	7.3	16.9	4.0	64.5	7.3	124
4–5	4.6	27.5	4.3	49.3	7.2	69
6 and over	6.3	21.4	4.7	62.0	6.7	192
All parities	7.5	21.0	4.4	60.5	6.5	385
Both categories						
0–3	11.4	25.2	6.1	51.6	5.6	734
4–5	14.3	29.3	3.9	47.5	5.0	461
6 and over	12.3	27.1	5.0	50.4	5.1	779
All parities	12.5	26.9	5.2	50.2	5.3	1974
SWEIDA						
Middle						
0–3	7.1	20.4	6.0	63.3	3.2	496
4–5	6.0	17.0	6.0	69.4	1.6	317
6 and over	8.8	16.0	8.6	64.5	8.2	501
All parities	7.5	17.9	7.5	65.2	2.4	1314
Low						
0–3	4.1	12.2	3.1	75.5	5.1	98
4–5	9.9	9.9	7.9	66.3	5.9	101
6 and over	5.6	9.6	7.1	71.7	6.1	198
All parities	6.3	10.3	6.3	71.3	5.8	397
Both categories						
0–3	6.6	10.0	5.6	65.3	3.5	594
4–5	6.9	15.3	6.5	68.7	2.6	418
6 and over	7.9	14.2	8.2	66.5	3.3	699
All parities	7.2	16.1	6.8	66.6	3.2	1711
RURAL ALEPPO						
Middle						
0–3	1.4	5.7	1.8	80.6	10.6	30
4–5	4.2[a]	7.3[a]	4.2[a]	75.0[a]	9.4[a]	9
6 and over	2.8	7.6	1.7	79.2	8.7	25
All parities	2.4	6.7	2.1	79.2	9.6	64
Low						
0–3	0.9	1.4	2.5	87.8	7.5	441
4–5	0.5	2.5	4.5	86.1	6.4	202
6 and over	1.1	2.7	3.4	83.7	8.1	624
All parities	0.9	2.2	3.2	85.5	8.1	1267

TABLE 8.D.11 (continued)

Residence, social status and parity	Percentage of EW with views on who should be sterilized					
	Husband	Wife	Either	Neither	No opinion	No. of EW responding
Both categories						
0–3	1.1	3.0	2.2	84.9	8.7	724
4–5	1.7	4.0	4.4	82.6	7.4	298
6 and over	1.6	4.3	2.8	82.3	9.0	913
All parities	1.4	3.8	2.8	83.3	8.6	1935

[a] Figures refer to fewer than 25 eligible women.

who disapproved of sterilization for both husaband and wife were 50.2% in Damascus, 66.6% in Sweida, and 83.3% in Rural Aleppo. In all three areas, sterilization was less popular among women of low social status than among those of middle status.

It is of interest to note that in all areas more women believed that, if sterilization was to be done, the wife rather than the husband should be

TABLE 8.D.12. REASONS WHY WIFE OR HUSBAND SHOULD BE STERILIZED, BY RESIDENCE, SOCIAL STATUS AND PARITY*

(a) Reasons wife should be sterilized

Residence, social status and parity	Percentage of EW giving indicated reason:						No. of EW approving steriliza- tion
	Husband would refuse	Reduce husband's sexual activity	Make husband physically weak	Woman is child bearer	Man's operation ineffective	Man is wage- earner	
DAMASCUS							
Middle							
0–3	22.1	3.1	15.9	41.8	9.5	7.6	158
4–5	33.1	3.5	14.8	33.0	11.3	4.3	115
6 and over	41.6	2.4	8.9	37.5	4.8	4.8	168
All parities	32.4	2.9	12.9	37.9	8.2	5.7	441
Low							
0–3	(35.0)	0.0	(30.0)	(15.0)	(15.0)	(5.0)	20
4–5	(10.5)	0.0	(42.1)	(31.6)	0.0	(15.8)	19
6 and over	37.5	2.5	7.5	40.0	5.0	7.5	40
All parities	30.4	1.3	21.5	31.0	6.3	8.9	79
Both categories							
0–3	23.6	2.8	17.4	38.8	10.1	7.3	178
4–5	29.9	3.0	18.7	32.8	9.7	6.0	134
6 and over	40.9	2.4	8.7	38.0	4.8	5.3	208
All parities	32.1	2.7	14.2	36.9	7.9	0.2	520

TABLE 8.D.12 (*continued*)

Residence, social status and parity	Percentage of EW giving indicated reason:						No. of EW approving steriliza-tion
	Husband would refuse	Reduce husband's sexual activity	Make husband physically weak	Woman is child bearer	Man's operation ineffective	Man is wage-earner	
SWEIDA							
Middle							
0–3	24.5	18.4	12.2	11.2	6.1	27.6	98
4–5	20.4	18.5	11.1	22.2	5.6	22.2	54
6 and over	26.0	9.1	14.3	20.8	7.8	22.1	77
All parities	24.0	15.3	12.7	17.0	6.6	24.5	229
Low							
0–3	(18.2)	0.0	(27.3)	(27.3)	0.0	(27.3)	11
4–5	(33.3)	(22.2)	0.0	0.0	0.0	(44.4)	9
6 and over	(42.1)	(5.3)	(10.5)	(15.8)	0.0	(26.3)	19
All parities	33.3	7.7	12.8	15.4	0.0	30.8	39
Both categories							
0–3	23.9	16.5	13.8	12.8	5.5	27.5	109
4–5	22.2	19.0	9.5	19.0	4.8	25.4	63
6 and over	29.2	8.3	13.5	19.8	6.3	22.9	96
All parities	25.4	14.2	12.7	16.8	5.6	25.4	268
RURAL ALEPPO							
Middle							
0–3	(15.4)	0.0	(15.4)	(69.2)	0.0	0.0	13
4–5	(28.6)	0.0	0.0	(71.4)	0.0	0.0	7
6 and over	(22.7)	0.0	(4.5)	(68.2)	0.0	(4.5)	22
All parities	21.4	0.0	7.1	69.0	0.0	2.4	42
Low							
0–3	0.0	0.0	0.0	(100.0)	0.0	0.0	5
4–5	0.0	0.0	(20.0)	(60.0)	0.0	(20.0)	5
6 and over	(35.3)	0.0	0.0	(58.8)	0.0	(5.9)	17
All parities	22.2	0.0	3.7	66.7	0.0	7.4	27
Both categories							
0–3	(11.1)	0.0	(11.1)	(77.8)	0.0	0.0	18
4–5	(16.7)	0.0	(8.3)	(66.7)	0.0	(8.3)	12
6 and over	(28.2)	0.0	2.6	64.1	0.0	5.1	39
All parities	21.7	0.0	5.8	68.1	0.0	4.3	69

* Figures in parentheses refer to fewer than 25 eligible women.

TABLE 8.D.12 (continued)

(b) Reasons husband should be sterilized

Residence and parity	Percentage of EW giving indicated reason:						
	Healthier	Easier	No hospi-talization necessary	Wife would refuse	Health of wife bad	Sharing in limiting pregnancy	Female operation might have complications
Damascus							
0–3	23.8	6.0	3.6	22.6	9.5	23.8	4.8
4–5	24.6	6.2	3.1	30.8	15.4	10.8	3.1
6 and over	26.0	7.3	3.1	25.0	22.9	13.5	0.0
All parities	24.9	6.5	3.3	25.7	16.3	16.3	2.4
Sweida							
0–3	38.5	5.1	5.1	20.5	5.1	7.7	5.1
4–5	24.1	15.8	0.0	37.9	3.4	13.8	3.4
6 and over	30.9	23.6	1.8	23.6	9.1	3.6	1.8
All parities	31.7	15.4	2.4	26.0	6.5	7.3	3.3
Rural Aleppo							
0–3	12.5	0.0	0.0	62.5	25.0	0.0	0.0
4–5	40.0	0.0	0.0	40.0	0.0	0.0	20.0
6 and over	28.6	0.0	0.0	42.9	28.6	0.0	0.0
All parities	25.9	0.0	0.0	48.1	22.2	0.0	3.7

* Figures in parentheses refer to fewer than 25 eligible women.

sterilized. The reasons given for this preference were as follows (Table 8.D.12(a)):

1. The husband would refuse to be sterilized. This opinion was expressed by 32.1% of women in Damascus, 25.4% in Sweida, and 21.7% in Rural Aleppo.

2. Wives are the childbearers. The proportions of eligible women giving this as a reason were 36.9% in Damascus, 16.8% in Sweida, and 68.1% in Rural Aleppo.

Other reasons were given by only a small minority of women. The influence of social status and parity on these responses was small.

Among women who thought the husband should be the one to be sterilized, the following reasons were given (Table 8.D.12(b)):

1. The wives should refuse to lose their fertility permanently because their husbands might want more children. This view was expressed by 25.7% of the women in Damascus, 26% in Sweida, and 48.1% in Rural Aleppo.

2. The husband was healthier.

3. The health of the wife was too poor for her to undergo the operation.

Timing Failure of Last Pregnancy

By age and family formation

Table 8.D.13 shows that the proportions of eligible women of middle social status who considered that their last pregnancy occurred sooner than they

419

TABLE 8.D.13. TIMING FAILURE OF LAST PREGNANCY, BY RESIDENCE, SOCIAL STATUS, AGE OF ELIGIBLE WOMAN, AND PARITY*

Percentage of EW who felt last pregnancy came too soon, at indicated parities:

Social status and age of EW	Damascus				Sweida				Rural Aleppo			
	1–3	4–5	6 and over	All parities	1–3	4–5	6 and over	All parities	1–3	4–5	6 and over	All parities
Middle												
<20	14.3	(100.0)	—	16.1	25.7	—	—	24.3	10.0	—	—	9.1
20–24	36.3	49.2	(83.3)	40.2	45.0	50.0	(100.0)	46.0	8.8	(12.5)	(10.0)	10.5
25–29	31.2	42.7	49.2	38.9	39.8	48.8	65.4	48.0	7.7	11.5	14.9	11.4
30–34	29.7	39.8	55.2	45.5	28.0	45.5	55.7	47.5	(0.0)	(15.0)	14.7	13.5
35–39	24.0	40.4	61.8	54.0	(19.0)	31.7	61.3	50.0	(0.0)	(33.3)	11.5	11.3
40–44	(6.3)	45.2	54.7	49.6	(20.0)	17.9	44.8	40.0	(0.0)	(20.0)	4.9	5.4
All ages	30.1	43.0	56.8	44.1	37.6	43.0	57.5	45.7	7.4	13.5	11.5	10.5
Low												
<20	(20.0)	—	—	(20.0)	(25.0)	(66.7)	—	(20.0)	(0.0)	—	—	—
20–24	(32.3)	(46.2)	(50.0)	37.5	(50.0)	—	—	(54.3)	6.6	16.1	(0.0)	7.9
25–29	(25.0)	(47.4)	(38.5)	36.5	(31.6)	46.7	(44.4)	42.4	4.0	8.3	12.0	7.6
30–34	(14.3)	(64.3)	54.7	52.7	(8.3)	46.7	45.7	40.3	(0.0)	3.7	12.0	9.5
35–39	(27.3)	(50.0)	45.3	43.7	(21.4)	(30.8)	48.2	41.0	(0.0)	(0.0)	9.7	8.3
40–44	(12.5)	(27.3)	48.3	41.6	(25.0)	(4.5)	41.2	33.9	(0.0)	(0.0)	2.9	2.5
All ages	24.7	37.8	48.4	41.9	29.3	36.6	44.2	39.2	4.1	6.4	8.3	6.8

* Figures in parentheses refer to fewer than 25 eligible women.

wished were as follows: 44.1% in Damascus, 45.7% in Sweida, and 10.5% in Rural Aleppo. For women of low social status, the rates were 41.9% in Damascus, 39.2% in Sweida, and 6.8% in Rural Aleppo. It is worthy of mention that there was a positive correlation between timing failure and each of the following: (a) parity (Table 8.D.13), (b) family size, and (c) pregnancy order (no tables shown for family size and pregnancy order). This was true for both social status groups. With regard to age, there was no consistent pattern.

By use of birth control

It is interesting to note that the percentage of eligible women who declared that their last child was a timing failure was higher for women who approved of birth control than for those who disapproved; the actual figures were 52.1% and 28.1%, respectively (table not shown).

By education

In Damascus, there was a tendency for timing failure to decrease with better education, while in Sweida the situation was almost the reverse (Table 8.D.14). In the rural areas, the number of eligible women whose education had progressed beyond the primary level was too small for valid conclusions to be drawn.

TABLE 8.D.14. TIMING FAILURE OF LAST PREGNANCY, BY RESIDENCE, EDUCATION OF ELIGIBLE WOMAN, AND PARITY*

Residence and parity	Percentage of EW at indicated educational level who experienced timing failure of last pregnancy				
	No school	Primary	Secondary	College +	All educational levels
Damascus					
0–3	27.9	29.4	36.5	(17.4)	29.1
4–5	38.5	49.0	54.8	(60.0)	43.7
6 and over	53.1	66.4	43.8	—	54.7
All parities	43.3	47.3	41.7	25.0	43.7
Sweida					
0–3	35.8	35.7	41.7	(0.0)	36.2
4–5	40.7	46.4	(36.4)	(100.0)	41.5
6 and over	50.7	56.6	(100.0)	(100.0)	51.4
All parities	44.4	43.4	42.6	(100.0)	44.2
Rural Aleppo					
0–3	5.7	(0.0)	—	—	5.6
4–5	8.8	(0.0)	—	—	8.7
6 and over	9.3	(33.3)	—	—	9.3
All parities	8.1	(7.7)	—	—	8.1

* Figures in parentheses refer to fewer than 25 eligible women.

Ideal Pregnancy Interval

Urban women preferred longer intervals between pregnancies than did rural women. An interval of 3 or more years is usually considered preferable from a health point of view and it was found that such an interval was preferred by 65.7% of women in Damascus, 77.3% in Sweida and only 22.6% in Rural Aleppo. The most widely preferred interval in Damascus and Sweida was 36–47 months, while in rural areas it was 1 year shorter, i.e., 24–35 months (Table 8.D.15).

TABLE 8.D.15. PERCENTAGE DISTRIBUTION OF ELIGIBLE WOMEN BY RESIDENCE, IDEAL PREGNANCY INTERVAL, AND FAMILY SIZE

Residence and ideal pregnancy interval (months)	Percentage of EW who specified the indicated ideal pregnancy interval and who had a family size of:							
	0	1	2	3	4	5	6 and over	All family sizes
Damascus								
<12	0.0	1.6	1.0	0.0	0.8	1.6	0.8	0.8
12–23	10.3	4.3	7.9	8.9	4.6	5.7	6.6	6.7
24–35	34.5	32.6	23.6	23.7	25.9	28.6	25.1	26.7
36–47	41.4	36.4	46.8	45.2	40.5	39.6	41.1	41.5
48 and over	13.8	25.1	20.7	22.2	28.2	24.5	26.4	24.2
No. of EW	145	187	203	257	259	245	650	1946
Sweida								
<12	0.0	0.0	0.5	0.5	0.0	0.0	0.0	0.1
12–23	2.6	1.8	2.1	1.0	1.2	0.5	0.9	1.2
24–35	25.6	27.4	25.6	18.7	18.9	22.9	19.0	21.4
36–47	47.9	46.4	49.7	53.0	53.9	55.6	55.5	52.9
48 and over	23.9	24.4	22.1	26.8	26.0	21.0	24.6	24.4
No. of EW	117	164	195	198	254	205	564	1897
Rural Aleppo								
<12	0.0	0.0	0.4	1.0	0.0	0.5	0.0	0.2
12–23	16.2	15.8	10.3	10.4	9.2	10.5	10.3	11.4
24–35	65.5	64.2	63.2	61.5	10.1	69.5	65.8	65.8
36–47	18.3	19.5	24.8	26.0	20.2	18.1	23.4	21.9
48 and over	0.0	0.5	1.3	1.1	0.5	1.4	0.5	0.7
No. of EW	197	190	234	192	218	210	670	1911

From Table 8.D.16, the following conclusions can be drawn: (a) the mean ideal pregnancy interval of the eligible women was influenced by both their own education and that of their husbands—the higher the educational level of either partner, the longer was the mean ideal pregnancy interval; (b) social status did not appreciably affect the mean ideal pregnancy interval; in Sweida, for example, the mean interval for women of middle social status was 37.7 months and for those of low social status it was 36.4 months; (c) the mean ideal pregnancy interval increased with increasing parity of the eligible woman's mother—for a parity of 2–3, it was 31.3 months, while for a parity of 4–5, the mean interval was 32.5 months.

TABLE 8.D.16. MEAN IDEAL PREGNANCY INTERVAL BY VARIOUS CHARACTERISTICS

Characteristic	Mean ideal pregnancy interval (months)	Number of EW
Husband's education		
No school	31.1	3354
Primary	34.8	1227
Secondary	35.3	656
College +	37.1	317
EW's education		
No school	31.5	4650
Primary	39.6	653
Secondary	38.3	214
College +	37.1	37
Age of EW		
<20	30.1	363
20–24	31.6	970
25–29	33.5	1110
30–34	33.5	1138
35–39	32.9	960
40–44	32.9	1013
Residence and social status		
Damascus		
Middle	36.0	1564
Low	34.8	382
Swelda		
Middle	37.7	1306
Low	36.4	391
Rural Aleppo		
Middle	26.0	660
Low	25.3	1251
Parity of EW's mother		
1	—	—
2–3	31.3	451
4–5	32.5	1127
6 and over	33.7	3497

Additional Children Wanted

The mean number of additional children wanted was very high in the rural area—much higher than in the urban areas. The mean number of additional children that eligible women wanted was 1.9 in Damascus, 2.5 in Sweida, and 5.1 in Rural Aleppo (Table 8.D.17). The mean number of additional children wanted was higher for women of low social status than for those of middle social status (table not shown), and increased with increasing ideal family size, but decreased slightly with actual family size.

In traditional communities like those under study, it is important to examine the sex of additional children wanted in relation to the sex of children already present in the family, if any. Tables 8.D.18 and 8.D.19 examine the number of

423

TABLE 8.D.17. MEAN NUMBER OF ADDITIONAL CHILDREN WANTED, BY RESIDENCE, PARITY, AND IDEAL FAMILY SIZE*

Residence and parity	Mean no. of additional children wanted by EW who specified an ideal family size of:							
	0	1	2	3	4	5	6 and over	All family sizes
Damascus								
1–3	—	—	1.09	1.35	1.98	(2.37)	(3.53)	1.76
4–5	—	—	(0.33)	(0.64)	0.92	(1.10)	(2.84)	1.14
6 and over	—	—	(3.17)	(0.86)	(1.54)	(1.86)	1.96	1.84
All parities	—	—	1.47	1.58	2.04	1.86	2.87	1.91
Sweida								
1–3	—	—	1.81	2.34	2.59	3.17	3.81	2.61
4–5	—	—	(0.73)	(1.44)	2.30	2.15	2.84	2.18
6 and over	—	—	(1.17)	(0.17)	1.79	2.03	2.84	2.25
All parities	—	—	1.66	2.24	2.52	2.58	3.16	2.52
Rural Aleppo								
1–3	—	—	—	(3.50)	4.38	3.67	6.21	5.23
4–5	—	—	—	(0.0)	(4.22)	(2.56)	4.25	3.83
6 and over	—	—	—	(7.00)	(3.18)	(2.53)	5.31	4.80
All parities	—	—	—	(4.50)	4.11	3.31	5.85	5.13

* Figures in parentheses refer to fewer than 25 eligible women.

additional boys wanted and the number of additional girls wanted in relation to the number of boys and the number of girls already present in the family, for all areas combined. The preference for males in this culture is apparent, as the number of additional boys wanted exceeded the number of additional girls wanted regardless of the composition of the family at the time. Moreover, the society was not a "planning" society, since the number of additional children wanted did not decrease as the number of children already present in the family increased.

TABLE 8.D.18. MEAN NUMBER OF ADDITIONAL BOYS WANTED, BY THE NUMBER OF BOYS AND THE NUMBER OF GIRLS ALREADY PRESENT IN THE FAMILY*

Number of boys already present in family	Mean no. of additional boys wanted by EW with indicated no. of girls in family							
	0	1	2	3	4	5	6 and over	All EW
0	2.30	2.25	2.04	1.90	(1.86)	(1.71)	(1.33)	2.19
1	1.96	1.90	1.79	1.74	(1.55)	(2.18)	(2.10)	1.88
2	2.15	1.72	1.82	1.73	(1.75)	(1.79)	(2.25)	1.86
3	(1.88)	1.53	1.75	1.95	(1.46)	(2.14)	(1.53)	1.73
4	(1.88)	(2.54)	2.93	(2.48)	(2.70)	(2.00)	(3.57)	2.62
5	(2.00)	(1.92)	(2.06)	(1.17)	(2.22)	(2.00)	(4.75)	2.05
6 and over	(3.00)	(2.00)	(1.86)	(2.00)	(3.36)	(2.50)	(0.80)	2.12
Totals	2.15	1.99	1.96	1.84	2.00	2.02	2.30	2.02

* Figures in parentheses refer to fewer than 25 eligible women.

TABLE 8.D.19. MEAN NUMBER OF ADDITIONAL GIRLS WANTED, BY THE NUMBER OF BOYS AND THE NUMBER OF GIRLS ALREADY PRESENT IN THE FAMILY*

Number of boys already present in family	Mean no. of additional girls wanted by EW with indicated no. of girls in family							
	0	1	2	3	4	5	6 and over	All EW
0	1.79	1.59	1.40	(1.08)	(1.67)	(0.00)	2.00	1.68
1	1.64	1.41	1.62	1.59	(2.40)	(2.33)	(2.50)	1.59
2	1.70	1.51	1.40	(1.68)	(1.57)	(1.78)	(2.00)	1.57
3	(1.08)	1.32	1.44	1.48	(1.36)	(2.56)	(0.89)	1.42
4	(1.14)	(1.19)	1.72	(1.83)	(2.20)	(2.18)	(3.50)	1.92
5	(1.33)	(1.20)	(0.85)	(0.78)	(1.56)	(2.40)	(5.33)	1.46
6 and over	(1.00)	(1.60)	(0.92)	(1.53)	(3.20)	(2.00)	(0.75)	1.65
Totals	1.69	1.45	1.43	1.50	1.96	2.16	2.41	1.63

* Figures in parentheses refer to fewer than 25 eligible women.

PART III: AN OVERVIEW OF THE STUDY

AN OVERVIEW OF THE STUDY

A. R. Omran

BACKGROUND

The collaborative study reported in this volume was designed to examine, in several developing countries, the health risks associated with certain patterns of family formation, including the number and spacing of pregnancies, maternal age, birth order, and family size. The possibility that such patterns may have been influenced by child loss was also examined and the opinions of the interviewed women on family formation and birth control were ascertained. Still another purpose of the study was to examine the social and cultural correlates of fertility and of family planning behaviour in various cultural settings.

The study was sponsored by the WHO Special Programme of Research, Development and Research Training in Human Reproduction, Geneva, and was coordinated by the WHO International Collaborating Centre for Epidemiological Studies in Human Reproduction, which is located in the Epidemiology Department of the University of North Carolina, Chapel Hill, USA. It was carried out in different cultural settings by research centres in ten countries. Studies in five centres (India, Iran, Lebanon, the Philippines, and Turkey) were completed earlier and reported in a previous volume.[1] The centre in China (Province of Taiwan), which withdrew from the collaborative study in 1972, subsequently completed the study independently with aid from the University of North Carolina and will report separately in 1980. Studies by the research centres in Colombia, Egypt, Pakistan, and the Syrian Arab Republic are reported in this volume.

Research Methods

Choice of strategy

The research strategies commonly considered in the study of family formation and health include (a) record linkage of birth certificates and child

---

[1] OMRAN, A. R. & STANDLEY, C. C., ED. *Family formation patterns and health.* Geneva. World Health Organization, 1976.

death certificates, (*b*) prospective household studies, (*c*) cross-sectional studies of children's health and development or of the mother's health, and (*d*) retrospective studies of certain disease conditions in relation to family formation.

For the current study, a cross-sectional approach was adopted involving a pregnancy history component in all countries. This decision was based on the following reasoning:

(*a*) record linkage, good as it may be for the study of childhood mortality, could not be used because of the absence of reliable and complete vital records (including recorded family formation data) in all countries;

(*b*) the prospective cohort approach was considered for every country, but because of the expense of this approach it could not be envisaged;

(*c*) despite their limitations, pregnancy histories could provide information on family formation, pregnancy wastage, child mortality, and family planning practices; the major advantage of this approach is the great saving in time and expense;

(*d*) the cross-sectional approach could provide a measure of current child health, growth and development, and IQ, as well as of maternal health; and

(*e*) the cross-sectional approach was particularly appropriate for collecting data on opinions and attitudes towards family formation and family planning, a major concern of all collaborating centres.

The cross-sectional approach and the retrospective pregnancy history analysis both have inherent limitations. Because of the importance of these limitations in the interpretation of the results of the collaborative study, they are briefly outlined in connexion with the appropriate study components.

Study components

The study components included:

(*a*) interviews with currently married women under age 45 (eligible women or EW);

(*b*) gynaecological examinations of all or subsamples of these women;

(*c*) paediatric examinations of all or subsamples of their children under the age of 5;

(*d*) IQ testing of their children aged 8–14 years (except in Egypt, where children aged 6–11 were tested).

Sampling

The main purpose of the study was to compare, within each of the countries, different patterns of family formation and their relations to health in various subcultures. Because of numerous constraints, it was impossible to select an area for the study that would represent a total population of a country, or a total culture, or a residential area within a country. Instead, in each

430

collaborating centre two or more samples of about 2000 EW each were selected from different urban, semi-urban, rural, or industrial groups. References to countries (Colombia, Egypt, etc.) in this chapter should be interpreted as references to these study populations (Tables 1A and 1B).

TABLE 1A. COLLABORATING CENTRES, STUDY AREAS, AND RESIDENTIAL GROUPS

Country	Collaborating institution	Study areas	Study populations
Colombia	The National School of Public Health, University of Antioquia, Medellin, Colombia	Nine neighbourhoods in Medellin	Old urban zone Newly settled zone
Egypt	Department of Epidemiology and Public Health, Assiut University and High Institute of Public Health, Alexandria University	Abnub district, Beni Muhammadeyat village, Kafr El Dawar industrial complex	Urban Rural Industrial
Pakistan	National Research Institute of Fertility Control, Population Division, Government of Pakistan	Two areas of Karachi: Nazimabad, and Malir/Saudabad	Urban Semi-urban
Syrian Arab Republic	Central Bureau of Statistics, Office of the Prime Minister, Damascus	Damascus, Sweida, Aleppo	Urban (large) Urban (small) Rural

Data collection

At the outset, a common research design was agreed upon by the participating investigators, and all collaborating centres used the same precoded interview questionnaires (appropriately translated into the local language and pretested locally)[1] and the same IQ test (Cattell & Cattell Culture-Fair Test), except for Egypt's investigators who used the Goodenough Draw-A-Man Performance Test. Although the clinical procedures used in the various centres were basically similar, they were carried out mostly in conformity with local patterns of practice. The collected data were analysed at WHO Headquarters in Geneva and at the WHO International Collaborating Centre in Chapel Hill, North Carolina.

Pooling of data from each centre, though desirable to enlarge sample sizes, especially for complex cross-tabulation, was rarely used in the body of the report. In this overview, data are pooled for fertility variables, pregnancy wastage, and childhood mortality. For this purpose, the residential groups were considered as clusters reflecting the major characteristics of the study areas. Nevertheless, pooling has been done with the proviso that, since no weighting was introduced in the process, the pooled data should not be considered as representative of the area as a whole.

---

[1] In addition, some of the questions were independently translated back into English to check the accuracy of the translation.

431

TABLE 1B. POPULATION COVERAGE

Country and residential group	Eligible women			Physical examination						IQ test children aged 8–14 years		
	Total in sample	Number inter-viewed	Percent inter-viewed	Women			Children under 5 years			Sample population	Number tested	Percent tested
				Sample population	Number examined	Percent examined	Sample population	Number examined	Percent examined			
Colombia												
Old urban zone	2747	2678	97.5	1306	1063	81.4	1141	943	82.6	1283	1074	83.7
Newly settled zone	2663	2601	97.7	1275	1147	90.0	1351	1234	91.3	1154	1025	88.8
		5279										
Egypt												
Urban	2200	2097	95.3	2097	1868	89.1	2195	1631	74.3	—	1172	—
Rural	2400	2145	89.4	2145	1504	70.1	2187	1678	76.7	—	548	—
Industrial	1232	619	50.2	619	338	54.6	—	—	—	—	1330	—
		4861										
Pakistan												
Urban	2500	2473	98.9	2473	2050	83.0	2367	1690	71.4	2947	2069	70.2
Semi-urban	2500	2389	95.6	2388	1753	73.0	2558	1397	54.6	3463	1325	38.3
		4862										
Syrian Arab Republic												
Urban (large)	2000	1975	98.8	1975	1214	61.5	2511	671	26.7	2954	1541	52.2
Urban (small)	2000	1711	86.0	1711	1116	65.2	2124	601	28.3	2395	1244	51.9
Rural	2000	1935	96.8	1935	1394	72.0	2840	953	33.6	2492	683	27.4
		5621										

TABLE 2. CHARACTERISTICS OF THE STUDY POPULATION BY RESIDENCE, SOCIAL STATUS, AGE, EDUCATION, AND OCCUPATION

Characteristics (indicators)	Colombia		Egypt			Pakistan		Syrian Arab Republic		
	Old urban zone	Newly settled zone	Rural	Urban	Industrial	Semi-urban	Urban	Large urban	Small urban	Rural
No. of EW interviewed	2669	2601	2145	2097	619	2389	2473	1975	1711	1935
Percent middle status	94	38	34	59	59	50	93	81	77	35
Mean age of EW	32	3.	—	—	—	31	31	31	32	30
Percent under 20 years	3	4	7	10	6	5	4	7	4	9
Percent illiterate EW										
Middle	4	2.	91	68	66	55	30	66	76	98
Low	35	4.	97	80	78	86	81	92	97	100
Total	6	3.	95	73	71	70	33	71	81	99
Percent illiterate husbands										
Middle	3	2.	57	14	12	7	4	33	39	59
Low	30	4.	88	50	14	64	62	94	96	96
Total	5	3.	78	29	12	36	8	45	52	84
Percent housewives										
Middle	87	8.	98	96	99	96	96	94	94	95
Low	95	9.	100	97	99	95	92	97	99	96
Total	87	9.	99	96	99	95	96	95	95	95
Percent professional husbands										
Middle	59	2.	22	40	10	69	60	20	37	32
Low	2	..	2	11	5	21	6	1	1	2
Total	55	1.	9	28	8	45	56	37	29	12

1. The Study Populations

The population groups and sample sizes covered by each collaborating centre are summarized in Table 1B.

The characteristics of the eligible women are shown in Table 2. According to local standards, the proportion of women who were of middle social status varied from less than one-half to more than two-thirds. In each area, so few of the women were of high social status that, for the purposes of analysis, they were included in the middle status group. The social status was determined according to a composite index, including family income, the education and occupation of the household head, and some measure of housing status. However, this index is culture bound and does not permit comparison between centres.

The fertility span from menarche to 45 years was represented, although unevenly. For instance, there were fewer women under age 20 in some of the groups than in others (Table 2).

As for education, most of the women were illiterate or had received only primary education. Relatively few women received secondary or higher education, while in all areas, most of the women married husbands more highly educated than themselves.

The great majority of women were housewives or engaged in low-paid jobs. The husbands were mostly skilled or unskilled workers, small landowners, or owners of small businesses. Except in the urban areas, few of the husbands were employed in professional jobs. In general, men and women living in urban areas were more educated and of higher social status than rural dwellers.

It should be noted that not all of the data for Egypt were available for analysis.

2. Family Formation Patterns and Social Characteristics

Most of the women in each area married at young ages (the mean ranging from 16 to 21 years); Columbian women married on the average at a later age (mean of 20 years) than women in the other three centres (Table 3).

As has been found before in many developing communites, fertility was relatively high in all the study areas. Completed fertility (mean parity at age 40–44) ranged from 5.6 in Colombia to 9.1 in Egypt. This differential was apparent whether fertility was measured as mean gravidity (number of pregnancies per woman), mean parity (number of live births per woman), or mean family size (number of living children). It is noteworthy that ideal family size as expressed by the eligible women was considerably less than the achieved family size, especially at age 40–44.

In every area, parity, family size, and ideal family size were all positively correlated with the EW's age, education, and social status.

It is of interest to report that in all areas the structure of most households was nuclear (husband, wife, and unmarried children). This variable was not,

TABLE 3. FAMILY FORMATION PATTERNS BY RESIDENCE AND SOCIAL STATUS

Characteristic	Colombia		Egypt			Pakistan		Syrian Arab Republic		
	Old urban zone	Newly settled zone	Rural	Urban	Industrial	Semi-urban	Urban	Large urban	Small urban	Rural
Mean age at marriage										
Middle	20.69	=0.02	—	—	—	17.3	18.5	18.31	18.71	17.07
Low	20.37	9.51	—	—	—	16.2	18.1	17.89	18.89	17.40
Total	20.68	9.70	17.0	17.6	18.0	16.7	18.3	18.23	18.76	17.29
Mean gravidity at age 40–44										
Middle	6.83	8.00	9.7	10.1	8.8	7.59	7.52	8.58	8.42	10.38
Low	6.23	9.75	8.7	10.5	8.8	8.58	8.36	9.23	8.31	9.33
Total	6.79	9.90	9.1	10.2	8.8	8.08	7.59	8.74	8.39	9.61
Mean parity at age 40–44										
Middle	5.65	6.58	8.8	9.0	8.6	6.63	6.60	7.23	7.47	8.97
Low	5.12	8.15	8.0	9.3	8.1	7.75	7.45	7.73	7.37	8.10
Total	5.63	7.65	8.2	9.1	8.4	7.18	6.67	7.36	7.44	8.33
Mean family size at age 40–44										
Middle	5.35	6.07	5.8	6.2	6.9	5.45	5.86	6.38	6.40	6.74
Low	4.77	7.46	6.1	7.0	6.9	5.92	6.48	6.66	5.99	6.29
Total	5.32	7.02	6.0	6.6	6.9	5.69	5.91	6.45	6.24	6.41
Mean ideal family size										
Middle	3.21	3.23	—	—	—	3.8	3.9	3.88	4.52	6.36
Low	3.20	3.21	—	—	—	4.0	4.2	3.89	5.03	6.51
Total	3.22	3.22	—	—	—	3.9	4.0	3.88	4.63	6.45
Percent nuclear families										
Middle	74.0	67.2	87.8	84.9	76.9	68.1	55.1	79.4	83.6	65.1
Low	67.3	67.5	96.0	84.0	82.3	74.5	70.4	73.5	83.6	60.9
Total	73.6	67.4	93.2	84.5	79.1	71.3	56.2	78.3	83.1	62.4

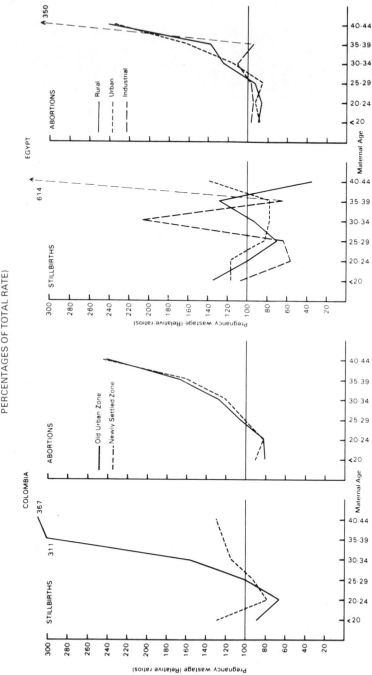

FIG. 1. PREGNANCY WASTAGE BY RESIDENCE AND MATERNAL AGE (RATES ARE PERCENTAGES OF TOTAL RATE)

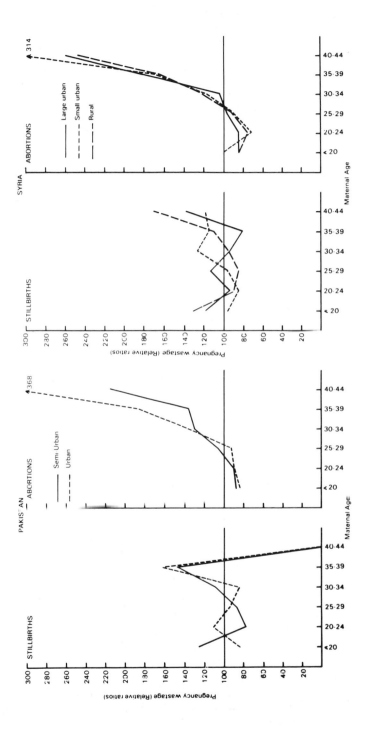

TABLE 4. PREGNANCY WASTAGE BY RESIDENCE

Country and residence	Number of pregnancies	Percent stillbirths	Percent abortions	Percent pregnancy wastage
Colombia				
Old urban zone	9 881	0.9	14.2	15.1
Newly settled zone	13 310	1.4	13.1	14.5
Egypt				
Urban	11 332	1.7	9.2	10.9
Rural	10 822	1.7	7.6	9.3
Industrial	2 825	2.0	8.7	10.7
Pakistan				
Urban	11 292	1.9	10.2	12.1
Semi-urban	12 921	2.3	9.1	11.4
Syrian Arab Republic				
Urban (large)	10 921	1.6	11.6	13.2
Urban (small)	9 383	2.7	7.9	10.6
Rural	11 263	2.0	9.1	11.1

however, used in the analysis, because it was realized during the surveys that, while these families were technically nuclear, they were often socially extended: some of the women in nuclear families might have been influenced in their fertility behaviour by relatives who were living outside the surveyed household, but in the same vicinity. All these communities were, in fact, in a stage of transition from extended to nuclear family structure.

3. Pregnancy Outcome and Family Formation

Information on pregnancy outcome was obtained by collecting from each eligible woman a detailed sequential pregnancy history dating from her marriage to the time of the survey. Pregnancies resulting in abortion (loss or termination of pregnancy occurring within 7 months of conception) or stillbirths (non-live births occurring 7 months or more after conception) were considered wasted. Stillbirth, abortion, and total pregnancy wastage rates by residence are shown in Table 4.

In several countries, most of the pregnancy wastage was made up of abortions. It was not possible to differentiate, from the retrospective pregnancy histories, between spontaneous and induced abortions. However, there is evidence from Colombia that induced abortion, although illegal at the time, was widely used.

For purposes of comparison, the pattern of pregnancy wastage (stillbirth and abortion) is expressed as a relative ratio. This is calculated by dividing the

438

pregnancy wastage rate of a specific component (such as birth order) by the rate for all components (total birth orders). Thus, the relative ratio of stillbirths among first order births is obtained as follows:

$$\frac{\text{Rate of stillbirths among first-order births}}{\text{Average rate of stillbirths among all birth orders (total)}} \times 100.$$

Pregnancy wastage and social characteristics

Pregnancy wastage varied by area, residence, and social status. Some of this variation was probably due to induced abortion. This may also explain some of the variation between centres. Variation in stillbirths was small.

Pregnancy wastage and maternal age

The pattern of pregnancy wastage, expressed as relative ratios by age to allow inter-area comparison, is given in Fig. 1. In most residential groups, pregnancy wastage ratios described a J-shaped relationship to maternal age. In most areas, 20–34 seemed to be the maternal age range in which there was the least pregnancy wastage. (However, in urban areas in Egypt and Syria, the pattern for stillbirths was uneven because of the small numbers). It is interesting to note that this pattern pertained not only to abortions, but also to stillbirths, a more reliable index of pregnancy wastage. It should be kept in mind, however, that abortion figures, which generally conform to the pattern, contain both induced and spontaneous abortions.

In most residential groups, higher rates of abortion were reported by the middle status women. The probable explanation is that middle status women resorted to induced abortion more frequently than low status women. Such a social differential was not, however, observed for stillbirth rates.

Pregnancy wastage and pregnancy order

For most residential groups, the relative ratios of pregnancy wastage (Fig. 2) showed an increase with pregnancy order. In some cases, there was also an increase in first order wastage.

Pregnancy wastage and pregnancy interval

In almost all study areas, both stillbirth and abortion rates per 100 pregnancies typically described a reversed J-shape with pregnancy interval, the highest risks being associated with intervals of less than 1 or 2 years, while minimal risks were associated with intervals of 3–5 years (Fig. 3). In all countries, the risks increased again for intervals of 6 or more years, probably because the women were older. Because the definition of pregnancy interval is the period between the end of the preceding pregnancy and the end of the index pregnancy, the interval could be some months shorter if the index pregnancy ended in abortion. Thus, some of the apparently increased risks of abortion with shorter pregnancy interval may be misleading.

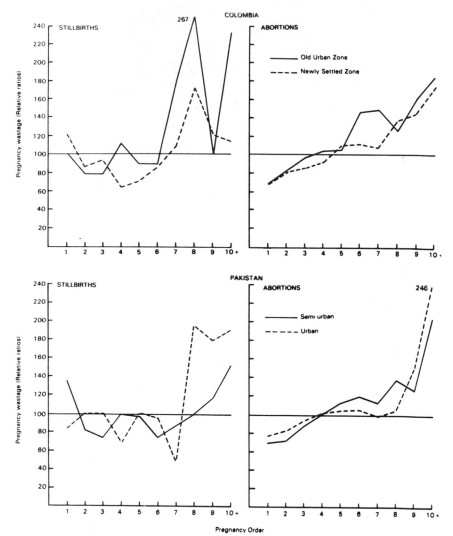

FIG. 2. PREGNANCY WASTAGE BY RESIDENCE AND PREGNANCY ORDER (RATES ARE PERCENTAGES OF TOTAL RATE)

Pregnancy wastage by outcome of preceding pregnancy

Several published reports have shown an increased likelihood of pregnancy wastage when the preceding pregnancy ended in abortion or stillbirth. This effect comes out clearly in Table 5. In the urban sample in Pakistan, for

440

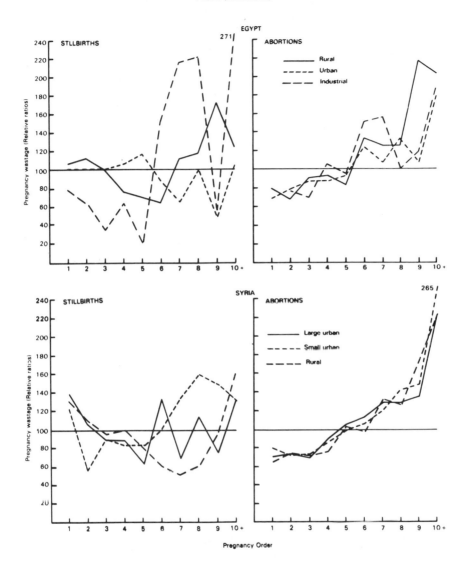

FIG. 2 (continued)

example, 18.2% of second pregnancies would end in fetal wastage if preceded by an abortion in the first pregnancy, whereas only 6.4% would have this poor outcome if the first pregnancy ended in a live birth. At higher levels of gravidity (e.g., gravidity 9) the results are even more dramatic with 50% of pregnancies being lost when preceded by an abortion compared with 12.4%

441

FIG. 3. PREGNANCY LOSS BY PRECEDING PREGNANCY INTERVAL

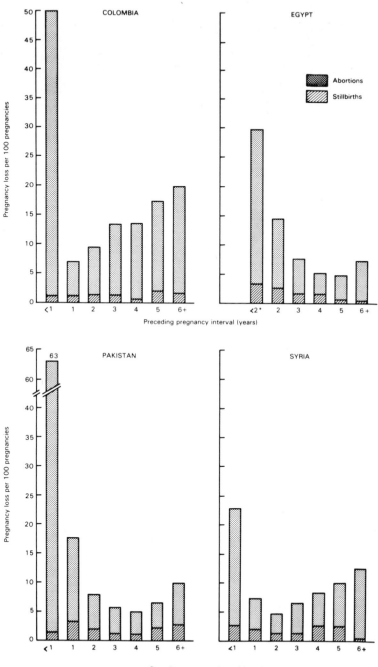

*For Egypt, the first two intervals are combined (<2)

TABLE 5. FETAL WASTAGE IN THE INDEX PREGNANCY BY GRAVIDITY AND OUTCOME OF THE PRECEDING PREGNANCY

(a) COLOMBIA

Residence and outcome of the preceding pregnancy	Total number of pregnancies	Percent fetal wastage by serial number of pregnancy (gravidity):							
		2	3	4	5	6	7	8	9
Urban									
Live birth	1564	6.5	7.6	7.1	14.4	14.4	12.7	19.0	14.3
Stillbirth	20	(—)	(—)	(—)	(—)	(—)	(—)	(—)	20.0
Abortion	211	20.0	15.8	17.9	30.0	29.4	15.0	34.8	11.1
Rural									
Live birth	1571	5.3	11.1	10.6	17.0	17.9	21.8	13.2	19.3
Stillbirth	12	(—)	(—)	(—)	(33.3)	(—)	(—)	(—)	(—)
Abortion	252	14.3	16.7	28.3	25.0	38.5	27.3	22.2	10.0

(b) PAKISTAN

Residence and outcome of the preceding pregnancy	Total number of pregnancies	Percent fetal wastage by serial number of pregnancy (gravidity):							
		2	3	4	5	6	7	8	9
Urban									
Live birth	1584	6.4	7.2	8.5	9.8	12.5	10.1	8.0	12.4
Stillbirth	24	(—)	(—)	(33.3)	(—)	(—)	(—)	(—)	(50.0)
Abortion	104	18.2	22.2	20.0	33.3	25.0	22.2	52.2	50.0
Semi-urban									
Live birth	1551	7.6	7.1	7.5	10.0	12.1	10.0	10.7	11.4
Stillbirth	39	(25.0)	(—)	(16.7)	(12.5)	(16.7)	(25.0)	(—)	(33.3)
Abortion	166	(33.3)	22.2	13.3	18.2	20.0	13.8	23.5	34.6

(c) SYRIAN ARAB REPUBLIC

Residence and outcome of the preceding pregnancy	Total number of pregnancies	Percent fetal wastage by serial number of pregnancy (gravidity):							
		2	3	4	5	6	7	8	9
Damascus									
Live birth	1241	8.6	5.4	9.6	11.3	10.2	14.8	7.2	11.5
Stillbirth	27	(—)	(28.6)	(25.0)	(33.3)	(—)	(25.0)	(100.0)	(—)
Abortion	128	12.5	13.3	25.0	—	33.3	8.7	29.2	26.7
Sweida									
Live birth	1140	5.9	7.6	3.8	5.9	7.4	7.6	8.5	8.0
Stillbirth	32	(20.0)	(20.0)	(20.0)	(—)	(—)	(100.0)	(16.7)	(66.7)
Abortion	97	(—)	18.2	30.8	(22.2)	47.1	16.7	(44.4)	23.5
Rural Aleppo									
Live birth	1122	3.7	7.2	8.5	8.3	8.1	10.1	5.8	9.0
Stillbirth	22	(0)	(20.0)	(—)	(40.0)	(50.0)	(—)	(—)	( )
Abortion	100	10.0	18.2	(—)	20.0	21.1	(—)	25.0	30.8

— = no wastage.
( ) = based on fewer than 10 preceding pregnancies with specified outcome.

when preceded by a live birth. This table also demonstrates the relative increase in pregnancy wastage with gravidity, whether the preceding pregnancy ended in a live birth or an abortion. Such patterns were noted for all centres.

Evaluation of the pregnancy wastage findings

A notable finding of this part of the study is that the risk of poor pregnancy outcome is lower for low parity groups, at maternal ages 20–29, and for pregnancy intervals of 3–5 years. This finding is in conformity with the results obtained in previous studies (see review in Part I).

Nevertheless, the following methodological problems should be considered, although they relate more to abortions than to stillbirths.

(*a*) Although the relationship of pregnancy wastage to family formation and social variables was probably greatly influenced by the selective use of induced abortion, it was not possible to separate spontaneous from induced abortions in this retrospective pregnancy history study.

(*b*) Underreporting of pregnancy outcome is usually a significant problem in retrospective history studies. In this collaborative study, women's pregnancy histories covered a period of up to 30 years; hence, underreporting was suspected to be likely, especially for the earlier pregnancies. Yet, in each area and for each residential group, the association of pregnancy wastage rates with family formation variables was the same for total pregnancies and for the last (and more easily remembered) pregnancies. This finding suggests that whatever underreporting occurred was more or less uniform (rather than selective for all pregnancies).

(*c*) The interaction between family formation variables is also a problem. Only for descriptive purposes were the family formation variables treated separately in the presentation, for in reality these variables interact closely with one another. For instance, a young multiparous mother is more likely to lose some of her pregnancies, not only because of her youth, especially if she is still in her teens, but because she may have repeated pregnancies at close intervals. To be able to disentangle these differences, stratification analysis of extremely large samples would be necessary.

(*d*) The nature of the samples also poses a problem, the samples comprising married women under the age of 45 rather than all women of reproductive age. Thus, pregnancies in older or unmarried women are not included. Furthermore, the more prolific women contributed disproportionately to the results; differences between such women and low gravidity women could have skewed the relationships.

(*e*) There was also the problem of selective survival. Women who lived to be interviewed could have been different in their social and family formation characteristics from women who died before the study but belonged to the same study population. It is also likely that women who died in this age span could have been those with higher pregnancy wastage and child loss.

(*f*) In certain situations, the strong relationship of poor pregnancy outcome

444

to short pregnancy interval could have been due partly to the effect of pregnancy wastage on the interval, rather than vice versa. This effect happens when a woman desiring a live birth experiences successive pregnancy losses.

(g) It was found in all areas and residential groups that the outcome of the index pregnancy was also affected by the outcome of the preceding one. In other words, a woman who lost a pregnancy was also more likely to lose the following one. The relationship of pregnancy wastage to gravidity, however, persists after controlling for this effect.

4. Child Mortality and Family Formation

Data on child mortality were obtained from the women through the detailed pregnancy history. Mortality rates were classified into the usual risk periods, namely, under 1 month (neonatal), 1–11 months (post-neonatal), and 1–4 years. In order to avoid confusing these rates with the conventional calendar rates, they are expressed as percentages of live births reported by eligible women. The details of mortality risks by birth order, maternal age, and birth interval are given in the body of the report.

For the purpose of this review, one index, namely, infant or under-one-year mortality is used. Cumulative as it is, this index is preferred to its components: neonatal (under month) and post-neonatal (1–11 months) mortality, particularly as, for deaths occurring many years previously, a mother's recall of whether the child died at 3 weeks or 5 weeks of life may not be accurate. In regard to the 1–4 years mortality, there is a problem of truncation, since children born less than 5 years before the interview would not have been exposed to the risk of death for the full 5 years; if they were only 2 years old at the time of interview, for example, they might die before reaching their fifth birthday. This problem is of small magnitude in the case of under-one-year mortality.

There is, however, a serious problem of another kind with the under-one-year mortality rates based on the experience reported by women aged up to 45 years. Obviously, the births on which these mortality rates are based occurred at different times, from less than 1 year to close to 30 years preceding the interview. During this long period, the risks of child mortality declined considerably in all areas. This decline, in turn, could have distorted the relationship between family formation variables and infant mortality. It is possible, for instance, that the relative risks for some early birth orders are exaggerated because these birth orders occurred at a time of higher risks of child mortality. To overcome this bias, at least in part, a cohort analysis was done, as shown in Tables 6 and 7.

Infant mortality and social class

As expected, infant mortality per 100 reported live births was higher in the low social status groups than in the middle status groups in virtually all populations.

445

TABLE 6. INFANT MORTALITY BY AGE AT INTERVIEW, MATERNAL AGE AT TIME OF INFANT'S DEATH, AND RESIDENCE*

Culture	Age at interview	Maternal age		
		<25	25–34	35–44
Colombia				
Old urban zone	<25	2.4	—	—
	25–34	2.1	1.6	—
	35–44	4.1	3.5	3.3
Newly settled zone	<25	2.8	—	—
	25–34	3.9	2.7	—
	35–44	5.9	4.4	4.1
Pakistan				
Semi-urban	<25	7.9	—	—
	25–34	7.5	6.5	—
	35–44	12.4	8.5	9.4
Urban	<25	3.1	—	—
	25–34	5.7	2.6	—
	35–44	7.1	5.0	5.7
Syrian Arab Republic				
Large urban	<25	6.5	—	—
	25–34	6.4	4.0	—
	35–44	9.0	5.7	3.7
Small urban	<25	6.9	—	—
	25–34	7.8	5.5	—
	35–44	12.1	8.7	6.4
Rural	<25	8.7	—	—
	25–34	11.0	7.7	—
	35–44	15.0	10.1	9.3

* No comparable data were available for Egypt.

Infant mortality and maternal age

Table 6 demonstrates the higher infant mortality experienced by the older cohorts. Mortality rates under 1 year among births occurring within the 10-year period preceding the interview (above the diagonal line in Table 6) were considered. In order to allow easy inter-area comparisons, these rates were converted into relative ratios with the rate for each total equalling 100. The results are given in Table 7 and Fig. 4.

Other investigations, reviewed in Part I, chapter 1, have most commonly found either a J-shaped or direct relationship between infant mortality rates and maternal age. In the present study, the J-shaped pattern was found in both Colombia and Pakistan. In the Syrian Arab Republic, the percentage of deaths of children under 1 year of age describes a reversed J-shape with maternal age,

TABLE 7. INFANT MORTALITY DURING THE 10 YEARS PRECEDING INTERVIEW, BY
MATERNAL AGE, BIRTH ORDER, AND DURATION OF PRECEDING PREGNANCY INTERVAL
(RELATIVE RATIOS)

Characteristic	Colombia		Pakistan		Syrian Arab Republic		
	Old urban zone	Newly settled zone	Semi-urban	Urban	Large urban	Small urban	Rural
Maternal age							
<20	117	109	134	103	169	130	131
20–24	74	81	91	108	104	98	95
25–29	70	109	101	76	82	93	98
30–34	157	91	69	95	91	118	85
35–39	135	138	133	151	84	105	116
40–44	230	84	242	151	0	102	74
Birth Order							
1	70	69	136	127	111	107	127
2	104	84	96	116	141	112	88
3	70	94	61	68	64	109	81
4	87	78	93	89	109	119	93
5	78	122	85	54	100	121	91
6 and over	187	131	113	159	89	74	104
Duration of preceding pregnancy interval (years)							
<1	346	276	45	216	143	169	148
1–2	100	88	152	119	91	109	92
2–3	88	88	98	100	75	28	63
3–4	71	76	41	111	66	52	63
4–5	50	91	47	35	0	22	134
5 and over	71	47	83	46	23	0	71

with high risks among infants born to mothers under 20 years of age, the rates decreasing steeply to a minimum somewhere between ages 20 and 34, then rising again to some extent. The relatively high risk associated with young maternal ages may be due partly to the higher risks of mortality among births occurring in the early years of the cohort when child mortality was higher than in the more recent years. Part of the risk may still be due to the young maternal age itself.

Infant mortality and birth order

In previous studies a reversed J-shaped relationship has been found between neonatal mortality rates and birth order, and a direct relationship for post-neonatal mortality rates. In the present study, a J-shaped relationship between mortality under 1 year of age and birth orders was found in Colombia and a U-shaped relationship in Pakistan. No distinct pattern was revealed in the Syrian Arab Republic. Because some of the first order births actually occurred in the early part of the 10-year period when mortality was high, only a part of their high risk of death can be attributed to being first order births. Conversely, the risks for sixth and higher order births may have been

FIG. 4. INFANT MORTALITY DURING 10 YEARS PRECEDING INTERVIEW, BY MATERNAL AGE, BIRTH ORDER, AND DURATION OF PRECEDING PREGNANCY INTERVAL (RELATIVE RATIOS)

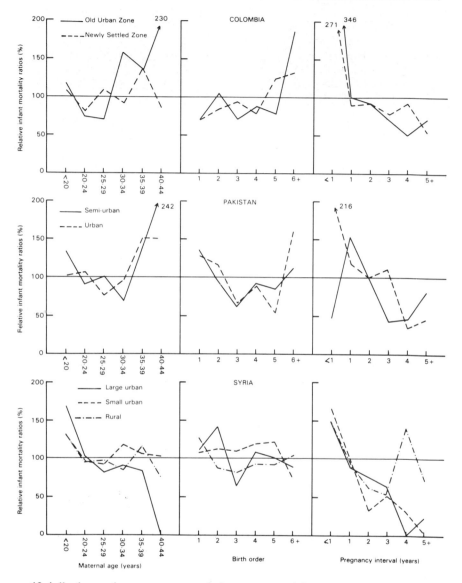

artificially lower because many of them occurred in more recent years after childhood mortality had declined.

Infant mortality and birth interval

As in earlier studies, the risk of under-one-year mortality was found to be high for births occurring within short intervals (less than 2 years) after previous births. In Rural Aleppo, a second increase in infant mortality occurred for intervals greater than 5 years (Fig. 4).

448

Evaluation of infant mortality and family formation

Despite cohort analysis, the relationship between infant mortality and family formation was still subject to some distortion, because some of the births exposed to the risk of mortality occurred earlier in the 10-year period preceding the interview. Hence, they were still exposed to higher risks than more recent births. Selective recall, although less likely to affect the last 10 years, could still have distorted both reported birth and reported death rates. A small problem of truncation may also have been present, since some of the children born less than 1 year before the interview could still have died before reaching the age of 1 year had they been observed for a longer period.

There is also the likelihood that certain environmental factors strongly related to mortality may have distorted the relationship of child mortality to family formation variables. While the effect of social status could be measured, that of other cultural, social, and environmental factors could not.

5. Family Formation and Child Health and Development

In a number of large-scale studies, it has been found that the more siblings a child has, the less adequate is his physical and intellectual development and the more prone he is to malnutrition and infection (see Part I, chapter 1). The data on child health were obtained from a medical and anthropometric examination of the children of the eligible women, as well as from a laboratory investigation of their blood and, for Egypt, of stools. In all countries, the women were asked whether their children under 10 years of age had experienced fever, diarrhoea, or cough (of more than 1 day's duration each) during the month preceding the interview. Weight and height were measured, and haemoglobin levels were determined for eligible women's children under 5 in all countries. This was supplemented for these children in all centres except the Syrian one with a paediatric examination and, in Egypt, with a parasitic infestation survey.

Height, weight, and haemoglobin

Using the frequency distribution of means, no consistent pattern emerged between weight, height, or haemoglobin in relation to family formation variables. However, the data from 3 of the centres were retabulated, classifying children as of low or high pregnancy order in relation to maternal age. The classification scheme is as follows:

Maternal age:	<20	20–24	25–29	30–34	35–39	40–44
Low pregnancy order for age:						
Colombia	1	1–3	1–5	1–7	1–7	1+
Pakistan	1	1–3	1–5	1–5	1–7	1–7
Syrian Arab Republic	1	1–3	1–5	1–7	1+	1+
High pregnancy order for age:						
Colombia		2+	4+	6+	8+	8+	—
Pakistan		2+	4+	6+	6+	8+	8+
Syrian Arab Republic		2+	4+	6+	8+	—	—

| Residence | Mean values for children of low and of high pregnancy order for given maternal age | | | | | |
| | Height (cm) | | Weight (kg) | | Haemoglobin (g/100 ml) | |
	Low	High	Low	High	Low	High
Colombia	65.8	64.0	7.2	6.6	11.1	10.8
Old urban zone	66.3	63.0	7.4	6.3	11.2	10.8
Newly settled zone	65.2	64.4	7.0	6.7	10.9	10.8
Pakistan	64.1	60.7	7.2	6.6	9.5	9.7
Semi-urban	59.6	59.2	6.3	6.2	9.4	9.7
Urban	66.0	63.0	7.6	7.1	9.5	9.7
Syrian Arab Republic	75.0	74.6	9.8	9.2	10.9	10.1
Large urban	74.6	(73.9)	9.9	(9.0)	10.9	(11.1)
Small urban	74.6	(74.0)	10.1	(9.3)	9.5	(9.4)
Rural	75.4	74.9	9.6	9.3	10.0	10.0

* Numbers in parentheses refer to fewer than 20 eligible women. No comparable data were available for Egypt.

The results are given in Table 8 for infants under 1 year of age. It is apparent that children of pregnancy orders classified as high for maternal age had somewhat lower mean heights and weights than those classified as low for maternal age. This difference is less marked for rural areas and for areas that still preserved a rural character. No consistent combined influence of maternal age and gravidity on haemoglobin was observed.

Infection

Paediatric examination of eligible women's children under 5 years of age revealed a prevalence of infection ranging from 20 to 50%, with a tendency to higher values in rural than in urban areas. The rate of infection among these children tended to rise with family size in both Colombia and Pakistan (Table 9). Intestinal parasitic infestation in both rural and urban areas of the Egyptian study revealed a distinct rise with family size.

It is interesting to note that, as reported by the mothers, the prevalence among children of fever and diarrhoea (each of more than one day's duration during the preceding month) tended to decrease with family size in several areas. This discrepancy between the clinical findings and the mothers' testimony could be explained by the possibility that the more children a woman had, the less likely she was to notice and/or remember their symptoms.

TABLE 9. FREQUENCY OF SELECTED CONDITIONS IN CHILDREN BY FAMILY SIZE

Percentage of children with various conditions in families of indicated size:

Residence	Fever[a]						Diarrhoea[a]						Infection[b]					
	1	2	3	4	5	6 and over	1	2	3	4	5	6 and over	1	2	3	4	5	6 and over
Colombia																		
Old urban zone	11	25	19	13	11	21	12	25	19	13	11	21	14	13	20	21	25	16
Newly settled zone	5	13	14	14	12	42	5	13	14	14	12	42	22	33	28	37	33	30
Egypt													1 & 2		3 & 4		5 and over	
Rural	20	20	15	16	15	12	20	17	14	14	13	10	50		46		48	
Urban	19	17	14	12	10	9	20	16	12	10	8	7	51		44		43	
Industrial	—		—		—		—		—		—		—		—		—	
	1 & 2		3 & 4		5 and over		1 & 2		3 & 4		5 and over		1 & 2		3 & 4		5 and over	
Pakistan																		
Semi-urban	49		52		52		38		36		32		29		30		33	
Urban	57		69		69		34		27		24		18		24		27	
	1	2	3	4	5	6 and over	1	2	3	4	5	6 and over						
Syrian Arab Republic																		
Large urban	47	43	46	43	44	45	57	45	39	29	40	35	Not available					
Small urban	50	42	38	34	38	38	48	39	28	32	35	33						
Rural	76	56	54	41	45	46	81	54	61	52	52	47						

[a] Children under 10 years, reported by eligible women.
[b] Children under 5 years, medically diagnosed.

451

TABLE 10. INTELLIGENCE QUOTIENTS OF CHILDREN AGED 8–14 YEARS IN DIFFERENT STUDY AREAS, BY RESIDENCE, BIRTH ORDER AND FAMILY SIZE*

Residence	No. in sample	Intelligence quotients of children of birth order:						Intelligence quotients of children in families of size:					
		1	2	3	4	5	6 and over	1	2	3	4	5	6 and over
Colombia													
Old urban zone	1072	112.72	110.18	106.42	106.74	106.44	104.27	(117.88)	113.37	112.76	110.54	108.38	105.13
Newly settled zone	1005	92.83	91.82	94.97	89.22	89.94	85.11	(76.20)	95.44	95.72	97.10	93.96	88.95
Egypt													
Rural	548	93.21	95.67	100.40	98.14	100.66	99.20	(98.99)	92.05	95.11	99.09	102.05	97.69
Urban	1172	103.39	101.12	103.05	100.36	99.41	101.70	(104.65)	102.80	102.36	101.91	100.98	101.46
Pakistan													
Semi-urban	1326	93.53	95.62	95.20	91.79	91.83	93.44	(96.14)	89.51	92.85	96.39	95.82	92.52
Urban	2067	105.07	105.02	104.63	102.97	104.89	103.17	(114.00)	110.21	106.69	106.73	103.53	103.14
Syrian Arab Republic													
Large urban	1525	109.05	107.89	106.47	108.28	102.43	105.20	(116.67)	(129.44)	110.71	108.92	107.80	105.51
Small urban	1237	102.66	101.00	103.91	102.46	102.30	101.69	(87.86)	(102.47)	101.19	102.38	102.19	102.46
Rural	635	84.75	83.65	82.78	84.37	84.44	84.04	—	77.50	77.12	79.97	81.48	85.64

* Figures in parentheses refer to fewer than 25 children.

Intelligence quotient and family formation

The Cattell & Cattell Culture-Fair Test was used (as a group test) administered to schoolchildren) by 3 centres to measure the IQ of children aged 8–14 years. The Goodenough Draw-A-Man Test was used in Egypt. Two problems became evident, however. First, the tests required some familiarity of children with forms and figures; hence, it was administered only to children attending schools. In some areas, the low rate of school enrolment meant that the test coverage was selective; these problems were compounded in some areas by the relatively small size of the samples. The raw scores in each area

TABLE 11. INTELLIGENCE QUOTIENTS OF CHILDREN BY BIRTH ORDER, RESIDENCE AND SOCIAL STATUS*

Residence and social status	Standard IQ score	
	Low birth order	High birth order
COLOMBIA		
Old urban zone		
High	115.7	108.8
Middle	110.8	106.2
Low	(101.6)	94.4
Newly settled zone		
Middle	101.9	93.9
Low	91.9	87.3
PAKISTAN		
Urban		
High	112.2	108.5
Middle	103.9	103.2
Low	(99.8)	96.5
Rural		
High	(100.0)	(00.7)
Middle	97.5	96.0
Low	93.4	90.1
SYRIAN ARAB REPUBLIC		
Large urban		
High	(123.6)	(120.0)
Middle	109.8	106.6
Low	104.2	103.0
Small urban		
Middle	103.5	102.6
Low	102.2	98.4
Rural		
Middle	90.6	86.6
Low	81.9	81.9

* Figures in parentheses refer to fewer than 25 eligible women. Comparable data were not available for Egypt.

453

were standardized according to the area's mean scores and standard deviations specific for age (Grant Dahlstrom—personal communication).

The results are summarized in Table 10. Except for Colombia, the pattern is not definite or consistent in relation to birth order or family size. This may be due to interactions of numerous variables with IQ. If, however, the combined effects of maternal age and birth order are considered (as previously done for weight and height), a more definite pattern emerges. A low birth order for a given age seems to be favourable to a higher IQ score. This is consistent in the 3 countries (data were not available for Egypt) and for all social and residential groups (Table 11).

It should be emphasized that in all areas and for all patterns of family formation the higher the social status of a child, the higher his or her IQ score.

TABLE 12. GYNAECOLOGICAL SYMPTOMS REPORTED BY ELIGIBLE WOMEN, BY RESIDENCE AND PARITY*

Symptom, country, and residence		Percentage of women reporting symptoms among EW of parity:						
		0	1	2	3	4	5	6 and over
Irregular periods								
Colombia:	Old urban zone	16	16	15	14	23	14	19
	Newly settled zone	28	24	20	22	24	28	24
Pakistan:	Semi-urban	37	22	23	24	22	23	38
	Urban	23	19	19	21	20	19	25
Syrian Arab Republic:	Large urban	31	21	26	23	20	15	22
	Small urban	32	33	28	29	27	23	30
	Rural	22	15	18	21	21	26	20
Discharge								
Colombia:	Old urban zone	33	42	43	41	40	37	34
	Newly settled zone	38	48	52	49	55	55	41
Pakistan:	Semi-urban	50	48	61	60	53	57	81
	Urban	40	39	48	53	47	51	49
Syrian Arab Republic:	Large urban	23	20	21	21	20	17	21
	Small urban	17	16	19	15	16	15	17
	Rural	16	17	15	14	15	22	17
Prolapse								
Colombia:	Old urban zone	0	2	3	2	2	4	4
	Newly settled zone	3	3	4	5	5	7	5
Pakistan:	Semi-urban	8	11	10	13	12	17	18
	Urban	2	8	8	13	16	16	15
Syrian Arab Republic:	Large urban	6	4	7	9	9	8	11
	Small urban	4	6	11	8	8	15	12
	Rural	11	11	11	15	16	18	17

* Comparable data were not available for Egypt.

There were also distinct differences between the IQ scores of children by residence, with the rural children scoring lower.

6. Family Formation and Maternal Health

The study questionnaire included inquiries about gynaecological symptoms of the women. In addition, gynaecological examination (usually conducted by a lady physican) was also done. (These data are not available for the Egyptian centre.) The frequency of gynaecological complaints (Table 12) varied among centres. The relationship of these complaints to parity was not consistent. Prolapse, however, which is the most serious condition and which may require surgical repair, was consistently reported more by women with high parity (4 or more) than by women with low parity (3 or less).

Gynaecological examination confirmed this positive relationship between prolapse and parity in all areas (Table 13). This relationship is examined

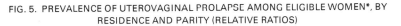

FIG. 5. PREVALENCE OF UTEROVAGINAL PROLAPSE AMONG ELIGIBLE WOMEN*, BY RESIDENCE AND PARITY (RELATIVE RATIOS)

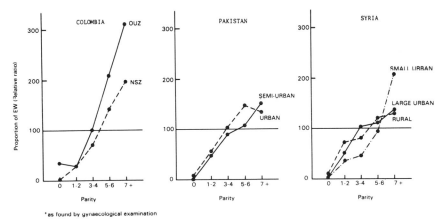

* as found by gynaecological examination

further in Fig. 5 where the relative ratios of prevalence of prolapse by parity are graphed. The relative ratios are the percentage of women with prolapse at each parity relative to the percentage for all parities. The increase in prolapse with increasing parity is found in each residential area. While some or all of this increase in prolapse can be attributed to birth injury, the cases of prolapse reported by or discovered in nulliparas could be due to congenital weakness of pelvic muscles and supporting tissues. Gynaecological examination also revealed a significant increase in infective and other diseases of the cervix, as well as in other diseases of the female genital organs, with parity and age in all areas.

The other gynaecological conditions (reported by the women or diagnosed by physicians) revealed only small or inconsistent variations with parity. Blood pressure measurement, which was carefully done in each area, showed that neither the mean systolic nor the mean diastolic blood pressure increased with parity, although both increased with age within each parity group.

455

TABLE 13. SELECTED GYNAECOLOGICAL FINDINGS IN ELIGIBLE WOMEN, BY RESIDENCE AND PARITY

Residence	Percentage of women with various findings among EW of indicated parity:																			
	Infective diseases of cervix					Uterovaginal prolapse					Other diseases of cervix					Other diseases of genital organs				
	0	1–2	3–4	5–6	7 and over	0	1–2	3–4	5–6	7 and over	0	1–2	3–4	5–6	7 and over	0	1–2	3–4	5–6	7 and over
Colombia																				
Old urban zone	0	2	4	7	6	3	2	8	18	25	7	18	19	13	22	50	57	71	75	75
Newly settled zone	2	7	5	9	13	0	5	13	27	38	6	21	21	22	17	34	50	58	65	77
Pakistan																				
Semi-urban	25	36	44	38	44	0	12	22	26	37	28	39	44	57	59	37	44	49	52	51
Urban	13	22	25	23	23	1	6	11	16	14	3	14	17	19	23	17	18	22	18	23
Syrian Arab Republic[a]																				
Large urban	4	11	15	16	16	0	5	10	11	13			—[a]					—[a]		
Small urban	5	7	10	11	11	0	1	2	3	7			—					—		
Rural	4	6	6	8	8	1	6	6	9	10			—					—		

[a] For the Syrian Arab Republic the figures for "infective diseases of cervix" include those for "other diseases of cervix" and "other diseases of genital organs"

7. Child Loss Experience and Family Formation

The child survival hypothesis stipulates that fertility level is positively related to child loss. Thus, it was assumed at the outset of the study that women who lost one or more of their children would, on the average, have higher fertility than those who did not, owing to what is called "replacement motivation". It was also possible that fertility would be high in communities with high child loss, even among women who themselves had not experienced such a loss, owing to what is called "insurance motivation". In other words, women in such communities would have more children as an insurance against possible or feared loss.

In order to examine these hypotheses, the fertility pattern, fertility ideals, and contraceptive use were investigated among women who had completed or who were close to completing their family formation (i.e., those aged 40 and over). It became evident in our analysis that fertility increased with child loss experience. But since this is a retrospective approach, the antecedent-consequence issue in the relationship of child loss to fertility at age 40 or over could not be ascertained. The relationship can go in either direction, i.e., high parity leads to high child loss and high child loss leads to high parity. As a partial solution to this problem, analysis was restricted to child loss among the first 3 live births for women aged 40–44 (Table 14).

Child loss experience and ideal family size

It is striking that the mean ideal family size, while reflecting the local cultural and residential pattern, did not change significantly with child loss in each group.

Child loss experience and fertility

Both mean gravidity and mean parity among women aged 40–44 increased progressively with child loss among the first 3 live births in all areas. Another relevant observation is that in all countries both the mean gravidity and, to a lesser extent, the mean parity of women who had no child loss among their first 3 live births were considerably higher than the corresponding mean ideal family size. This is consistent with an element of insurance motivation, namely, that fertility is high in this group because of expected high child loss. It may also be due, of course, to the lack of availability of fertility regulation methods.

Child loss experience and family size

With regard to mean family size, there was a negative association with child loss. This pattern was persistent in all areas and within each residential (and social) group. Using the mean ideal family size for each group as a measure of the level of fertility that women in the group would like to achieve on the average, we can see that women in each child loss category have achieved an actual family size much larger than what they considered ideal. This may again be a reflection of insurance motivation by all women.

457

TABLE 14. FERTILITY IDEALS AND PERFORMANCE AT AGE 40–44, BY CHILD LOSS AMONG THE FIRST 3 LIVE BIRTHS*

Mean ideal family size and fertility patterns among EW[a] with indicated child loss:

Residence	Mean ideal family size[b]			Mean gravidity			Mean parity			Mean family size		
	0	1	2–3	0	1	2–3	0	1	2–3	0	1	2–3
Colombia												
Old urban zone	3.6	3.4	3.6	7.6	8.8	(10.0)	6.4	7.4	(8.0)	6.2	5.9	(6.0)
Newly settled zone	3.4	3.2	3.2	9.5	10.7	(9.2)	8.0	8.7	(7.7)	7.7	7.0	(5.2)
Egypt												
Rural	3.8	4.0	4.2	8.8	9.3	10.1	8.0	8.6	9.4	6.0	5.7	5.0
Urban	3.7	3.7	3.7	9.3	10.8	10.5	8.3	9.6	9.7	6.7	6.4	4.9
Industrial	3.6	3.5	(3.8)	9.1	10.0	(8.8)	8.4	9.0	(8.6)	7.3	6.7	(5.3)
Pakistan												
Semi-urban	4.0	4.0	4.0	8.2	8.7	9.0	7.3	7.9	8.3	6.8	5.8	4.1
Urban	3.9	3.9	4.1	7.8	8.6	9.1	6.9	7.6	8.1	6.6	6.0	5.3
Syrian Arab Republic												
Large urban	4.1	4.0	4.1	8.7	10.3	(10.8)	7.2	8.9	(9.1)	6.9	7.1	(5.8)
Small urban	4.8	5.0	5.0	8.6	9.1	10.0	7.6	8.3	8.9	7.1	6.3	6.0
Rural	6.6	6.5	6.0	9.5	10.7	10.6	8.2	9.2	10.0	7.5	6.9	5.6

* Figures in parentheses refer to fewer than 25 eligible women.
[a] Excluding women with fewer than 3 live births.
[b] All ages.

Child loss experience and contraception

One might attempt to test the child survival hypothesis by determining whether women who have lost a child were less likely to use family planning methods than women who have not. While the approval and use of contraception varied from one centre and residential group to another, the data

TABLE 15. APPROVAL AND USE OF BIRTH CONTROL, BY CHILD LOSS AMONG THE FIRST 3 LIVE BIRTHS*

Residence	Proportion of women approving/using birth control among those with indicated child loss:					
	Approval of birth control (%)			Ever use of birth control (%)		
	0	1	2–3	0	1	2–3
Colombia						
Old urban zone	96.6	94.6	91.7	93.2	94.0	91.7
Newly settled zone	94.1	92.4	83.3	88.6	81.9	80.0
Pakistan						
Semi urban	91.5	94.3	85.6	42.6	37.3	31.3
Urban	91.7	89.5	84.7	67.9	64.2	44.1
Syrian Arab Republic						
Large urban	76.6	73.0	62.5	58.6	57.6	42.2
Small urban	68.1	59.2	49.4	38.5	28.5	(25.3)
Rural	13.4	19.6	13.4	3.7	(4.6)	(3.8)

* Figures in parentheses refer to fewer than 25 eligible women. Comparable data were not available for Egypt.

consistently show that women who had lost one or more of their first 3 live births were less likely to approve of or to use contraception than women with no child loss. The negative attitude was more pronounced with higher child loss (Table 15). These findings are of importance in the preparation of educational and motivational material for family planning, which clearly should stress the increased chances of child survival that now prevail.

Child loss experience and subsequent birth interval

The duration of the birth interval following the death of a child was found to be several months shorter in all areas than the interval following the birth of a child who had survived his first year of life. This finding (table not given) reflects the biological effect of child survival, namely a longer period of post-partum amenorrhoea, especially with prolonged lactation. It could also be due (at least in part) to the wilful postponement of another pregnancy until the suckling child has become older.

TABLE 16. OPINIONS ON FAMILY FORMATION AND HEALTH BY RESIDENCE

Percentage of women agreeing with opinions in left-hand column

Opinion	Colombia[a]		Egypt			Pakistan		Syrian Arab Republic		
	OUZ	NSZ	Rural	Urban	Industrial	Semi-urban	Urban	Large urban	Small urban	Rural
A child's health is better in a small family	80.3	89.6	91.7	93.4	82.2	98.9	94.0	89.8	97.0	94.6
The mother's health is better in a small family	80.7	87.4	91.3	93.2	82.2	99.0	94.1	90.2	96.9	94.9
A child's health is better when the birth interval is 3 years rather than 1 year	81.5	92.4	95.2	94.7	79.6	98.5	95.8	93.1	97.8	94.8
The mother's health is better when the birth interval is 3 years rather than 1 year	84.3	91.6	94.8	94.6	78.4	98.5	96.0	93.8	97.8	94.9
A decrease in child mortality would result in fewer children being born										
Illiterate	67.7	63.3	52.8	73.7	36.4	62.3	63.7			
Primary education	67.1	69.6	77.7	80.9	38.7	64.9	65.4	78.4[b]	75.1[b]	44.5[b]
Secondary or higher education	71.3	81.6	83.3	92.6	—	71.8	64.8			
Contraception is beneficial to the mother's health	85.1	91.5	81.1	90.9	97.6	99.5	98.1	99.2	97.1	97.9
Contraception is beneficial to the child's health	94.6	98.5	42.8	66.7	97.8	99.9	99.4	99.3	99.1	94.8

[a] OUZ = old urban zone; NSZ = newly settled zone.
[b] These percentages are from Syria's total sample (responses by educational level were not available).

Comment

Our data support the child survival hypothesis and reflect the existence of the replacement motivation, the insurance motivation, and the biological motivation. Most of the differences are statistically significant.

8. Opinions on Health, Family Formation, and Birth Control

An important part of the interview survey was directed at determining knowledge, attitudes, and practices in relation to birth control, as well as the opinions of the interviewed women on family formation and health. The details of this survey are given in the separate country reports. By way of illustration,

TABLE 17. TIMING FAILURE OF LAST PREGNANCY, BY RESIDENCE, SOCIAL STATUS, AND PARITY*

Residence and social status	Percentage of EW who felt that their last pregnancy came sooner than they had wanted, at parity:			
	1–3	4–5	6 and over	All parities
COLOMBIA				
Old urban zone				
Middle	33.5	55.4	63.8	43.0
Low	44.1	48.4	65.9	51.4
Newly settled zone				
Middle	42.2	58.3	58.4	48.3
Low	54.5	60.5	69.1	61.8
PAKISTAN				
Semi-urban				
Middle	17.8	44.8	54.5	39.4
Low	22.7	39.2	35.5	42.9
Urban				
Middle	34.6	46.7	55.3	43.8
Low	33.3	38.7	53.9	45.0
SYRIAN ARAB REPUBLIC				
Large urban				
Middle	30.1	43.0	56.8	44.1
Low	24.7	37.8	48.4	41.9
Small urban				
Middle	37.6	43.0	57.5	45.7
Low	29.3	36.6	44.2	39.2
Rural				
Middle	7.4	13.5	11.5	10.5
Low	4.1	6.4	8.3	6.8

* No comparable data were available for Egypt.

461

however, the main hypotheses on health and family formation are summarized in Table 16.

For the first 4 questions in the table, the women were asked whether the health status would be better, worse, or the same in specified patterns of family formation. Almost all women in some areas and an overwhelming majority of them in others believed that a planned family (one with few, well-spaced pregnancies) promotes better maternal and child health and enhances the ability of a mother to provide child care.

Women were also asked whether a decrease in childhood mortality would result in fewer children being born. In each country a majority of the women felt that a decrease in childhood mortality would lead to declining fertility, with the proportion of affirmative answers increasing with educational level.

Of women who approved in principle of birth control, an overwhelming majority in each of the countries did so because they believed it was beneficial to the mother's or the child's health. When those who were opposed to the principle of birth control were asked if they were willing to use contraception on medical advice to protect their own or their child's health, the proportion of women who were willing to do so varied from a fifth in Pakistan to up to 90% in Colombia.

Timing failure of last pregnancy

One of the ways to discover an unmet need for family planning in conservative societies is to ask women if their last pregnancy came sooner than

TABLE 18. TIMING FAILURE OF LAST PREGNANCY, BY RESIDENCE AND EDUCATION*

| Residence | Percentage of EW at indicated educational level who experienced timing failure of last pregnancy: | | | | |
	No school	Primary	Secondary	College or higher	All levels
COLOMBIA					
Old urban zone	51.7	46.6	32.7	32.7	43.5
Newly settled zone	59.1	56.1	45.7	(80.0)	57.0
PAKISTAN					
Semi-urban	40.9	43.7	38.0	31.6	41.2
Urban	45.2	45.4	41.0	42.3	43.9
SYRIAN ARAB REPUBLIC					
Large urban	43.3	47.3	41.7	25.0	43.7
Small urban	44.4	43.4	42.6	(100.0)	44.2
Rural	8.1	(7.7)	—	—	8.1

* Numbers in parentheses refer to fewer than 25 eligible women. No comparable data were available for Egypt.

462

they had wanted. An affirmative answer to this question may be an indication that the pregnancy was not wanted.

Over one-third of the women in all areas (with the exception of the rural area in Syria) felt that their last pregnancy came sooner than they had wanted (Table 17). The prevalence of timing failure in the last pregnancy was higher among the low than among middle status women in Colombia. The reverse was true of the Syrian Arab Republic, while in the Pakistan the difference was small (for the total population). In all areas, the prevalence of timing failure increased consistently with parity, indicating an unsatisfied need for family planning. On the other hand, the prevalence was negatively associated with the women's education, suggesting that the more educated women are more successful planners than the less educated women (Table 18).

A Concluding Remark

In this overview, it has been possible to select a few of the most salient findings from each section of the study. The results of the study confirm, on the whole, earlier findings on the relationships between family formation patterns and health. This study has been the result of considerable collaborative efforts among the participating centres, to which the credit should primarily belong.

WHO publications may be obtained, direct or through booksellers, from:

ALGERIA: Société Nationale d'Edition et de Diffusion, 3 bd Zirout Youcef, ALGIERS
ARGENTINA: Carlos Hirsch SRL, Florida 165, Galerias Güemes, Escritorio 453/465, BUENOS AIRES
AUSTRALIA: *Mail Order Sales:* Australian Government Publishing Service, P.O. Box 84, CANBERRA A.C.T. 2600; *or over the counter from* Australian Government Publishing Service Bookshops *at:* 70 Alinga Street, CANBERRA CITY A.C.T. 2600; 294 Adelaide Street, BRISBANE, Queensland 4000; 347 Swanston Street, MELBOURNE, VIC 3000; 309 Pitt Street, SYDNEY, N.S.W. 2000; Mt Newman House, 200 St. George's Terrace, PERTH, WA 6000; Industry House, 12 Pirie Street, ADELAIDE, SA 5000; 156–162 Macquarie Street, HOBART, TAS 7000 — Hunter Publications, 58a Gipps Street, COLLINGWOOD, VIC 3066 — R. Hill & Son Ltd, 608 St. Kilda Road, MELBOURNE, VIC 3004; Lawson House, 10–12 Clark Street, CROW'S NEST, NSW 2065
AUSTRIA: Gerold & Co., Graben 31, 1011 VIENNA I
BANGLADESH: The WHO Programme Coordinator, G.P.O. Box 250, DACCA 5 — The Association of Voluntary Agencies, P.O. Box 5045, DACCA 5
BELGIUM: Office international de Librairie, 30 avenue Marnix, 1050 BRUSSELS — *Subscriptions to World Health only:* Jean de Lannoy, 202 avenue du Roi, 1060 BRUSSELS
BRAZIL: Biblioteca Regional de Medicina OMS/OPS, Unidade de Venda de Publicações, Caixa Postal 20.381, Vila Clementino, 04023 São Paulo, S.P.
BURMA: *see* India, WHO Regional Office
CANADA: *Single and bulk copies of individual publications (not subscriptions):* Canadian Public Health Association, 1335 Carling Avenue, Suite 210, OTTAWA, Ont. K1Z 8N8. *Subscriptions: Subscription orders, accompanied by cheque made out to the* Royal Bank of Canada, OTTAWA, Account World Health Organization, *should be sent to the* World Health Organization, P.O. Box 1800, Postal Station B, OTTAWA, Ont. K1P 5R5. *Correspondence concerning subscriptions should be addressed to the* World Health Organization, Distribution and Sales, 1211 GENEVA 27, Switzerland
CHINA: China National Publications Import Corporation, P.O. Box 88, BEIJING (PEKING)
COLOMBIA: Distrilibros Ltd, Pio Alfonso Garcia, Carrera 4a, Nos 36–119, CARTAGENA
CYPRUS: Publishers' Distributors Cyprus, 30 Democratias Ave Ayios Dhometious, P.O. Box 4165, NICOSIA
CZECHOSLOVAKIA: Artia, Ve Smeckach 30, 11127 PRAGUE I
DENMARK: Munksgaard Export and Subscription Service, Nørre Søgade 35, 1370 COPENHAGEN K
ECUADOR: Libreria Cientifica S.A., P.O. Box 362, Luque 223, GUAYAQUIL
EGYPT: Osiris Office for Books and Reviews, 50 KASR El Nil Street, CAIRO
EL SALVADOR: Libreria Estudiantil, Edificio Comercial B No 3, Avenida Libertad, SAN SALVADOR
FIJI: The WHO Programme Coordinator, P.O. Box 113, SUVA
FINLAND: Akateeminen Kirjakauppa, Keskuskatu 2, 00101 HELSINKI 10
FRANCE: Librairie Arnette, 2 rue Casimir-Delavigne, 75006 PARIS
GERMAN DEMOCRATIC REPUBLIC: Buchhaus Leipzig, Postfach 140, 701 LEIPZIG
GERMANY, FEDERAL REPUBLIC OF: Govi-Verlag GmbH, Ginnheimerstrasse 20, Postfach 5360, 6236 ESCHBORN — W. E. Saarbach, Postfach 101610, Follerstrasse 2, 5000 KÖLN I — Alex. Horn, Spiegelgasse 9, Postfach 3340, 6200 WIESBADEN
GHANA: Fides Enterprises, P.O. Box 1628, ACCRA
GREECE: G. C. Eleftheroudakis S.A., Librairie internationale, rue Nikis 4, ATHENS (T. 126)
HAITI: Max Bouchereau, Librairie "A la Caravelle", Boite postale 111-B, PORT-AU-PRINCE
HONG KONG: Hong Kong Government Information Services, Beaconsfield House, 6th Floor, Queen's Road, Central, VICTORIA
HUNGARY: Kultura, P.O.B. 149, BUDAPEST 62 — Akadémiai Könyvesbolt, Váci utca 22, BUDAPEST V
ICELAND: Snaebjørn Jonsson & Co., P.O. Box 1131, Hafnarstraeti 9, REYKJAVIK
INDIA: WHO Regional Office for South-East Asia, World Health House, Indraprastha Estate, Ring Road, NEW DELHI 110002 — Oxford Book & Stationery Co., Scindia House, NEW DELHI 110001; 17 Park Street, CALCUTTA 700016 (*Sub-agent*)
INDONESIA: M/s Kalman Book Service Ltd. Kwitang Raya No. 11, P.O. Box 3105/Jkt., JAKARTA
IRAN: Iranian Amalgamated Distribution Agency, 151 Khiaban Soraya, TEHERAN
IRAQ: Ministry of Information, National House for Publishing, Distributing and Advertising, BAGHDAD
IRELAND: The Stationery Office, DUBLIN 4
ISRAEL: Heiliger & Co., 3 Nathan Strauss Street, JERUSALEM
ITALY: Edizioni Minerva Medica, Corso Bramante 83–85, 10126 TURIN; Via Lamarmora 3, 20100 MILAN
JAPAN: Maruzen Co. Ltd, P.O. Box 5050, TOKYO International, 100–31
KOREA, REPUBLIC OF: The WHO Programme Coordinator, Central P.O. Box 540, SEOUL
KUWAIT: The Kuwait Bookshops Co. Ltd, Thunayan Al-Ghanem Bldg, P.O. Box 2942, KUWAIT

LAO PEOPLE'S DEMOCRATIC REPUBLIC: The WHO Programme Coordinator, P.O. Box 343, VIENTIANE
LEBANON: The Levant Distributors Co. S.A.R.L., Box 1181, Makdassi Street, Hanna Bldg, BEIRUT
LUXEMBOURG: Librairie du Centre, 49 bd Royal, LUXEMBOURG
MALAWI: Malawi Book Service, P.O. Box 30044, Chichiti, BLANTYRE 3
MALAYSIA: The WHO Programme Coordinator, Room 1004, Fitzpatrick Building, Jalan Raja Chulan, KUALA LUMPUR 05–02 — Jubilee (Book) Store Ltd, 97 Jalan Tuanku Abdul Rahman, P.O. Box 629, KUALA LUMPUR 01–08 — Parry's Book Center, K. L. Hilton Hotel, Jln. Treacher, P.O. Box 960, KUALA LUMPUR
MEXICO: La Prensa Médica Mexicana, Ediciones Cientificas, Paseo de las Facultades 26, Apt. Postal 20–413, MEXICO CITY 20, D.F.
MONGOLIA: *see* India, WHO Regional Office
MOROCCO: Editions La Porte, 281 avenue Mohammed V, RABAT
MOZAMBIQUE: INLD, Caixa Postal 4030, MAPUTO
NEPAL: *see* India, WHO Regional Office
NETHERLANDS: Medical Books Europe BV, Noorderwal 38, 7241 BL LOCHEM
NEW ZEALAND: Government Printing Office, Publications Section, Mulgrave Street, Private Bag, WELLINGTON 1; Walter Street, WELLINGTON; World Trade Building, Cubacade, Cuba Street, WELLINGTON. *Government Bookshops at:* Hannaford Burton Building, Rutland Street, Private Bag, AUCKLAND; 159 Hereford Street, Private Bag, CHRISTCHURCH; Alexandra Street, P.O. Box 857, HAMILTON; T & G Building, Princes Street, P.O. Box 1104, DUNEDIN — R. Hill & Son, Ltd, Ideal House, Cnr Gillies Avenue & Eden St., Newmarket, AUCKLAND I
NIGERIA: University Bookshop Nigeria Ltd, University of Ibadan, IBADAN
NORWAY: J. G. Tanum A/S, P.O. Box 1177 Sentrum, OSLO 1
PAKISTAN: Mirza Book Agency, 65 Shahrah–E–Quaid–E–Azam, P.O. Box 729, LAHORE 3
PAPUA NEW GUINEA: The WHO Programme Coordinator, P.O. Box 5896, BOROKO
PHILIPPINES: World Health Organization, Regional Office for the Western Pacific, P.O. Box 2932, MANILA — The Modern Book Company Inc., P.O. Box 632, 922 Rizal Avenue, MANILA 2800
POLAND: Składnica Księgarska, ul Mazowiecka 9, 00052 WARSAW (*except periodicals*) — BKWZ Ruch, ul Wronia 23, 00840 WARSAW (*periodicals only*)
PORTUGAL: Livraria Rodrigues, 186 Rua do Ouro, LISBON 2
SIERRA LEONE: Njala University College Bookshop (University of Sierra Leone), Private Mail Bag, FREETOWN
SINGAPORE: The WHO Programme Coordinator, 144 Moulmein Road, G.P.O. Box 3457, SINGAPORE I — Select Books (Pte) Ltd, 215 Tanglin Shopping Centre, 2/F, 19 Tanglin Road, SINGAPORE 10
SOUTH AFRICA: Van Schaik's Bookstore (Pty) Ltd, P.O. Box 724, 268 Church Street, PRETORIA 0001
SPAIN: Comercial Atheneum S.A., Consejo de Ciento 130–136, BARCELONA 15; General Moscardo 29, MADRID 20 — Libreria Diaz de Santos, Lagasca 95 y Maldonado 6, MADRID 6; Balmes 417 y 419, BARCELONA 22
SRI LANKA: *see* India, WHO Regional Office
SWEDEN: Aktiebolaget C. E. Fritzes Kungl. Hovbokhandel, Regeringsgatan 12, 10327 STOCKHOLM
SWITZERLAND: Medizinischer Verlag Hans Huber, Länggass Strasse 76, 3012 BERN 9
SYRIAN ARAB REPUBLIC: M. Farras Kekhia, P.O. Box No. 5221, ALEPPO
THAILAND: *see* India, WHO Regional Office
TUNISIA: Société Tunisienne de Diffusion, 5 avenue de Carthage, TUNIS
TURKEY: Haset Kitapevi, 469 Istiklal Caddesi, Beyoglu, ISTANBUL
UNITED KINGDOM: H.M. Stationery Office: 49 High Holborn, LONDON WC1V 6HB; 13a Castle Street, EDINBURGH EH2 3AR; 41 The Hayes, CARDIFF CF1 1JW; 80 Chichester Street, BELFAST BT1 4JY; Brazennose Street, MANCHESTER M60 8AS; 258 Broad Street, BIRMINGHAM B1 2HE; Southey House, Wine Street, BRISTOL BS1 2BQ. *All mail orders should be sent to* P.O. Box 569, LONDON SE1 9NH
UNITED STATES OF AMERICA: *Single and bulk copies of individual publications (not subscriptions):* WHO Publications Centre USA, 49 Sheridan Avenue, ALBANY, N.Y. 12210. *Subscriptions: Subscription orders, accompanied by check made out to the* Chemical Bank, New York, Account World Health Organization, *should be sent to the* World Health Organization, P.O. Box 5284, Church Street Station, NEW YORK, N.Y. 10249. *Correspondence concerning subscriptions should be addressed to the* World Health Organization, Distribution and Sales, 1211 GENEVA 27, Switzerland. *Publications are also available from the* United Nations Bookshop, NEW YORK, N.Y. 10017 (*retail only*)
USSR: *For readers in the USSR requiring Russian editions:* Komsomolskij prospekt 18, Medicinskaja Kniga, MOSCOW — *For readers outside the USSR requiring Russian editions:* Kuzneckij most 18, Meždunarodnaja Kniga, MOSCOW G-200
VENEZUELA: Editorial Interamericana de Venezuela C.A., Apartado 50.785, CARACAS 105 — Libreria del Este, Apartado 60.337, CARACAS 106 — Libreria Médica Paris, Apartado 60.681, CARACAS 106
YUGOSLAVIA: Jugoslovenska Knjiga, Terazije 27/II, 11000 BELGRADE
ZAIRE: Librairie universitaire, avenue de la Paix Nº 167, B.P. 1682, KINSHASA I

Special terms for developing countries are obtainable on application to the WHO Programme Coordinators or WHO Regional Offices listed above or to the World Health Organization, Distribution and Sales Service, 1211 Geneva 27, Switzerland. Orders from countries where sales agents have not yet been appointed may also be sent to the Geneva address, but must be paid for in pounds sterling, US dollars, or Swiss francs.

Price: Sw. fr. 44.—   Prices are subject to change without notice.   C/1/81